"A product of many years of deliberation, scholarly conversation, and refinement, Glas' *Person-Centered Care in Psychiatry* is his vision of a psychiatry which is both scientifically and humanistically rigorous. Optimistic in temperament and outlook, Glas' work builds a psychiatry that is equally comfortable with molecules, brains, people, relationships, institutions, and societies."

– John Z. Sadler, MD, The Daniel W. Foster, M.D. Professor of Medical Ethics, Professor of Psychiatry & Clinical Sciences, UT Southwestern, Dallas, TX

"Gerrit Glas is a distinguished and well-known philosophical thinker who is also a practicing clinician. Philosophers working in the mental health research field are rarely equipped to say much of value about practice, and the practitioners who write are not often persuasive on the philosophical background, especially on complex issues to do with normativity, contextual influences and personhood. This makes Glas's work exceedingly rare and especially welcome."

– Jennifer Radden, D.Phil. Oxon., Professor emerita of Philosophy, University of Massachusetts Boston

"Gerrit Glas' synthesis of the Dutch philosopher Herman Dooyeweerd's work with the more familiar philosophical systems of Sören Kierkegaard and Paul Ricoeur, brings a refreshingly original slant to contemporary debates about the role of science in person-centred psychiatry."

– Professor Bill (K.W.M.) Fulford, Fellow of St Catherine's College and Director of the Collaborating Centre for Values-based Practice, University of Oxford

PERSON-CENTERED CARE IN PSYCHIATRY

One of the paradoxes about psychiatry is that we have never known more about and better treated mental disorders, yet there exists so much unease about the practice of mental healthcare. Patients feel still stigmatized, psychiatrists are struggling with their roles in a rapidly changing system of healthcare, there is lack of consensus about what mental disorders are and what the focus of psychiatry should be. Person-Centered Care in Psychiatry: Self- relational, Contextual and Normative Perspectives offers a distinctive approach to two important linked conceptual issues in psychiatry: the relation between self, context, and psychopathology; and the intrinsic normativity of psychiatry as a practice.

Divided into two parts, this book shows how the clinical conception of psychopathology and psychiatry as normative practice are intrinsically connected, and how the normative practice approach can be conceived as a natural extension of the analysis of the web of relations that sustain illness behavior as well as professional role fulfilment.

Person-Centered Care in Psychiatry brings these topics together for the first time against the backdrop of unease about scientistic tendencies within psychiatry in an interconnected discussion that will be of interest to academics and professionals with an interest in the philosophy of psychology, psychiatry, and mental healthcare.

Gerrit Glas is a practicing psychiatrist and professor of philosophy at the Vrije Universiteit and the Amsterdam University Medical Centre. His main interest is in conceptual and normative issues at the intersection of psychiatry, philosophy, neuroscience, and society.

PERSON-CENTERED CARE IN PSYCHIATRY

Self-relational, Contextual, and Normative Perspectives

Gerrit Glas

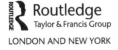

Routledge
Taylor & Francis Group

LONDON AND NEW YORK

First published 2019
by Routledge
2 Park Square, Milton Park, Abingdon, Oxon OX14 4RN

and by Routledge
52 Vanderbilt Avenue, New York, NY 10017

Routledge is an imprint of the Taylor & Francis Group, an informa business

British Library Cataloguing in Publication Data
A catalogue record for this book is available from the British Library

Library of Congress Cataloging-in-Publication Data
Names: Glas, Gerrit, 1954- author.
Title: Person-centered care in psychiatry : self-relational, contextual, and
normative perspectives / Gerrit Glas.
Description: Abingdon, Oxon ; New York, NY : Routledge, 2019. |
Includes bibliographical references and index.
Identifiers: LCCN 2019007116 (print) | LCCN 2019007856 (ebook) |
ISBN 9780429242960 (Master E-Book) | ISBN 9780367197384 (hardback : alk.
paper) | ISBN 9780367197391 (pbk. : alk. paper) | ISBN 9780429242960 (ebk)
Subjects: | MESH: Person-Centered Psychotherapy | Mental Disorders--therapy
Classification: LCC RC480.5 (ebook) | LCC RC480.5 (print) | NLM WM
420.5.N8 | DDC 616.89/14--dc23
LC record available at https://lccn.loc.gov/2019007116

ISBN: 978-0-367-19738-4 (hbk)
ISBN: 978-0-367-19739-1 (pbk)
ISBN: 978-0-429-24296-0 (ebk)

Typeset in Bembo
by Taylor & Francis Books

CONTENTS

List of illustrations   *ix*
Preface   *x*

1   Psychiatry in need of philosophy   1

PART 1
Self, context, and psychopathology   **19**

2   Self-relatedness, psychopathology, and the context: A clinical
     perspective   21

3   Self-relatedness, psychopathology, and the context: The
     concept of disease   44

4   Self-relatedness, psychopathology, and the context: The
     concept of self   62

PART 2
Psychiatry as normative practice   **79**

5   Being a professional: Self-relatedness and normativity   81

6   Toward a normative practice approach for mental healthcare   99

7   Psychiatry in contexts   124

8   Philosophical backgrounds   150

9   Conclusion: Future prospects   168

References   *193*
Index   *212*

ILLUSTRATIONS

Diagrams

2.1 The professional pays attention to relations [1] – [5]   22
5.1 The professional relates in different ways to his/er own
    professional fulfilment [A] – [E]   82
5.2 Aspects of the professional role, domains, and competencies   87
6.1 Psychiatry as normative practice   106
7.1 Contexts, professional roles and the object of psychiatry   125
7.2 Meso-level and types of influence   134
7.3 Macro-level and types of influence   140

PREFACE

This book finds its roots in my work as a practicing psychiatrist, supervisor, and academic philosopher. It has been written out of concern for both my patients and the next generation of psychiatrists. Many patients feel lost and alienated in the systems of care that we have built for and around them, by the categories we use, and by the frameworks of understanding we have developed. Young colleagues also sometimes feel lost and alienated when they are confronted with the widely diverging expectations surrounding their professional role, the bureaucracies they will belong to, and the tensions and ambiguities within themselves and in their interactions with patients, colleagues, managers, representatives of the legal system, patient organizations, funding agencies, and the government.

I will start in practice, in the encounter with the patient, in the web of relationships within which both the patient and we, as professionals, find ourselves. These relationships shape not only interactions between the patient and the professional but also those between the patient and his or her illness and the professional and his or her professional role. This book is an attempt to define and understand the nature of these relationships, especially how they affect both the illness role and the professional role. I argue that patients do not coincide with their illness roles. Psychiatrists are not merely dealing with manifestations of psychopathology, but with what patients, from the earliest manifestation of their problems, do with these problems in the context of their lives, in their relationships with others, in their encounters with professionals, and within the system of mental healthcare. I correspondingly argue that professionals do not coincide with their professional roles, that they are more than merely bundles of skills and knowledge, and that they must adapt and define their role in relation to who they are as persons and in the context of mental healthcare and society. Their identity as professionals crystallizes at the intersection of medical professionalism, the private sphere of patients, and public responsibility.

I focus more specifically on two important interlinked themes in psychiatry: the relationships among self, context, and psychopathology and the intrinsic normativity of psychiatry as a practice. Written against the background of the scientistic tendencies of present-day psychiatry, it is argued in Part I of this book that psychiatry needs a clinical conception of psychopathology alongside more traditional scientific conceptions. In addition, I argue that this clinical conception of psychopathology must be based on a fundamental rethinking of the intertwinement between the patient as person, illness manifestations, and the context of the patient. Thus, the patient's illness is conceived as the product of this intertwinement, rather than the outward manifestation of a broken mechanism within the patient.

In Part II, I analogously show that self- and context-related factors have a large impact on the professional role and on one's professional identity. I argue that an analysis is needed of the normative aspects of the relationships that sustain and frame professional role fulfilment. This analysis culminates in the normative practice approach (NPA), which distinguishes between qualifying, conditioning, and foundational rules, principles, and norms. The analysis also suggests that differences between contexts are based on different constellations of norms and normative principles, as well as different definitions of the aims of mental healthcare.

The normative practice approach enables us to locate and resist scientistic defenses of the legitimacy of psychiatry and to replace them with a positive account that provides clinicians (and scientists) with the conceptual tools they need to justify what they do in broader contexts. I argue that the professional role is ultimately morally qualified. Knowledge and skills are, of course, foundational to psychiatric practice, but they do not provide the principles that characterize, or qualify, the professional relationship as a moral relationship. The same holds for the legal, economic, and social aspects of (mental) healthcare. These aspects are guided and determined by conditioning norms and principles. These norms and principles are a sine qua non for professional practice, but they do not qualify professional practice in a deeper sense. They do not, in other words, denote the purpose, or telos, of this practice.

The main thrust of the argument demonstrates that psychiatry needs a normative account of its legitimacy, in which we recognize normative dimensions beyond those that sustain the expert role. In other words, psychiatrists should not defend the legitimacy of their profession along scientistic lines, by referring solely to the scientific basis of their expert role. Instead, they should provide a more holistic account in which justice is done to the broader social, legal, and economic contexts of professional activity. The analysis of this inherent normativity begins within clinical practice; it extends to the concept of disease, as well as to wider domains of psychiatric care and the sociology of professions. Finally, it culminates in an analysis of the implicit normativity of healthcare institutions in general in terms of their tasks and duties for the provision of mental healthcare.

Precursors of the ideas in this book originated long ago, in discussions with Henk Jochemsen, Sytse Strijbos, and Jan Hoogland in the 1990s. These ideas were further developed in interactions and intellectual exchanges with other colleagues and friends, especially Maarten Verkerk, Henk Geertsema, Derek Strijbos, and

Leon de Bruin. This work was written in the context of the "Science beyond Scientism" research project, funded by the Templeton World Charity Foundation. This project included an analysis of scientistic tendencies within psychiatry and a structural analysis of psychiatry as a normative practice. I thank René van Woudenberg (principal investigator), Jeroen de Ridder, Rik Peels, Gijsbert van den Brink, Lieke Asma, Naomi Kloosterboer, Hans van Eyghen, Josephine Lenssen, and other members of the Theoretical Philosophy Group of the Vrije Universiteit for their comments and fruitful collaboration. I would also like to thank members of the Normative Practices Discussion Group at the Vrije Universiteit—especially Govert Buijs, Jan van der Stoep, Christine van Burken, Bert Loonstra, Perry Huesmann, and Corné Rademaker—for their valuable comments on the early drafts of some of the chapters. Special thanks also go to the members of the steering committee of Redesigning Psychiatry, an ambitious group of designers, philosophers, and psychiatrists who combine organizational design, innovation in psychiatric care, and conceptual research to develop more humane mental healthcare: I thank Matthijs van Dijk, David van den Berg, Nynke Tromp, Sander Voerman, Philip Delespaul, Femke de Boer, Beatrijs Voorneman, Tonnie Staring, Joost Baas, Eddo Vedders, Paul Hekkert, and Marc van der Gaag for many inspiring insights and discussions. I am grateful for my collaboration with many other colleagues who helped me to focus and clarify my thoughts: Jeroen Geurts, Hanneke Hulst, Gerben Meynen, Benjamin Drukarch, Linda Douw, Tineke Abma, Henk de Regt, and Sander Griffioen. Ideas for this book were especially fostered by my clinical work and my work as supervisor and director of residency training in the Dimence Groep (Dimence Group), a large mental health hospital in the Netherlands. I tested many of my thoughts in discussions with colleagues at this institute—especially Sabine Raams and Elnathan Prinssen—and with members of the board of the hospital, Herma van der Wal and Ernst Klunder, who also facilitated a six-month sabbatical in 2015 and recently supported and helped set up the project Werken met Waarden (Working with Values) in the hospital.

1

PSYCHIATRY IN NEED OF PHILOSOPHY

1.1 Paradoxes and concerns

One of the paradoxes of the current state of mental healthcare is that we have never known more about mental disorders and simultaneously been more uncertain about the science as well as the practice of psychiatry.

This is remarkable. Psychiatry as a science is flourishing. Over the last three decades, there has been an enormous increase in empirical research on the genetic, neurobiological, psychological, and social determinants of mental disorder. At the same time, mental healthcare has improved significantly, at least in most Western countries. There are more treatments and there exists much more refined differentiation in the way healthcare is delivered. Reform in legislation and in the organization of care has led to greater patient autonomy, more control over the process and outcomes of therapy, more transparency in decision making, and more patient participation at all levels of policymaking.

Yet, these improvements have not diminished the unease about psychiatry, as a science and as a practice. Psychiatry as a science is haunted by discussions about a proper system for diagnosis and classification. There is no consensus on what mental disorders "are." Researchers have discovered many determinants of mental illness, but most of them lack specificity and are related to more than one psychiatric disorder. In addition, scientific leaders have differing views on where psychiatry as a science should be heading; for example, toward a variant of biomedical reductionism and a reunion with neurology (Insel & Wang 2010) or toward a science of the mind-brain-in-context as a branch of complexity theory (Thompson 2007), to mention only two extremes.

No wonder psychiatrists are struggling with their professional roles and their identity. Some of them see the prototypical psychiatrist as a hospital-based medical specialist with a focus on the neural underpinnings of mental problems. Others prefer a role as networker and negotiator at the interface between science and society. Still others look for hybrid constructions, in which the psychiatrist is a mix of expert, negotiator, and health advocate.

With respect to mental healthcare as a practice, there are also many tensions and uncertainties. The field is struggling with its acceptance in society. There is strong agreement about the need for evidence-based psychiatric treatment. However, despite this need and all the efforts to fulfill it notwithstanding, treatment results have not dramatically improved over the last two or three decades. This also holds for stigmatization. An enormous amount of effort has been put into anti-stigma programs. Nevertheless, stigmatization has hardly decreased. People with mental disorders still hide their problems. They still feel that having a mental problem is something they should feel ashamed and culpable of.

It is the aim of this chapter to show that most of these practical, conceptual, and moral concerns can be grouped together under three fundamental themes. A second purpose is to highlight one dominant response to the challenges, which is scientistic. The scientistic response seems attractive and convincing at first glance, but it is, in fact, inadequate, as I will show. The final goal of this chapter is to briefly introduce the philosophical framework I work within, which draws on core ideas developed by the Danish philosopher Sören Kierkegaard (1848), the French philosopher Paul Ricoeur (1990), and the Dutch philosopher Herman Dooye-weerd (1953–1958). Ricoeur and Dooyeweerd belong, together with Karl Jaspers, to the first and most vocal opponents of scientism. From Kierkegaard and Ricoeur, I borrow the notions of self-relatedness and self-referentiality to investigate the nature and implicit normativity of the patient's relationship to his or her illness and the professional's attitude toward the fulfillment of his or her professional role. Dooyeweerd's systematic philosophy functions as a conceptual resource for the formulation of a heuristic framework of normative principles that play a role within the different contexts of psychiatry. Other philosophers who significantly influenced my ideas about the normative aspects of professional and institutionalized practices are Alasdair MacIntyre (1984) and Charles Taylor (1989).

1.2 Fundamental conceptual issues and their inner connection

Instead of presenting an exhaustive list of the current practical, conceptual, and moral problems in psychiatry and providing arguments on how to conceptually group them together, I simply suggest that most of these problems belong to three general conceptual themes. I indicate these themes briefly here and provide more detail in the remainder of this chapter:

1. The nature of psychopathology, especially considering its context dependence and its relatedness to the self.
2. The value-ladenness of psychiatry as a clinical practice.
3. The role and status of scientific knowledge, especially in view of the nature of clinical knowledge.

1.2.1 Self-relatedness and context dependence of psychopathology

Mental illnesses do not exist in and of themselves. They are neither Kantian things-in-themselves—beyond what we can grasp with our senses—nor are they material entities (things, events, or processes) located somewhere in space-time; and neither are they only mental constructions that help us organize the world. However, mental illnesses do indeed exist. They exist not only in the mind of the psychiatrist, but first in the lives of the patients who experience them. Terms such as psychosis, anxiety, depression, and addiction refer to a variety of categorically distinct phenomena within the patient, including feelings, thoughts, inclinations, and non-intentional behaviors. These phenomena occur in patterns or regular combinations of features. These regularities and patterns form the basis for psychiatric nomenclature.

The science of psychopathology attempts to grasp these patterns and regularities by relating them to explanatory factors (determinants, risks, and vulnerabilities). The search for patterns, regularities, and explanatory factors inevitably leads to simplifications. Individual details are put between brackets. Like any other science, psychopathology focuses on general patterns. This is what we call "abstraction": the carving out of a pattern and regularity as a first step toward the discovery and formulation of explanatory hypotheses. In philosophy of science, abstraction is usually referred to as "reduction." I use both terms to refer to the same cognitive act of carving out an aspect, part, or set of features of the object under study. Ideally, this carving out is determined by a hypothesis or theory. Abstraction is the first stage in the testing of this hypothesis or theory.

A well-known issue in this context concerns the transition from abstraction to reification. Abstraction, as we have seen, refers to the artificial pulling out and setting aside of an aspect, part, or set of features in order to explain patterns or regularities. Ideally, there is no moment during the process of abstraction that the artificiality of this process and of the abstracted entity is ignored. Reification, however, "forgets" this artificiality. Instead of viewing the aspects, parts, or sets of features as being divorced of their holistic context, it considers them as things in themselves and sometimes even as the whole thing.

To reify means to make (*facere*) a thing (*res*) of something. For example, in the field of psychopathology, one might say that panic disorder "is" a disturbance in the brain's serotonin metabolism. The presence of this disturbed serotonin metabolism is indeed an important empirical finding in patients with panic disorder. The disturbance forms a part of panic disorder as a clinical phenomenon. However, the entire clinical picture involves much more than altered serotonin levels. To assert that panic disorder essentially consists of a disturbance of the brain's serotonin metabolism is to commit a mereological fallacy, as Bennett and Hacker (2003) would refer to it. A mereological fallacy is a logical error which occurs when a part (from the Greek *meros*) is treated as if it were the whole. In this case, the serotonin abnormalities (a part) are being taken as an adequate description of panic disorder (the whole). Mereological fallacies usually lead to reification of the abstracted part and to an abstract view of the entire phenomenon, in this case, panic disorder. However, every patient suffering from panic disorder can tell that it involves much more than altered serotonin levels. Reification is also sometimes referred to as "substantialization" (making a substance of something) or "absolutization" (making something absolute, a thing-in-itself, apart from its relationships with other things), or, in German, *Verdinglichung* (making a concrete thing of an abstract entity).

From the above, it is no large step to understand why, during the process of abstraction, scientists tend to put between brackets both the context in which psychopathology evolves and the relationships among the symptoms and the self of the patient. After all, these relationships are important sources of individual variation in the presence and expression of symptoms, and variation is an impediment to the reconstruction of patterns and regularities, which is the goal of the process of abstraction. The scientist is usually not interested in the way depression affects a person's self-image or interferes with highly personal contextual issues, such as functioning as a parent. However, these factors are, of course, crucial in the clinical treatment of depression.

The tendency to abstract from the context and from the patient as a person is further enhanced by psychiatry's indebtedness to the somatic concept of disease, which focuses on states within the individual, i.e., on symptoms and underlying causal processes, determinants, and latent variables. Symptoms are typically seen as the expression of an individual's state, which is viewed as the disease in the proper sense. This strategy of conceptualizing disease does not leave much room for a contextually sensitive and self-relational view of psychopathology. When abstraction subsequently culminates in reification, the separation between psychopathology, on the one hand, and context and self, on the other, becomes a fact.

What do I mean by a contextually sensitive and self-relational view of psychopathology? With respect to context sensitivity, it is, to begin with, clear that the nature and severity of psychiatric symptoms are often at least partially determined by environmental factors. Problems in memory and attention may long remain unnoticed, but not in situations that are cognitively demanding. The delusions of a computer game addict differ from those of an elderly widow. It is, furthermore, important to notice that the mental healthcare system itself is also a major contextual contributor to variation in the presence and expression of symptoms. The availability of facilities, treatments, and other forms of support shapes the way patients present their complaints. The context sensitivity of the expression of psychiatric symptoms is even more evident when examined from a developmental perspective. Children must learn to verbalize what they feel. Behind every symptom, mental or bodily, doctors must presuppose a socialization process that exerts much influence on the expression of symptoms.

The adjective "self-relational" refers to the fact that patients relate to their symptoms and that symptoms have an impact on how a patient relates with him or herself, with his or her disorder, and with their environment. Later in this book, I discern different ways of self-relating. For now, it is sufficient to recognize two points: First, that mental problems almost always have an impact on how the patient relates to him or herself; and second, that there are some symptoms that intrinsically refer to aspects of the self. I believe the first point is obvious. Persons who under normal circumstances have an average level of self-confidence may feel totally insufficient when depressed. In such cases, depression interferes with the way one relates to oneself. The second point, the immediate and intrinsic reference to aspects of the self, is particularly relevant for the understanding of emotions and certain dispositions (e.g., character traits). For example, anxiety not only points to danger outside myself but also to something *in* me, i.e., to an aspect of myself that is vulnerable toward the kind of threat that provokes the anxiety. Emotions have an intrinsic self-referentiality: They refer intrinsically to an aspect or aspects of the person experiencing them. This self-referring occurs alongside reference to the object of emotion, which is typically external to the person experiencing the emotion. Anger refers to situations in which I feel insulted or attacked. But the fact that a situation can have such an impact on me indicates also something about me, i.e., that I can be insulted and attacked on this point. Much of the variation in the expression of emotion depends on the enormous spectrum of human vulnerabilities. Most of these vulnerabilities are, of course, within the range of normality.

One of the greatest problems in current psychopathology is that leading systems of diagnosis and classification such as the International Classification of Diseased (ICD) and the Diagnostic and Statistical Manual of Mental Disorders (DSM) offer little room to do justice to the context sensitivity of symptoms and the self-relational aspects of psychopathology. These classification systems play a crucial role in diagnosis and treatment planning, but they can hardly be said to capture all that the individual patient needs. What patients need is often not so much determined by the nature and the severity of the symptoms as by the impact of these symptoms on the self-image of the patient and on context-dependent demands. One of the reasons for lack of satisfaction with the mental healthcare system is the blindness of most current diagnostic systems to the context-boundedness of mental problems and to their embedding in the I–self relationship of the patient.

1.2.2 The value-ladenness of clinical practice

Psychiatry is both a science and a practice. As a practice, it refers to norms, preferences, criteria, interests, and values. In the typical case, two people meet: the professional and the patient. The two parties communicate based on their own explicit and implicit assumptions. These assumptions play a role in what is said and left unsaid. Ideally, the patient and the professional succeed in establishing a shared view, or reconstruction, of the patient's problems and their possible solutions. This reconstruction entails an idea about what is most urgent and needs immediate attention. It provides a coherent picture of all relevant factors contributing to the patient's problem. The collaborative effort of patient and physician ideally leads to a 3-D view of what is going on and what should be done (Glas 2010). This 3-D view offers perspective; it identifies what is in the foreground and what is in the background; it sheds light on the relevance of the different elements that play a role in the patient's situation. Ms. A with panic disorder suffers immensely from the intensity of the anxiety, but her primary reason for seeking help is her agoraphobia, which prevents her from going to work. She doesn't dare leave her home unaccompanied and thus fears losing her job. Here, the efforts of the therapist are directed first at the agoraphobia. Mr. B with moderately severe depression has recurrent suicidal thoughts that disturb him, but he suffers most from lack of sleep and waking early in the morning. He feels exhausted, and the exhaustion is so intense that it leads to a disquieting experience of powerlessness and lack of control. The psychiatrist, therefore, first focuses on restoration of a normal sleeping pattern. These preferences are based on what people deem valuable. Ms. A prefers exposure therapy for her agoraphobia because having work is an important value in her life. Mr. B values normal sleep above alleviation of his suicidal thoughts because exhaustion gives him an intense experience of lack of control.

Norms, preferences, interests, values—they not only play a role at the level of practical decision making but also in a broader sense. They are present in implicit working models in the minds of clinicians (and patients), e.g., in the ideas they have about the nature of mental disorder and the proper role of the psychiatrist. Values help shape one's ideas about professionalism and professional identity. They are transmitted via residency training programs, role models, and culture in the organization. Values determine one's responses to the institutional dynamics within mental healthcare and to the societal role of psychiatry. These issues are dealt with in more detail later in this book. We will also systematize the different normative aspects at stake here. For now, it is enough to note that the practice of psychiatry is value laden in many respects.

The value-ladenness of psychiatric practice seems obvious. There is, nevertheless, much unease about it. Why is that? Why is it that even within the psychiatric community, there is so much ambivalence about the fact that value negotiation is at the heart of psychiatric consultation (Woodbridge & Fulford 2004)? Why are ethics and moral reasoning still so underrepresented in residency training programs?

I suggest that it is the underlying model of medical practice that plays a role here. What seems decisive is the assumption that medical problems have a hard, objective core and a soft, subjective margin. Under this model, scientific knowledge about the origin, course, and treatment of diseases belongs to the objective core, whereas values, preferences, patient interests, and clinical intuitions belong to the soft margin. Insofar as practices are built on this underlying assumption, they are inclined to favor evidence-based treatment protocols and to distance themselves from the soft aspects of psychiatry. This occurs by either ignoring these aspects or by describing them as belonging to a prescientific form of psychiatry.

Clearly, the objective-core-soft-margin concept of psychiatric care easily leads to a technical conception of professionalism. Let me briefly outline this technical—or even better, technicistic—conception as a contrast to the idea of psychiatry as a person-centered and value-oriented practice (an idea defended in this book). I am aware that I am sketching an extreme and that, in daily practice, the positions are seldom as pronounced as depicted here. Nevertheless, pointing out an extreme at one end of the spectrum helps clarify the idea of person-centered and value-oriented psychiatry at the other end of the spectrum. According to proponents of the technicistic view, it is the task of the professional to apply scientific knowledge as purely and detachedly as possible by using techniques (pharmacotherapy, psychotherapy, and so on). The knowledge itself is value free, and the application of it should be as well, according to this view. This is because the applications have been tested, usually by randomized clinical trials. The technicistic approach fits well with a primordially economic and legal view of the relationship between patient and psychiatrist. In the most extreme variant of this approach, the professional relationship adopts the form of a meeting between "strangers," i.e., between neutral parties collaborating based on a contract concerning the goods each party supplies to the other (Veatch 1983). This contract is founded on legal rules and obligations, *not* trust.

Adherents of the technicistic approach are inclined to work with a reductionist (and reified) concept of mental disorder. The reason for this is obvious: It is much easier to maintain that disorders can be brought under control and subjected to technical manipulation (in the form of medication or psychotherapy) when they are conceived as circumscript, identifiable states within an individual, rather than the expressions of highly contingent interactions within the individual and between the individual and the context. This is why reductionism in one's conception of psychopathology is conceptually and practically related to a technicistic view of the psychiatrist's professional role and to a disregard for the value-ladenness and person-centeredness of psychiatric practice.

In summary, why is the value-ladenness of psychiatry a main source of unease about psychiatry? This is because of the dominance of the objective-core-subjective-margin model. This model favors an objectivistic and abstract (i.e., reified and scientistic) conception of disease and a technicistic view on the professional role. Both are difficult to reconcile with a conception of psychiatric practice that puts value negotiation at the center of clinical practice.

1.2.3 The role and conceptual status of clinical knowledge

There is one other fundamental issue that needs to be addressed in the context of this brief overview of practical, conceptual, and moral concerns about present-day psychiatry: the role and status of clinical knowledge, especially in relation to scientific knowledge. How does clinical knowledge relate to scientific knowledge? Are they identical? And, if not, how do they differ? And is this difference important? What kind of knowledge is clinical knowledge? The problem here is how to adapt scientific knowledge—which typically focuses on general patterns and largely invariant causal mechanisms—to the clinical way of knowing, which aims at individual patient characteristics.

There is an extensive, albeit scattered, corpus of texts on the nature of clinical knowledge (Montgomery 2005; Norman 2000; Schon 1983; Toulmin 1976). Most of these texts are concerned with clinical knowledge as an epistemic problem. My scope here is broader, because of the interconnection between the epistemic problem and the previous two issues, i.e., the context-bound and self-relational aspects of psychopathology and the idea of psychiatry as a value-laden practice.

The unease about the nature of clinical knowledge when compared with scientific knowledge seems less obvious than the previous two concerns. However, I believe that the issue is no less important. With every new finding in the basic sciences (molecular biology, genetics, and neuroscience) the distance between science and clinical knowledge seems to increase. There is clearly a tension here, a tension that is known as the "problem of translation." Representatives of the basic sciences suggest that medicine needs translational scientists (see, for instance, Zerhouni 2005). Appealing and seemingly self-evident as this may sound, it is nevertheless not so clear what the term "translational" means (Austin 2018; Francken & Slors 2017; van der Laan & Boenink 2015). Does it imply that there is, first, scientific knowledge and only subsequently a (non-scientific) translation to clinical practice? If so, what are the rules for translation? Or should the translation process itself be viewed as part of the science? If so, are there scientific standards for translation? What does translation mean, given that the basic sciences aim at general patterns and universal causal mechanisms, whereas clinical practice focuses on individual cases and tailor-made treatments?

From the clinical side, there are worries about the clinical relevance of current explanatory models and classification systems. Diagnostic tools are more than ever based on scientific evidence. However, the strong emphasis on scientific evidence has led to a flattened concept of disease (i.e., atheoretical lists of symptoms) and to diagnostic categories that, although being increasingly intersubjectively reliable, cannot keep pace with the degree of conceptual adequacy and validity that is required in the clinical context.

This issue touches the role of evidence-based medicine (EBM), which more than two decades ago was launched as the new paradigm for clinical care in medicine and psychiatry (Sackett et al. 1996; Sackett et al. 1997). EBM promised to be the umbrella under which the connection between science and clinical practice could be made (Geddes & Harrison 1997). Clinicians were supposed to act based on EBM's hierarchical scale of evidence, which put meta-analyses of randomized clinical trials (RCTs) at the top of the hierarchy and expert opinion and clinical experience at the bottom. In other words, clinical judgment and implicit forms of knowing scored lowest in EBM's hierarchy of evidence. No wonder many clinicians began to feel a tension between treatment protocols that are based on the kind of science EBM favors and their usual way of practicing, which is based on case-oriented clinical judgment informed by clinical experience. Let us take a closer look, however.

At first sight, the EBM approach indeed doesn't seem to be capable of doing justice to the tailor-made assessments of individual patients that is at the heart of clinical work (Gupta 2014; Miles & McLoughlin 2011). This is because the EBM approach tends to abstract from individual patient characteristics. However, a further qualification is in place here. Sackett et al. (the founders of the EBM methodology) explicitly mention clinical experience as an information source for clinical decision making. Evidence-based medicine consists of "the conscientious, explicit and judicious use of current best evidence in making decisions about the care of the individual patient. It means integrating individual clinical expertise with the best available external clinical evidence from systematic research" (Sackett et al. 1996). Evidence itself does not direct the decision-making process; it should be weighed against clinical experience and patient values (Sackett et al. 1997). This is a remarkable statement given that the writings of Sackett et al. are almost entirely devoted to the weighing of scientific evidence and hardly say anything about the other two components in the decision-making process: clinical judgment and balancing with patient values. Thornton (2007, pp. 205–207) rightly remarks that it is unclear how Sackett's statement about the weighing of evidence can be combined with the very idea of a hierarchy of evidence that places RCTs at the highest and clinical judgment at the lowest rank.

Thus, the problem we are left with is how the dominant EBM paradigm is dealing with clinical knowledge (or judgment). The unease clinicians experience is a consequence of the mismatch between the generality of explanatory frameworks and treatment protocols, on the one hand, and the need for tailor-made assessment and treatment of the individual case, on the other. The underlying philosophical issue concerns the nature of clinical knowledge, which is the epistemological blind spot of psychiatry. Science aims at universals, whereas clinical knowledge uses universals to focus on individuals. Clinical competence lies within the skillful combining of pieces of knowledge about universals (patterns, mechanisms, causal pathways, and explanatory frameworks). The clinician attempts to detect the relevance of each of these pieces, separately and in combination with other pieces, for the understanding of the patient's problem. This clinical competence is person sensitive (to coin a new term), context sensitive, and value sensitive and should, therefore, be rooted in character and virtues. The theory of clinical knowledge psychiatry needs is not merely epistemic; it has a broader scope in that it attempts to connect the epistemic distinctness of clinical knowing with competencies such as empathy, context sensitivity, and moral discernment.

1.3 Why scientism cannot be the answer

The previous section discussed three important conceptual issues in psychiatry. This section connects these issues by relating them to scientism as a prevailing paradigm in psychiatry.

1.3.1 Scientism and the connection between the three main conceptual issues

The connection between these three issues may be recognized as being based on a fairly typical and, in fact, dominant attitude toward to the epistemic and normative challenges psychiatry is facing. This attitude is scientistic. Scientism is the view that all truth is based on science and on science alone. All other knowledge is mere opinion and, therefore, insufficiently founded. Scientism can also entail ontological claims, such as that the only things that exist are things that can be described and explained by science.

Scientism seems like an extreme position, but it is nevertheless ubiquitous in psychiatry, especially in academic circles (Insel & Wang 2010; Kandel 1998). Its proponents assert that psychiatry should:

- seek its legitimacy by relying on facts and on science alone
- return to a predominantly biomedical approach to disease
- embrace neuro-realism, with its thesis that mental disorders are brain disorders
- strive for the uncovering of the causal chains underlying mental disorder.

The relationship between these suggestions and the three conceptual issues can be stated as follows. The scientistic approach to psychiatry gives radical priority to scientific knowledge at the expense of everyday and clinical experiences with disease. This point is related to theme (3) (see 1.2): the nature of clinical knowledge in comparison with scientific knowledge. The scientistic approach assigns to the clinician the role of a "neutral" technical expert. This relates to theme (2) (see 1.2): the value-ladenness of psychiatry. Scientism views psychopathology as the ultimate result of dysfunctional neural machinery, conceptually distinct from the person and his or her context. This is an answer to the first theme, i.e., how to account for the self-relational and context-bound aspects of psychopathology.

Scientism is also behind some of the phenomena already addressed in this chapter, such as the transition from abstraction to reification, the negligence of the context in psychiatry's concept of disease, the objective-core-subjective-margin idea of psychopathology, and the way the hierarchy of evidence is construed in the EBM approach.

1.3.2 Abstraction, scientism, and the order of knowing

This book develops an anti-scientistic, person-centered approach to psychiatry. To support this thesis, I will mainly use philosophical arguments. The main reason why the scientistic approach fails is that it uncritically reverses the order of knowing; it forgets that scientific knowledge is always secondary to everyday understanding, and that its meaning can only be formulated in relation to this everyday form of understanding.

Does this imply that everyday knowledge is more solid and trustworthy than scientific knowledge? Of course not. It is *because* of science that we know more about the world and can trust our inferences about it. However, there are fundamental qualities within our experience and knowledge of the world that disappear under the abstracting, reductionist gaze of the scientist, and these fundamental qualities can never be regained by science. What disappears in the act of scientific knowing are at least three aspects:

- the individual identity of the object
- the wholeness of the object
- the web of relationships between the object and the world (relationships that codetermine the identity of the object).

In the act of abstraction, the object is viewed from a particular angle. Thus, the scientist focuses on a particular aspect or combination of aspects of the object, or between the object and other classes of objects. By focusing on an aspect of the object, both the individuality and the wholeness of the object are lost, or, less dramatically, put between brackets. The individuality disappears because the scientist focuses on general patterns, regularities, and common (causal) factors. The wholeness is lost because concentration on one aspect implies that other aspects are ignored. The coherence between the object and the world (the web of relations) also fades to the background due to the artificial isolation of one aspect or one type of relationship between the object and the world. This artificial isolation is typically brought about by experimental design. In fact, it is the experimental design that helps the scientist focus on a particular aspect or type of relationship.

Therefore, there is always an intrinsic one-sidedness in the way the scientist knows. This is not something to deplore. It is simply how science works, and it has proved its enormous importance for the unraveling of patterns, regularities, determining factors, and laws. However, things go wrong when scientists believe they can uncover the ultimate truth about the object or reveal what the object "really" or "fundamentally" is. Such claims were earlier referred to with the terms absolutization, substantialization, and/or reification. All these terms refer to what occurs when experimental results and scientific findings are isolated, when the role of abstraction in the production of these results and findings is forgotten, and when theoretical knowledge about aspects of an object is identified with knowledge or truth about the object as a whole.

Scientism cannot be the answer for psychiatry, first of all because clinicians and scientists think differently. Clinicians try to find effective and efficient solutions to the practical problems of individual patients. Scientists aim to discover lawful patterns or mechanisms that explain specific phenomena in groups of patients. Their use of the term "cause" is different. A clinician may say: "Your depression was caused by a severe loss: the death of your wife." The scientist would say something like: "We know severe loss predicts depression. We also know that severe loss interferes with the neural mechanisms mediating the stress response. Your depression is probably caused by an abnormality in the functioning of these neural mechanisms." The clinician focuses on loss as an existential and psychological reality (with, of course, concomitant biological aspects), whereas the scientist focuses on neural mechanisms as an aspect of bereavement and depression.

A scientistic approach to psychiatry is at odds not only with the epistemology of clinical knowledge but also with the object of psychiatry. Psychiatric illness is typically context bound and self-referential in its expression. In the scientistic approach to psychiatry, this context-boundedness and self-referentiality are put aside and ignored. Psychiatric disorder is seen as the expression of an underlying dysfunction or a malfunctioning of one of the (neural) processes mediating thinking, feeling, perceiving, and planning and organization of behavior. This dysfunction forms the heart of the illness; it *is* the illness according to the scientistic view. If context-boundedness and self-referentiality play a role at all, it is only a secondary one, as factors that mold and reshape the core manifestations of brain dysfunction.

1.3.3 An example: Kandel and LeDoux on psychotherapy

Many psychiatrists don't recognize this scientism at the heart of their profession. After all, the dominant biomedical model does acknowledge that not only biological but also psychological and social factors are important in the genesis of mental disorder. These factors are called "etiological" and are distinguished from the pathogenesis, i.e., the causal path that leads from neural dysfunctioning to behavior. This so-called "final common pathway" is clearly biological, whereas etiological factors may also entail psychological and social factors.

It is questionable, however, whether this distinction precludes scientism. Let me illustrate this with an example: What Kandel and LeDoux say about the biological underpinnings of the effects of psychotherapy. Eric Kandel and Joseph LeDoux are reputed scientists and both have written about the biological underpinnings of the effects of psychotherapy (Kandel 2006; LeDoux 1996; 2015). Kandel says about psychotherapy that it only works insofar as it produces changes in gene expression and altered anatomical patterns of interconnection between nerve cells:

> Insofar as psychotherapy or counseling is effective and produces long-term changes in behavior, it presumably does so through learning, by producing changes in gene expression that alter the strength of synaptic connections and structural changes that alter the anatomical pattern of interconnections between nerve cells of the brain. (Kandel 1998, p. 460)

LeDoux describes psychotherapy as "just another way to rewire the brain" and as "just another way of creating synaptic potentiation in brain pathways that control the amygdala" (LeDoux 1996, pp. 263, 265; see also LeDoux 2012).

Both quotations are crypto-scientistic in the sense that they make the effectiveness of psychotherapy crucially dependent on structural, i.e., long-term, changes at a biological level. Changes that are not structural or long term don't count. They don't count for the patient, because they are not real. And they don't count for the understanding of how psychotherapy works. The crucial term in the quote of LeDoux is the adverb "just," which suggests that psychotherapy is "nothing else" or "nothing more" than a means to rewire the brain. The Kandel quotation is written in a similar, although subtler, vein. It relates the effectiveness of psychotherapy to learning processes that are based on changes in gene expression that produce altered strengths in synaptic connections. The complexity of the formulation should not detract from the ultimate message, which is that the real changes occur at the level of nerve cells and their interconnections.

It is tempting to agree with these formulations. However, let us also realize what these statements don't state, but merely *imply*: that the real change is in the brain and not in what the patient feels, thinks, or does. The real change is not that the patient has greater control over his or her life or is better able to understand what is going on. The real change is what neuroscience has proved to be the case. Patients may say that they feel better, understand more, and are now able to take responsibility for their lives, but the scientist knows what "in reality" has occurred, and that this is best described and conceptualized in neural terms.

The scientism of these statements is subtle but pervasive. It turns the gaze of the clinician one-sidedly toward what is going on in the brain. It leads to an essentialist conception of behavioral change, a decontextualized approach to psychopathology, and a lack of awareness of normative issues that are intrinsic to mental healthcare.

1.4 A person-centered approach: Philosophical resources

At this critical juncture, we turn to philosophy to see how it can help us develop a novel way of thinking about psychiatry. Instead of a scientistic, abstract, and reified concept of mental disorder, we need an embedded, relational, context-sensitive, normative and—in short—person-centered concept of psychopathology. But this other, person-centered concept of psychopathology also needs a different professional—not the scientist-clinician or clinical scientist who is promoted by leaders in the field, but professionals who, besides knowing their science, are open minded with respect to the individuality of the case and to the value-sensitive matters that arise during consultation. It also requires a rehabilitation of clinical knowledge as a way of knowing in its own right.

Are there philosophical resources that can help us develop an alternative? I think there are. In this work, I make especial use of ideas originating in the philosophies of Sören Kierkegaard (1848), Paul Ricoeur (1990), Charles Taylor (1989), and Herman Dooyeweerd (1953–1958). Another important source for the idea of normative practices is Alasdair MacIntyre (1981), whose idea of "goods that are internal to practices" aligns with Dooyeweerd's idea of the structural "givenness" of normative principles. With respect to the status of clinical knowledge, I also rely on empirical and philosophical literature on "tacit knowledge" (Gascoigne & Thornton 2014; Polanyi 1958).

From Kierkegaard, I borrow the notion of "self-relatedness" and his method of analyzing the bewildering variety of ways of self-relating. The self is a relational category, according to Anti-Climacus, the pseudonymous author under whose name Kierkegaard published his *Sickness unto Death*. It is "a relation which relates to itself, or, that in the relation which is its relating to itself. The self is not the relation but the relation's relating to itself." Anti-Climacus further refers to the self as the "positive third." The self can only be positive because it is established by something else outside itself (Kierkegaard 1848/1980, SKS IV, p. 129). Later in the text, this "something else" is called a power in which the self is "transparently" grounded (Kierkegaard 1848/1980, SKS IV, pp. 130, 161, 164, 242).

These are, of course, very difficult formulations. For now, it is sufficient to see that for Kierkegaard, the self is not a thing (an "entity" or substance) nor just an illusion, but a "relation which relates to itself." When the self relates to itself, this is meant to mark the contrast with relating to something else, for instance a situation or another person. I am a self when I relate to something of myself, for instance, something I did, or thought, or felt. When I relate to this doing, thought or feeling as a part (or aspect) of myself, I am a self, my "self." In other words, it is in the way I am relating to myself that I show who I am and who it is that I call my "self." I do not discuss here at length what Anti-Climacus means by "the power outside itself." The expression can be taken to point to the role of important others (and to Kierkegaard's religious mind, ultimately, the divine). We humans do not begin with ourselves; others begin with us. They are important for the opening up of our selfhood. This concern for others is of course a fundamental fact of life from its earliest beginnings, as developmental psychology has shown. Charles Taylor (1989) has elaborated on this theme in his social and moral philosophy by emphasizing the importance of recognition by the other to the formation of a sense of self and of identity.

Kierkegaard's notion of self-relatedness is important for the understanding of psychopathology as a clinical phenomenon. It is legitimate to abstract from this self-relatedness when one is doing science; however, in a clinical context, we need the concept in a very fundamental way. This is because patients relate to their problems. This self-relating often becomes part of the illness history, even to the point that self and psychopathology can hardly be disentangled any more. It is important for both for the clinician and the patient to know whether one is dealing with symptoms that are straightforward expressions of a disorder or with reactions of the patient to these symptoms, including the impact of the comments of others on illness manifestations. Self-relatedness is, practically speaking, important for the understanding of differences in the way people face their psychiatric problems. Some people panic at the slightest feeling of being out of control; others courageously resist their symptoms, even when they are intolerably intense or frightening.

The notion of self-relatedness is of course not unknown in psychiatry. Clinicians pay attention to it under different headings: "attitude of the patient toward the illness," ""insight," "denial," "self-dramatization," and "somatization." These terms express that patients have a relationship or attitude toward their problem. The idea that people relate to themselves is, of course, also well known in psychotherapy. Discrepancies between what people say and how they implicitly relate to themselves are grist to the mill of psychodynamic psychotherapy. Work on "the self" consists of attempts to lay bare the internalized relationships between self and object representations and to reshape them in the context of a sufficiently intense therapeutic relationship (Kernberg 1984). In family therapy, there is the expression that a family or "system" may push someone into the role of an "identified patient."

The novel element in Kierkegaard's use of the notion of self-relatedness is at least twofold. On the one hand, there is his sensitivity to the inherent ambiguities and complexities of self-relating (and the richness in the way he brings these ambiguities and complexities to the attention of his readers); on the other hand, there is the way in which he connects self-relatedness (as a structural dimension that is given with our existence) with deeper normative and existential considerations and concerns (see also Glas 2017b). Kierkegaard's phenomenology of forms of self-relatedness *avant la lettre* serves, therefore, as a stepping stone toward a normative analysis of illness behavior and of professionalism.

Along this path, we will also meet Paul Ricoeur and his distinction between identity in terms of *idem* (sameness) and *ipse* (oneself or self-reference). Idem refers to the features by which an entity, event, or person can be identified, either individually or as an exemplar of a more general category. The *ipse* (or *soi* in French) refers to "who I am." Who I am is not what I think of myself, a form of self-consciousness, or the ego that posits itself rationally (as in Descartes). It is a self that "finds itself" in its own language, acts, and narratives. In other words, the self is always mediated; it needs a detour via its manifestation in the world to find itself (Ricoeur 1990, pp. 2–3, 16–19). The self is not a substance (or entity) (idem, p. 118ff.), or a predicate (idem, p. 34); neither is it an objectifiable event (idem, p. 48). It is "who I am" while speaking, acting, and interacting. Ricoeur uses the term "self-referentiality" (or sui-reference) to indicate what he means: the implicit referencing of a speech act, act, or narrative to the "I" or self of the person who is speaking, acting, or narrating (idem, pp. 48–53, 57, 118–125). This referencing is implicit, which means that references to aspects of who one is are implied in the act or narration; or, as I am inclined to add, in one's emotions, gestures, thoughts, fantasies, and attitudes.

Idem and *ipse* may overlap, as in the notion of character. Character refers, on the one hand, to the constant features (idem) of a person's personality that may help to identify that person (i.e., the type of character he or she has). Character refers, on the other hand, to who one is (*ipse*). The concept then does not aim so much at identifiable qualities; instead, it addresses a normative dimension of personhood: the implicit or explicit answer to the question of who I am for myself, for others, and in the world; who I wish and strive to be; and who I am in the light of life's ambiguities and of my strengths and shortcomings. According to Ricoeur, the self is inscribed in the *idem*. This is what the notion of character shows. The self is not a free-floating relation; it is anchored. That is, the self-referential aspects of my feelings and doings are anchored in identifiable features of my behavior and speech.

In this book, I frequently make use of the notion of self-reference, or self-referentiality, as I call it: the implicit referencing to who one is in one's emotions, gestures, attitudes, and interactions. In Chapter 2, I add to the complexity of Ricoeur's concept of self-referentiality by outlining three forms of self-referentiality (primary, secondary, and tertiary) (see also Glas 2017a).

To delineate the contextual dimension of psychopathology, the illness role, and the professional role, I use and elaborate on the work of Herman Dooyeweerd (1953–1958). Dooyeweerd provides a framework of normative principles that originally were developed for the analysis of what he calls "differentiated societal relationships." From his philosophy, I borrow the idea of practices with an intrinsic normativity and the type of analysis in terms of different types of constitutive principle (foundational, qualifying, and conditioning principles) (more on Dooye-weerd in Chapter 8.2). The intrinsic nature of these principles is emphasized in a different way by Alasdair MacIntyre, who describes professional (and other) practices as determined by "goods that are internal to practice" (MacIntyre 1981, p. 187). I make use of McIntyre's account of practices as embodying virtues and connect it with Dooyeweerd's analysis of practices as determined by normative structures (and principles). To enable the transition from the analysis in terms of self-relatedness to this analysis in terms of normative structures, I also refer to the work of Charles Taylor (1989), who describes the moral subject as intrinsically connected to "the good." Selfhood consists of the way one relates to these goods. Self-relatedness is, in fact, an embodiment of goods in the life of historically situated and contextually sensitive subjects. Dooyeweerd's philosophy also offers other important insights for the person-centered and clinical approach to psychopathology and psychiatry defended in this book. These ideas will be spelled out in the relevant context (also in Chapter 8.2).

1.5 Outline of the argument

The line of argument of this book runs as follows: In the first part (Chapters 2–4), I draw on and expand the concepts of self-relatedness and self-referentiality to describe and analyze the way the patient relates to him- or herself. The general thrust of this part of the book is that psychiatry needs a clinical conception of psychopathology, alongside the more usual scientific approaches to psychiatric dis-order. This clinical conception of psychopathology recognizes that the self of the patient is involved in the illness and that contextual factors contribute to the form and the content of illness manifestations. Psychopathology cannot be seen apart from the way the patient relates to the illness. This self-relating may occur consciously (explicit) or subconsciously (implicit). Implicit forms are indicated with the term "self-referentiality." Psychopathology is also influenced by social and cultural influ-ences and by the patient's attitude toward these influences. Further analysis of the complexity of self-relatedness, self-referentiality, and context-related interactions naturally brings us into contact with the value-laden aspects of being ill.

In the second part of the book (Chapters 5–8), I apply a similar analysis of the different aspects of self-relatedness to the professional. There are implicit (self-referential) and explicit (self-relational) ways in which the self of the pro-fessional is involved while fulfilling her job. The professional's relationship and engagement with her role is shaped by the many different contexts in which she works. By unraveling the different aspects of this contextually sensitive self-relatedness, we identify the thread that leads to an analysis of the normative structure of clinical practice. Tensions and ambiguities in one's professional role fulfilment make us sensitive for the kinds of value and norm that are at stake.

At this point, Dooyeweerd's theory of modal distinctions and his analyses of the structures of different types of social relationship will prove to be helpful in a heuristic way. The framework that I develop has been introduced earlier and has become known as a "normative practice approach" (NPA) (Jochemsen & Glas 1997; see also Glas 2018). With this framework for a normative analysis in mind, it is not only possible to resist the scientistic defense of the legitimacy of psychiatry but also—and even more importantly—to replace it with a positive account that provides clinicians and scientists with the conceptual tools to explain what they do in their communication with other stakeholders. In this part of the book, I outline how an analysis of the normative structure of mental healthcare would look if it considered that psychiatry has not one but many contexts. I explore this route by making a distinction between mental healthcare at an individual (doctor–patient) level, at an institutional level, and at a societal level. Mental healthcare has different purposes in these different contexts.

In the final chapter of the book (Chapter 9) the perspective developed throughout the book will be compared with other value-sensitive accounts of psychiatry. It is investigated how these other accounts add to the precision and validity of the NPA, and, conversely, how the other concepts and accounts may gain focus and coherence in light of the NPA. Attention will be paid to values-based practice, values-based healthcare, the recovery movement, precision medicine, personalized medicine, P-4 medicine, and person-centered psychiatry. The implications of these views for residency training will be sketched. The chapter ends by elaborating on the existential dimension of professionalism. Openness of the professional about his or her own role fulfilment requires the ability to communicate about the self-referential and self-relational aspects of professional role fulfilment. Tensions and ambivalences with respect to this openness and sensitivity in the current system of mental healthcare will also be addressed.

PART 1

Self, context, and psychopathology

2

SELF-RELATEDNESS, PSYCHOPATHOLOGY, AND THE CONTEXT: A CLINICAL PERSPECTIVE

2.1 The clinical contribution to psychopathology: Self-relatedness and contextuality

This chapter argues that psychiatry needs a clinical concept of psychiatric illness alongside other, scientific concepts of disease. The clinical concept of psychopathology considers that psychiatric symptoms and syndromes are intrinsically self-related and context bound. This approach is, contrary to what one might expect, not common. Psychopathological conditions are usually conceived as expressions of biological dysfunction and/or psychological vulnerability. The clinical conception does justice to the fact the psychiatric illness is also the result of ingrained patterns of interaction between the patient as a person, these dysfunctions and vulnerabilities, and all conceivable sorts of contextual factors. Recognizing these patterns of interaction and their multifaceted nature is of great importance for understanding psychiatric illness and for planning and monitoring treatment.

This chapter first develops a clinical perspective in the form of a model of the web of relationships in which psychopathology evolves, and, more particularly, of the interactions among the person, his or her psychopathology, and the context (shown in Diagram 2.1). The scheme with the web of relationships will also be used and expanded in later chapters.

Next, building on an earlier work of the author (Glas 2017a), a distinction is introduced between different ways of accounting for the self in relation to psychopathology, i.e., in terms of self-relatedness, self-referentiality (implicit, non-conscious), self-awareness, and self-interpretation. I also distinguish among different types of self-referentiality (e.g., first-, second-, and third-order forms of self-referring).

The counterpart of these distinctions is a set of contextual distinctions. These distinctions are only briefly announced in the final section of this chapter and will be more broadly discussed in Chapters 5 and 6. In Chapter 5, I will describe how a similar of web of relationships can be discerned with respect to the professional and the way he or she relates to his or her professionalism. In Chapter 6, I will further elaborate on the distinction between micro- (individual), meso- (institutional), and macro- (societal) levels of analysis of the context.

The main aim of this chapter is to provide a framework that elucidates that, at a clinical level, psychopathological conditions are not more or less separate and separable states of affairs within the patient. They are, instead, always embedded in relationships—including the I–self relationship. I argue that it is often not so much the condition "itself" (which, in fact, is an abstraction) that is the target of intervention but rather the way in which the patient deals with the illness. This "dealing with" is an intricate phenomenon; it is not only influenced by the personality of the patient but also by the illness "itself" and by contextual factors. All these factors together form a web or network of relationships that influences and shapes the way symptoms are expressed and dealt with.

This chapter gives only an outline of the clinical perspective on psychopathology. The theoretical background and underpinnings of some of the distinctions I make are provided in Chapter 3, in the sections on the I–self relation.

2.2 The diagram

Let us focus on Diagram 2.1, which offers a schematic outline of the different relationships that play a role both within the patient and between the patient and the professional during the clinical encounter.

The patient has a problem, looks for help, and visits the professional. This is the initial situation. When I refer to a professional, I have a psychiatrist in mind and not a nurse, psychologist, or psychotherapist. This is for the sake of argument. It is the

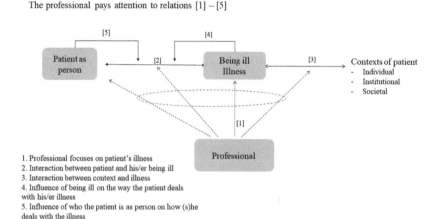

The professional pays attention to relations [1] – [5]

1. Professional focuses on patient's illness
2. Interaction between patient and his/er being ill
3. Interaction between context and illness
4. Influence of being ill on the way the patient deals with his/er illness
5. Influence of who the patient is as person on how (s)he deals with the illness

DIAGRAM 2.1 The professional pays attention to relations [1] - [5]

psychiatrist who most urgently feels the tension between classical disease-oriented and clinical approaches to psychopathology, and it is this tension that I want to address. I focus, therefore, on a prototypical psychiatrist, with knowledge of evidence-based guidelines and treatment protocols and with sufficient psychotherapeutic sophistication to address the relational complexity of the clinical situation.

Let us consider the following common situation more closely. I give no more detail than is needed to make some initial distinctions:

> Jeremy is a 23-year-old male art history student. For the past couple of months, he has suffered from depressive complaints. Jeremy enters the consulting room and begins to describe his experience. He states that he finds it difficult to finish his academic studies. He is almost a year behind now, and he feels bad about the lack of progress. The psychiatrist, Sue, listens to what he says. She pays attention to his physical appearance, his psychomotor behavior, and the tone of his voice. She asks some questions, aiming at clarification and more precision. Sue checks whether Jeremy's condition fulfills the criteria of a psychiatric disorder (major depressive disorder, especially). While doing so, she gets a feeling for the contact between Jeremy and herself. She asks Jeremy about his own interpretations of what is going on. She asks about what friends and relatives have said about his situation. In doing so, she shows her interest and her eagerness to know Jeremy better, and she weighs the opinions of others against her own professional impressions. Thus, she develops an image of Jeremy as a person and the role of depression in the story of his life.

This brief description gives an impression of how multifaceted the activities of the clinician are. Sue listens and observes. She applies scientific knowledge when she asks for more detail. She uses common-sense understanding to estimate the impact of Jeremy's condition on his life (e.g., on his relationships, his self-image, and his career). However, she also implements psychotherapeutic skills by probing for deeper meanings and for underlying patterns that signify what kind of person Jeremy is. She displays communicative and organizational competence. Sue is working within a limited timespan; nevertheless, she strikes a balance between what Jeremy himself needs to tell her and what she needs to know from a professional point of view.

All these elements together—knowledge, skills, and attitudes—form a peculiar mix, which is difficult to characterize from an epistemological point of view. Clinical diagnostic expertise at least entails certain affective, cognitive, and action-related dispositions and much explicit and implicit knowledge. The psychiatrist is listening as a professional, with a professional purpose, not as a friend or neighbor. Professional knowledge and expertise are crucial for this listening. It is Sue's intention to understand what is happening to Jeremy and to do something about it, according to the standards of the profession. One of these standards is that the psychiatrist must act on the basis of a diagnosis (i.e., a state-of-the-art statement about the condition of the patient and its possible causes). Requirements of such diagnostic statements are that they must refer to conditions that are abnormal (i.e., fulfill the criteria for "disorder" that are sufficiently well-established in the profession and usually reflective of a dysfunction or dysregulation at some level). In the next chapter, we will see that there is much discussion about the concept of and the criteria for psychiatric disorder and about the concept of dysfunction.

The above may suffice to explain the arrows that are grouped together as relation [1] in the diagram. The arrows indicate that the professional focuses her attention on how Jeremy deals with his illness [2], on how contextual factors influence the clinical picture [3], on the impact of the illness on Jeremy's relating to his illness [4], and to the impact of Jeremy's personality on how he relates to his "being ill" [5]. I deliberately use the expression "being ill," instead of disorder or disease, to indicate that the professional aims primarily not at a scientific concept of disorder or disease but at illness manifestations that are much more intertwined with the person of the patient and with the context. "Being ill" in the diagram primarily refers to the patient's experiences and his or her reports about the symptoms and signs. What must be emphasized from the start is that disorders don't exist on their own. The uninterrupted line around "being ill" could give the impression that I am reifying "illness," but that is not what the diagram aims to express.

We now turn to the next arrow, which is directed at the relationship between Jeremy as a person and his illness [2]. Relation [2] refers to the way Jeremy relates to his condition of "being ill." It may very well be the case that Jeremy has something different in mind when he relates to his illness than the psychiatrist. For instance, Jeremy may put emphasis on distress, such as feelings of tenseness or palpitations, and on impediments to his functioning, such as fatigue and lack of concentration. By contrast, the clinician may be inclined to focus on criteria for diagnosis and classification and on possible risk factors, such as suicidality. Discrepancies in the definition of the problem are, of course, a source of much dissatisfaction and conflict in the consulting room. These discrepancies should be addressed and resolved as quickly as possible. Being able to not only inform the patient about what is going on but also successfully negotiate what needs to be done is a core competency for the psychiatrist.

Relation [2] is bidirectional. Jeremy interprets what is going on and tries to cope with his illness. However, being ill also influences Jeremy as a person. For example, Jeremy may feel powerless against his depressive mood and the concomitant worries, and he has the strong impression that he is incompetent as a student and insufficient as a person. "I am a failure," he says to his psychiatrist. He is demoralized and does not seem very much inclined to offer resistance against his symptoms. Jeremy's demoralization is a major factor to reckon with.

A cautionary note should be added at this point. Demoralization is a complicated example because it may have different sources. It can be the immediate expression of the depression itself, but it may also reflect a hitherto latent aspect of Jeremy's premorbid personality and the impact of it on Jeremy's coping with the illness. Expert opinion entails the ability to weigh the evidence for each of these options in the individual case. I will discuss this issue in a moment.

Jeremy's symptoms do not stand on their own; they are influenced by the context [3]. This is our next point. Jeremy is a student with somewhat one-sided interests and with only a few friends who have similar interests. He has never had an intimate relationship. Some of his friends are regular cannabis users. Most of them have a relaxed and somewhat passive attitude toward the exigencies of life. They are not very career oriented or competitive. In Jeremy's social niche, there is a tendency to view depressive feelings as a largely normal reaction to a world that is run by big money and to a society that does not seem to need more than superficial communication. His friends tend to be skeptical toward psychiatry and cultivate a quasi-artistic outlook on life.

This brings us to relation [4], which is of considerable importance in the everyday evaluation of mental disorder. This relation refers to the influence of the patient's condition on the way the patient deals with the illness. People who have an anxiety disorder tend to deal with their anxiety in an anxious way. Likewise, patients with depression are inclined to relate in a depressive way to their depression. This is also the case with Jeremy, as we have seen. The depressive feelings are so strong that he thinks he will never be able to conquer them. He is demoralized.

Relation [5], finally, represents the influence of a broad range of person-bound factors on the way the illness is dealt with. It is easiest to think here of the patient's personality, temperament, or character. There is, however, more to this relation than personality. Personal values are important for one's ethos and general outlook on life, as well as all kinds of concern rooted in one's significant life events and in one's cultural and/or religious background. Jeremy's view on life is somewhat detached and not very positive. He thinks only few people can understand his core concerns as an artist. He sees himself primarily as an unrecognized painter. There is a discrepancy between his slightly inflated self-image and what can realistically be expected in terms of recognition of his work by the public. Jeremy tends to attribute this lack of recognition to the public's ignorance and not to personal factors (e.g., lack of talent, insufficient strategies in selling his art). His decision to study the arts was a second, ambivalent choice. In this study, he turns out to be an underachiever.

I add one remark with respect to the relative contribution of relationship [5]. There is a tendency in psychiatry to focus on personality as a negative, limiting factor. However, positive factors also need to be mentioned in this context. Contemporary psychiatry is beginning to discover the value of these factors. In psychology, there already exists a large body of literature on the importance of character strengths and virtues such as openness, kindness, endurance, perseverance, gratitude, empathy, the capacity to forgive, and hope (Cloninger 2004; Peterson & Seligman 2004; Slade 2009). Positive psychology, the psychology of well-being, the recovery movement, acceptance commitment therapy, and mindfulness exercises—diverse as they are—are all expressions of a new way of thinking about mental problems, a way of thinking that is not one-sidedly focused on abnormality, but instead attempts to make use of positive resources in the patient and in his or her environment.

The diagram, although already rather dense, still only describes partially what occurs within the patient and between the psychiatrist and the patient. It is quite common for all these relations to play some role in the manifestation of a particular symptom. Not explicitly drawn in the diagram, or discussed so far, are other interactions, reflecting, for instance, the influence of the context on the patient as a person and on his or her relating to the illness. Contexts, in other words, affect not only the immediate manifestation of illness but also the patient as a person, his or her interpretations and expectations about the illness and its treatment, and his or her ability to cope with the illness.

Let us shed light on this complexity by focusing on Jeremy again. I already alluded to the question of how his demoralization can best be explained. Is it predominantly an impact of the depression on himself [2] or on his coping with the depression [4], as was suggested above? Or do we need to think of influences "located" in one of the other relations? After all, demoralization could also straightforwardly reflect how severe the illness is [1]. It could be explained by contextual influences such as, in Jeremy's case, socioeconomic disadvantages and the influence of friends [3]. Personality factors might also be involved: Jeremy's self-image is somewhat inflated; as a self-declared artist, he is ambivalent about attempts to adapt to a life that is less "artistic" and special [5].

For treatment planning, it is crucial to know what kind of demoralization Jeremy has. Proper assessment requires more biographical and contextual detail. It appears that he was the only child of a divorced and recurrently depressed mother and that he has grown up with all the worries of a lonely and sensitive child of a parent who could hardly take care of herself. His talent for painting nourished his self-image, but it was not something that he could easily share with his peers. His dream of making a career as a painter has not come true. The study of art history was a rational, but ambivalent choice and does not give him the prospect of a job in the near future. Relationships with his friends are somewhat shallow; he has never dared enter into a more lasting relationship. Jeremy knows that his reclusiveness will limit him when he applies for a job. His weak self-confidence is also compromised by difficulties in finishing his master's thesis and lack of social support. There are simply no others who could help him try to resist his demoralization—a clear example of contextual influence on a patient's relation to his illness.

The psychiatrist must know all this in order to weigh the relative contribution of each of these factors and to properly address Jeremy's attitude toward his illness. This weighing and communicating requires a high level of interpretative and communicative skill.

The incompleteness of the diagram is no weakness, I think. It is sufficient for the diagram to function as a stepping stone and to give an impression of the number and subtlety of the interactions and relations within the patient and between the patient and the professional. The different items in the diagram (being ill, patient as person, context, professional role) are not separate building blocks, with relations between them as secondary byproducts. What the professional observes is usually the result of an interaction, in which the interacting "entities" themselves continuously evolve and are co-shaped by the interactions. Jeremy's demoralization may serve as an example of an interaction between self-image, depression, and the socioeconomic and societal context.

These interactions and their assessment are on the table of every clinician in the contact with every patient. Clinicians are not treating disorders, or even patients with disorders, but the effects of interactions between the patient as a person, illness manifestations, and contexts at different levels.

Let us focus now on the relationship between psychopathology and the self.

2.3 Self-relatedness and psychopathology

Patients relate to their illness. They have thoughts, feelings, and wishes about it and take a stance on it. This self-relating-to-the-illness may become so dominant that it is difficult to distinguish it from the illness "itself." Illness and relating-to-the-illness at least overlap and often (more or less) merge. Most current and widely accepted (scientific) conceptions of psychiatric disease completely disregard this self-relational dimension of psychopathology. They see the relationship between self and psychopathology as secondary, at best.

The absence of reflection on the self-relational aspect of psychopathology is a blind spot. The central claim of this chapter is that psychiatry must develop a clinical concept of psychopathology that is intrinsically self-related (and contextrelated). This clinical concept can function alongside other, more scientific (and limited) conceptions of psychopathology.

This section fleshes out how the notion of self can be related to psychiatric illness. I limit the discussion to the introduction of several distinctions and the illustration of their use in clinical practice. The theoretical background and rationale for these distinctions are given in the next chapter.

2.3.1 Self-relatedness, self-referentiality, self-awareness, and self-interpretation

For a better understanding of the relationship between psychiatric conditions and the self, it is helpful to distinguish between four different ways of conceiving of the self and the relations in which the self is involved in psychopathology. These four different ways of conceptualizing the self specify the ways in which psychopathological conditions are related to and signify aspects of the self, even in instances in which the individual is not aware of this signifying. These different ways of speaking about the self in the context of psychopathology are also needed to better understand the layeredness of psychopathological phenomena.

First, there is the concept of self-relatedness. This is a general concept that refers to the fact that I, as a person, am related (and relating) to myself, i.e., to an aspect of myself, an aspect of me as a person. Self-relatedness refers to the fact that persons have a relationship, not only with the world and others, but also with themselves. Self-relatedness stretches out in time, and its instantiations are part of a process. For instance, John may make a condescending remark about someone. Afterwards, John may regret what he did. He thinks: "What a bad person I am." The thought: "What a bad person I am" is a thought of John about himself as a person; it is a way in which John relates to himself or to an aspect, or instance, of his functioning. By giving a negative qualification about what he did, John takes a stance toward himself. Whether his self-evaluation is right is not the issue. What is relevant is that John adopted a stance toward what he did and that it took some time to do this. This stance taking occurs continuously in our daily activities, implicitly and explicitly, and it is referred to by psychologists as "self-regulation." If we stay close to this common-sense notion of self-related-ness, this definition remains unproblematic. However, the definition changes when we delve a bit deeper and question what is meant by terms such as "self," "stance," "attitude," "person-as-a-whole," and "self-regulation" (see the next chapter).

The second concept is that of self-referentiality, which refers to the fact that certain mental phenomena—such as emotions, gestures, speech acts, social inter-actions, and attitudes—implicitly refer to a self, i.e., to an aspect of the person experiencing the emotion or displaying the gesture, speech act, social interaction, or attitude (Ricoeur 1990). For instance, my anger says something about the situation that elicited it, but it simultaneously contains a message about me. Let us say that my anger is caused by the brutality of someone else. Here, my anger refers primarily to this brutality. At the same time, however, it also refers to me, to an aspect of who I am. It indicates, for instance, that the aspect of myself that is under attack is an aspect that is important and valuable enough for me to be upset about. After all, someone's brutality could be such that I don't care about it or don't deem it threatening enough to defend myself.

Self-referentiality implies that there is something, an emotion in this case, that refers to a self, myself, or an aspect of myself. The self-referring capacity of emo-tions, gestures, speech acts, and social interactions often remains implicit. The person experiencing the emotion does not notice it, neither do bystanders. The other important feature of self-referential phenomena is that it is the phenomenon itself—and not the person "behind" the emotion—that has the capacity to refer to the self or to aspects of it. Self-referentiality is, therefore, a *symbolic* concept. It is the phe-nomenon itself that refers and not the agent who "performs" the emotion, gesture, interaction, or speech act. Self-referring typically occurs spontaneously and implicitly. It is in the way we implicitly reveal something about ourselves. Self-referentiality is not lost, however, when the person experiencing an emotion (or displaying a gesture, etc.) becomes aware of what is expressed. Emotions, gestures, interactions, and attitudes don't lose their self-referring capacities when a person becomes aware of having them. However, becoming aware of the meaning of our self-referential expressions and doings may initiate a reaction or chain of reactions that ultimately may change the self-referential meaning of the emotion or gesture. This is how our mental life becomes layered and how our expressions and interactions develop multiple overlapping and gradually changing meanings.

Third, self-awareness is awareness of an aspect of my self or of myself as a whole; self-awareness is a state of mind in which an aspect of my self or I myself become the object of consciousness. At a certain point in time, I notice that I am angry. Because it is me who is angry, the recognition of being angry is a form of self-awareness. It is—in the default case—an awareness of the anger itself and of its meaning at the same time. It is an awareness of the fact that I am angry and of what the anger is about.

Fourth and finally, I discern self-interpretation. Self-interpretation concerns the way in which I understand, perceive, or value myself. It is a secondary valuation of self-awareness. Self-interpretation is needed where the initial awareness of an expression or utterance is unclear or ambiguous. I may feel hurt by someone without initially knowing why. On further reflection, I may discover why I felt hurt. I may realize how the other person subtly awakened my latent feelings of inferiority or threatened my precious ideas and feelings about someone I love. The anger again reveals a threat to something that is important for me, and further reflection (or discussion with others) makes me aware what it is in me that is threatened: my territory, my love for someone, my self-esteem, or—more intricately—my image of what others think about me.

2.3.2 Grief as an example

The relevance of these distinctions is demonstrated by the methods that fuel psychotherapeutic practice. Helping the patient understand and interpret what he or she is feeling, desiring, and doing forms a substantial part of the therapist's job. Frequently, feelings are initially distorted, suppressed, or simply not noticed by a patient. They are self-referential, but the person is not aware of them.

For instance, grief may be masked by unrest and irritability. Unrest and irritability are dispositions together with their instantiations. Unrest manifests itself as a tendency to remain constantly busy; irritability as a tendency to react impatiently and dysphorically. Both have all kinds of behavioral, mental, bodily, and interactional instantiations. Therapists initially attempt to raise awareness in the patient of these tendencies and their instantiations. Identifying hitherto unrecognized tendencies and their instantiations allows progress from unnoticed, self-referential tendencies and behaviors to tendencies and behaviors of which the patient is aware. The next step is to explore whether these tendencies and behaviors mean something and, if so, what. Do they mask sadness, or ambivalence, or a certain vulnerability of one's self-image, or combinations of these? Attempts to answer such questions facilitate progression from self-awareness to self-interpretation.

The distinction between self-referentiality and self-awareness is important because dispositions, feelings, and emotions may signify something about a person, even if the person experiencing the emotion is not aware of this signifying. The distinction between self-awareness and self-interpretation (or self-understanding) makes sense because self-awareness does not automatically imply self-interpretation. Interpretation goes a step further than awareness: It requires the ability to reflect on what is going on, to recognize what emotions mean, and to put this recognition into a larger perspective about what is going on.

Nevertheless, this is still an idealized description. Therapeutic practice and real life are, in fact, far richer and more intricate. The distinctions between self-referentiality, self-awareness, and self-interpretation are conceptually clear enough, but, in practice, they are difficult to implement. And the transitions—from self-referentiality to self-awareness to self-interpretation—tend to be less sharp than their descriptions suggest. Self-referential and unconscious irritability and unrest are usually conscious to some extent. It would, after all, be difficult not to notice their signs. Let me illustrate this with an example:

> Ronald is a middle-aged man who lost his wife to cancer. Ronald initially feels sadness, unrest, and heightened irritability. He pushes these feelings away, however. He immerses himself in work and works harder and harder. Relatives and friends ask whether they can help "because you seem so tense and distressed." Ronald is not very willing to concede this. "Yes, I was sad," he says, "and my life has changed enormously. But I like my work, I felt better after a couple of months. Now that you ask me, I am indeed a bit distressed. I don't worry about that; however, a couple of decent nights' sleep will make me feel better again. I can cope with what has happened." (et cetera).

Let us assume that Ronald is dissimulating and that his relatives and friends are right in thinking that there is something more serious going on. The case shows how grief is initially felt for a short span of time and then suppressed, probably via coping mechanisms such as avoidance, denial, and rationalization. Rationalization is an interesting boundary case. It is clearly a form of self-interpretation, but it mainly functions at the level of self-awareness, by neutralizing and avoiding distressing aspects of grief. When Ronald says that there is "nothing to worry about" and that "a couple of decent nights' sleep will suffice," he gives an interpretation of his condition that also serves as a rationale for his lack of awareness of his own manifestations of grief. This (partial) lack of awareness exists together with an intact referencing function of the grief itself, as embodied and exemplified by the unrest and irritability. This intact self-referring, after all, enables relatives and friends to recognize what is going on. Lack of self-awareness is not a static given, however. It may wax and wane, depending on the context. A talk with a sensitive friend may temporarily lead to more openness and some sharing of his feelings of sadness. Later on, reading about grief and interactions with other bereaved persons may help Ronald to gradually process the grief.

In summary, what I initially described as a clear-cut case in which self-referential but unconscious tendencies and feelings come to awareness and subsequently are interpreted appears to represent a much more complex amalgam of different levels of conscious awareness, with an important role for contextual and personal factors smeared out over a certain period of time. Non-conscious inclinations and emotions are, as it turns out, not completely unconscious. Coping mechanisms and self-interpretation exert their influence not only at the level of self-reflection but also at the level of (self-) awareness. Combined with interactions with relatives and friends and different ways of self-relating over time, all these factors together form a dynamic interplay that initiates changes in self-awareness and self-interpretation.

2.3.3 Self-referentiality and self-awareness

This section further explores the interface between self-referentiality and self-awareness by delving somewhat deeper into the definition of these concepts and by adding some remarks about action tendencies and the role of implicit forms of self-relating. By doing so, I can give a better impression of the fluidity of transitions and the dynamic nature of the phenomena that concern us.

As I have said, it is very possible for a feeling or emotion to be both self-referential and conscious. The self-referential aspect refers to the signifying aspect that is *intrinsic* to and *implicit* within the emotion. Self-referentiality is not a form of relating, or stance taking, but a form of self-signifying within the stream of our affective reactions and attitudes. This is important to note, because there is a tendency in some branches of psychology to think that emotions mean something because of the appraisals and judgments that they entail and that give an interpretation of a particular state of affairs in the world. On this account, emotions can only mean something about oneself insofar as we can make ourselves the object of such appraisals and judgments (more about this in the next chapter). This is not what is meant by the notion of self-referentiality.

What I am advocating is that the meaning of emotions (and other self-referential activities) is given with their implicit self- (and object-) directed *signifying role*. Self-awareness and self-interpretation come conceptually later, although they may temporally coincide with self- (and object-) directed referring. Conscious interpretations, appraisals, and judgments matter, of course. They are important for the unraveling of the meaning of emotions. Self-referential meaning also tends to coincide with the content of appraisals and other forms of emotional evaluation. But the two are nevertheless conceptually distinct. Appraisals and judgments can probably best be viewed as confirmations or further specifications of meanings that already existed in the implicit mode, at least in everyday situations. This may be different in psychopathology and psychotherapy. Ronald's rationalizations, for instance, exemplify how conscious interpretation may follow a route that deviates from the implicit self-referring aspect of emotions. It is because of these deviations that I put so much emphasis on the distinctions between different ways of speaking about the self in the context of psychopathology.

Self-referentiality is not an easy concept, but neither is self-awareness. I adopt a pragmatic stance and avoid using distinctions too rigidly, particularly the distinction between tacit and explicit forms of self-awareness. Self-awareness can exist as a tacit, non-thematic, bodily anchored perception of what is going on when I am relaxed or immersed in some activity. It can also exist as thematic, explicit, and observational awareness of aspects of myself. This awareness emerges when one consciously focuses on particular aspects of the self. Sartre would call this kind of consciousness "positional consciousness"; it is a consciousness that takes an observational or interpretative stance toward aspects of myself (Colombetti 2014, Chapter 5; Legrand 2007; Zahavi 2005). We will see that these forms are extremes on a continuum.

I am, moreover, inclined to consider awareness as a concept with a double meaning (double in the sense that it refers both to the fact *that* one feels and to *what* one feels, tenseness and the absence of fatigue, for instance, or, unrest and the absence of anger). The "what" of the awareness does not necessarily need to be a particular theme or object, since that would rule out non-thematic content as part of the concept of self-awareness. There is a non-thematic "what" in some forms of self-awareness. I am referring to situations in which I am in a global feeling state or mood, situations in which the feeling or mood does not have a thematic object but is sufficiently crystallized that I can identify my condition as pleasant or unpleasant, elated or depressed, disgusting or rewarding. One can be aware of oneself and identify what one feels without knowing exactly what it is that the feeling is about. One may say: "No, I was not upset, but tense," or "I don't know exactly why, but I felt irritated and tired; it was not sadness," without knowing where the tension, or irritation or tiredness, come from and what it means.

We are also touching on the boundaries of self-referentiality here. There are forms of self-awareness that are not self-referential; for instance, certain bodily feelings and pain. The awareness of numbing, aching, choking, and other sensations is usually located somewhere in the body. Such feelings express an awareness *of* oneself, more specifically of aspects of one's body. However, they are not *about* oneself. They are not referring to who one is as a person or to aspects of oneself as a person. These specifications leave us with an enormous range of forms of self-awareness. There are, on the one hand, non-self-referential forms of self-awareness, such as bodily feelings; there are borderline cases with limited self-referentiality, such as elementary, bodily feelings and sensations that give only a faint impression of how the subject's self is affected. Slight touches of sadness are an example. On the other hand, there are cases of self-awareness that refer to the deepest layers of the personality or self. The awareness of belonging to someone might be an example. More complicated are situations in which non-self-referential bodily feelings announce the advent of a feeling or emotion: a wave of nausea announcing disgust about something, feelings of compression in the stomach preceding one's worries about a public performance or worries that are both object and self-directed.

Action tendencies play an important role in deciphering the meaning of implicit self-referential phenomena. In real life and in psychotherapy, self-referential behaviors (gestures, emotions, attitudes, and interactions) are not only recognized on the basis of their reference to objects and to aspects of the self, but also on the basis of the action tendencies they embody. Emotions are "felt tendencies" according to Arnold (1960). These tendencies are inclinations or dispositions to act in certain ways (Frijda 1986, Chapter 2.8). Anger, for instance, is characterized by the tendency to punish someone for his or her actions; it is a readiness to action that announces itself in, for instance, the clenching of one's fists or in cherished fantasies about how one will punish the other. Action tendencies are important for emotion recognition, especially in emotions with a low felt intensity. Sometimes one does not feel the anger, but only notices one's clenched fists or one's fantasies. Spontaneous inclinations and concomitant action plans may be more revealing about one's emotional state than what one knows from introspection. Grief, for instance, may be recognized when people show a tendency to withdraw from social interaction and from engaging in meaningful activities. Such withdrawal is often first observed by others and not by the person him- or herself.

To complicate matters even further and to anticipate what will be discussed in the next sections, I must add that emotions are sometimes primarily recognized based on secondary reactions to them (e.g., reactions to the tendency to withdraw). Ronald, the person who did not recognize his grief, was working excessively hard. In his case, working hard could be interpreted as an attempt to counteract pervasive feelings of loss and disconnectedness. It is a reaction to the felt tendency to withdraw and to give up one's life. It was the combination of signs of distress, excessive working, and unconvincing rationalizations that prompted the suspicion of his friends that Ronald was denying the severity of his loss. Each of the three in itself provided insufficient grounds for their worries, but together, they were enough to give reason to suspect a problem.

2.3.4 Primary, secondary, and tertiary self-referentiality

Does what has been said so far mean that it does not matter whether we are aware of our emotions? We have seen that explicit, conscious awareness and implicit, self-referential meaning do not exclude one another. Self-referential signifying usually remains preserved in cases in which the subject becomes aware of the meaning of the signifying. I also suggested that interpretations of emotion often come after the fact (*post hoc*). However, it would be premature to conclude from this that the self-referential aspects of our functioning do all the signifying work and that self-awareness and interpretation are, at best, the icing on the cake. I suggest that self-awareness and self-interpretation may specify the meaning of emotion and inform strategies for self-regulation and self-management.

In this section, I explore another related aspect: the potential self-referential meaning of one's secondary reactions to emotions, whether the latter are self-referential or not. By proceeding in this way, I will also broaden our perspective again, that is, to psychopathology in a wider sense. It is especially in the field of psychopathology that the secondary (and tertiary) reactions to one's initial responses become important. One of the difficulties in the clinical assessment and scientific study of psychopathology is that there are so many secondary reactions to the initial layer of affective, cognitive, and behavioral responses. It is sometimes difficult to disentangle these later layers from the primary phenomena.

Let me give a brief example, still in the sphere of everyday experience: Hiding one's face may be a primary response that is part of the emotion of shame. However, it may also be a secondary reaction, for instance when one becomes aware of the blushing of one's cheeks. The blushing would then be the primary emotional response and hiding one's face would be the secondary reaction to the awareness of blushing. The blushing often has a self-referential quality: The person who is blushing feels embarrassed about something. This self-referencing of the immediate emotional reaction I call, from now on, primary self-referential (instead of merely self-referential). However, the hiding of the face, as a secondary reaction, also has self-referential potential. For instance, it may signify that the person who is blushing hates to feel unmasked by his or her blushing and tries to avoid this by hiding the face. The hiding of the face would then indicate that he or she doesn't want to be exposed to others who might see the embarrassment and wonder what provoked it. Such secondary reactions are self-referential as well. For instance, they may refer to proudness on the part of the blushing person or to latent feelings of guilt. The person who hides his or her blushing would then do so because he or she is too proud to allow others to notice the blushing, or because of guilt feelings about what has caused the shame and concern that others will become aware of the cause. The blushing still occurs, but the emotional meaning of the blushing is denied or hidden. This denial and hiding reveals a secondary form of self-referentiality. It signifies something about the person, a vulnerability for feelings of inferiority, humiliation, and/or guilt—a vulnerability of which the person may or may not be aware but to which the secondary reaction refers. The referentiality of these secondary reactions I call secondary self-referentiality.

The example shows that there is a complex dynamic among self-referentiality, self-awareness, and self-interpretation. Clinical psychopathology has a similar complexity. Patients may initially be aware of their primary symptoms and signs and subsequently deny or downplay them, even to the extent that the initial illness manifestations are no longer felt. The secondary reactions then dominate the clinical picture. This may occur based on some trait or aspect of one's personality, although not necessarily. If the denying (secondarily) refers to a personality trait, it may indicate that the patient is vulnerable to certain self-perceptions or perceptions by others. Self-referential, secondary reactions to symptoms and signs of illness may have other sources, however. They are constantly changing, moreover. People may become aware that they are denying their illness manifestations and do something about it. They may figure out why they do this and try to change their attitude and behavior.

So far, I have focused on cases in which the emotional reactions and illness manifestations are self-referential. Is it possible to imagine conditions in which this primary self-referentiality is lost? I think that such conditions exist, not only secondary to coping processes (such as denial and suppression) but also as part of the psycho(patho)logical process itself. We could see such cases as belonging to a broader class of psychological phenomena in which self-referentiality is lacking. Cases of loss of self-referentiality are then a subclass of the group of psychological conditions without self-referentiality.

Lack of self-referentiality is not uncommon. I already mentioned bodily feelings as an example, but there are other conditions, normal and psychopathological. Elementary perceptions (*qualia*) belong to the normal end of the spectrum of non-self-referential phenomena. On the pathological end, we encounter clouded consciousness, confusion, severe apathy, and extreme forms of panic in which the panic attacks come out of the blue as a storm of senseless physical sensations. This list is certainly not exhaustive. All these conditions are marked by lack of self-referentiality. Patients react to these conditions, and these reactions may again say something about the person (i.e., insofar as the reacting itself implicitly refers to an aspect of who the person is).

The same holds for cases of loss (instead of lack) of self-referentiality. In such cases, an initially self-referential psychological condition transforms into a non-self-referential one. I am inclined to suggest that these conditions are not common, but, nevertheless, they do exist. Depression may, for instance, evolve into a prolonged, severe psychotic depression and, especially in elderly patients, end in a state that is marked by feelings of emptiness, alienation, apathy, and repetitive and contextless thoughts. Other examples are found at the severe end of the spectrum of obsessive compulsive disorder, in chronic cases in which compulsive rituals gradually lose their meaning and obsessive thoughts become empty. Likewise, panic disorder may begin as a form of severe anxiety with self-referential elements, gradually evolving into a condition in which the anxiety is just there, pointless, absorbing everything, without transparency, and without what philosophers have called "aboutness" (i.e., self-evident reference to an aspect of the self or the world). The patient may be fully aware of his or her condition. He or she may also have all sorts of explanation for the condition. However, the awareness and the explanations do not (usually) alter the senseless quality of the feeling itself. It is in such cases also that it makes sense to address the secondary self-referential aspects of the patient's mental state. Despite the meaninglessness of their symptoms, patients still adopt an attitude toward them, and this attitude (or stance) may self-referentially signify who one is in one's being ill. Dealing with these secondary self-referential implications of one's stance toward one's being ill is of crucial importance in clinical practice, both in diagnostic assessment and in treatment plan design.

Patients, in short, relate to what they are feeling, doing, or inclined to do. They relate to their being ill, whether there is (*primary*) self-referential meaning in this being ill or not. Their way of dealing with their condition sometimes shows courageous persistence, in other cases, a lack of hope and trust; sometimes autonomy and perseverance, in other situations, dependence and lack of initiative. Patients may or may not be aware of this. All forms of self-relating, whether patients are aware of it or not, may have, or acquire, a *secondary* self-referential meaning. Awareness and interpretation of the self-referential quality of one's relating to one's illness may also change the original meaning—or meaninglessness—of one's condition. It seems plausible to assume that at least some change will take place when symptoms are placed in a context and related to one's sense of who one is. The original phenomenon may become less urgent, for instance, or more differentiated, easier to deal with, understandable, or tolerable. However, there are cases in which the primary psychopathological phenomenon is psychologically impenetrable and successfully resists attempts to change or interpret it. Delusion is an obvious example. Altered body image in anorexia nervosa and irrational obsessions are other examples. Most complex are those situations in which the aspect of the self that is secondarily referred to influences the course, intensity, and quality of the original phenomenon. Personality problems with an impact on the original problem are an example of this. For instance, consider a patient with depression and strong self-dramatizing tendencies. The sadness and depression have straightforward primary self-referential meanings. However, the self-dramatizing attitude of the patient toward the illness makes the picture more difficult to interpret. This attitude refers to a secondary form of self-referentiality, i.e., the patient's stance toward his or her problem. This stance in turn is not something as such; rather, it colors and influences the illness "itself," to the extent that the depression in *sensu stricto* can no longer be distinguished from its dramatized version. The patient is making a drama of his or her depression, and the sadness thus takes on a theatrical color.

I have distinguished so far between two dimensions in the understanding of self-referentiality: an immediate, primary self-referential dimension of transparent phenomena (emotions, gestures, attitudes, and interactions) and a secondary, self-referential dimension that manifests in the way the patient relates to his or her condition. Before I finish this section, I would like to briefly discuss a third form of self-referentiality: This *tertiary* self-referentiality results from the internalization of moments of self-understanding in the course of time. Patients accumulate over time moments of self-interpretation that are integrated into their identities as persons with mental health problems. This occurs all the time, of course, especially in chronic cases, when psychiatric illness has exerted an enduring influence on the patient's life. In such cases, prolonged support, psychoeducation, and adequate psychotherapy may also contribute to the patient's insight into the illness and its long-lasting impact on the patient's identity.

This insight will be internalized and become second nature, as it were. It evolves into a tacit form of self-knowledge (i.e., into a tertiary form of self-referentiality), which manifests itself in the way the patient has integrated or failed to integrate the fact of being ill into the project of his or her life. This third form of self-referentiality is especially important in patients with considerable illness histories (e.g., people with chronic depression, bipolar disorder, personality disorder, addiction, and schizophrenia). In these cases, it is not so much self-referentiality, which, via self-awareness, amounts to self-understanding. It is, in fact, the other way around: A specific form of self-interpretation ("me as a person with chronic, incurable disease, but nevertheless personal qualities that give me a life with sufficient fulfilment") has been internalized and evolved into an implicit interpretation of who one is. This implicit self-interpretation reveals itself in the way the patient relates toward the illness and toward others, including the mental healthcare system and its representatives. One can think of patients who manifest a certain wisdom about their illness. These patients realize that their illness will not go away; nevertheless, they have learned to cope with it. Other cases concern persons who have internalized their role as a victim or as a patient with unexplained medical problems and thus identify themselves in terms of their struggle for recognition by doctors, the legal system, and governmental agencies. Note again that we need a time dimension to understand the layeredness of the different self-referential forms of signifying, the awareness and interpretations of these forms, and the secondary reactions to the awareness and interpretation of one's illness. It is by reconstructing the course of the illness over time that we untangle the different layers of these complex conditions.

Second- and third-order self-referentiality inform mental healthcare workers not only about the weaknesses of the patient but also about their inner strengths and creativity in dealing with the illness. Approaches such as the recovery movement in psychiatry are putting this dimension on the agenda and give suggestions about how to make use of it in a therapeutic context (Slade 2009). This seems a fruitful approach that finds its philosophical rationale in the kind of analyses given above.

Textbox 2.1 gives an overview of the different forms and meanings of addressing the self in clinical practice.

---

1   Self-relatedness: Relating to oneself (processual)
2   Self-referentiality: Implicit reference to aspects of the self:

    a   Primary self-referentiality: Immediate, implicit reference of a gesture, emotion, attitude, or interaction to aspects of the self

    b   Secondary self-referentiality: Self-referentiality in one's relation to one's gestures, emotions, attitudes or interactions (whether primary self-referential or not)

    c   Tertiary self-referentiality: Self-referential meaning of internalized attitudes towards the illness or aspects of it

3   Self-awareness: Being aware of one's gestures, emotions, attitudes, or interactions
4   Self-interpretation: Interpretation of gestures, emotions, attitudes, or interactions; identifying what they mean in a broader context.

I believe the above gives an adequate impression of the variety and complexity of clinical reality. The distinctions that were introduced were first and foremost meant to facilitate a conceptual grasp on a reality that is intrinsically fluid, dynamic, and only partially transparent.

2.3.5 Self-relatedness and the three forms of self-referentiality in practice

I will finish this section by showing how the distinctions that have been introduced so far (self-relatedness; primary, secondary, and tertiary self-referentiality; self-awareness; and self-interpretation) fit within the general scheme depicted in Diagram 2.1 and discussed in Section 2.2 (for another example, see Strijbos & Glas 2018).

I do this by referring to the following new case:

> Peter is a 31-year-old web designer who has recently developed panic disorder without clear and immediate reference to objects or himself. In other words, his panic does not entail concrete or coherent concerns about his body or person, such as concerns about suffering a medical emergency of losing control. The

panic is a storm of meaningless physical sensations. Peter goes to his general practitioner who, after physical examination, reassures him that physically there is nothing wrong. The GP asks whether there are psychosocial stress factors. Peter explains that he is living alone after having broken up with his girlfriend and that his working situation is not very stable. However, these stress factors have been present for a couple of years and do not seem to have disturbed him too much so far. After the consultation, the panic does not disappear; in fact, it worsens. The symptoms are so overwhelming that Peter thinks that he will die or lose his mind if he leaves home unaccompanied. He realizes that his condition could lead to a vicious circle of increasing helplessness. However, he does not resist his increasing incapacity and dependence on others. The course of events suggests a relationship between the severity of the symptoms, their paralyzing effects, Peter's passive attitude, and his personality (or self). The panic disorder ties in with his long-standing feelings of insufficiency, which have led to apathy. It is in dealing with his complaints that certain aspects of Peter's personality become manifest, particularly tendencies to passivity and to conflict avoidance.

I will now quote each sentence and indicate to which relations and distinctions each refers. Numbers between brackets refer to the numbers in Diagram 2.1. Italic terms refer to the ways different forms of self-relatedness can be addressed (self-relatedness, self-referentiality in its different variants, self-awareness, and self-interpretation):

> "Peter … has recently developed panic disorder without clear and immediate reference to objects or himself … his panic does not entail concrete or coherent concerns about his body or person …"

These sentences refer to Peter's being ill [1]. The manifestations of the illness are *non-self-referential*.

> "His panic is a storm of meaningless physical sensations."

The term "sensations" refers to what Peter feels (*self-awareness*); what Peter feels is *non-self-referential*.

> "Peter goes to his general practitioner who … reassures him that … there is nothing wrong."

Peter's behavior—going to the doctor—suggests that he interprets his problems as medical. This is a specimen of *self-interpretation*. The complaints are situated in a medical context [3]. The general practitioner tries to reassure him, which is a way to alter Peter's stance towards his complaints (reference to relation [2]). The reassurance is cast in the form of an *interpretation* ("physically" there is "nothing wrong").

> "The GP asks whether there are psychosocial stress factors."

This is probing whether contextual factors play a role in the genesis of the illness [3].

> "Peter explains that he is living alone after having broken up with his girlfriend and that his working situation is not very stable."

Peter and his doctor try to identify possible contextual factors [3].

> "However, these stress factors have been there for years and do not seem to have disturbed him too much so far."

This is a (self-)interpretation.

> "After the consultation the panic ... worsens. The symptoms are so overwhelming that Peter thinks he will die or lose his mind ..."

This can be interpreted as an instance of relationship [2]: immediate influence of the disorder on the patient's image of himself. Later in the course of the illness, this self-image may consolidate and influence Peter's relationship to his illness [5]. It might well be, moreover, that Peter begins to anticipate the possible occurrence of panic attacks and that this anticipatory anxiety becomes part of the panic disorder and influences his relating to the illness [4].

> "Peter thinks he will die or lose his mind ..."

These are examples of self-relating (he thinks, he evaluates), as well as self-awareness (the feelings are overwhelming) and self-interpretation ("I cannot stand this; I will die or become mad").

> "He realizes that his condition could lead to a vicious circle of increasing helplessness."

This refers to a deeper form of self-interpretation that builds on self-awareness and which takes the relations [2], [4], and [5] into account.

> "The course of events suggests a relationship between the severity of the symptoms ..."

... reference to the illness [1].

> "their paralyzing effects ..."

... reference to the influence of the illness on Peter's relation to the illness [4].

> "Peter's passive attitude ..."

… predominantly a reference to the interaction between personality and illness [2].

> "… and his personality (or self): The panic disorder ties in with longstanding feelings of insufficiency …"

… refers to *self-awareness* and to influence of the personality on dealing with the illness [5].

> "which have led to apathy."

This is a crucial point in the diagnosis: Will the apathy be seen as merely the result of the interaction between the different factors or as the result of a process of internalization and consolidation that has transformed it into a personality characteristic? In the latter case, the attention of the clinician may shift to Peter's personality, which occupies then the place of the original "disorder" [1].

> "It is in dealing with his complaints …"

… refers to relation [2].

> "that a secondary form of self-referentiality becomes manifest, which reveals an aspect of his personality, i.e., a tendency to passivity and conflict avoidance."

… this is another way of describing relation [5].

The secondary form of self-referentiality is, so to say, the flipside of relationship [5]. Relationship [5] refers to how the patient's personality (tendency to passivity and avoidance) affects how the patient deals with the illness. *Secondary self-referentiality* describes the same phenomenon, but now from the inside; i.e., from the side of relationship [2] by indicating how, in Peter's way of dealing with the illness, aspects of his personality implicitly become manifest. Tertiary self-referentiality refers then to the situation in which these secondary forms of self-referring have become internalized. This presupposes that the forms of self-relatedness in which this self-signifying is implicated have become structural features of Peter's personality.

The above description does not provide a very clear example of *tertiary self-referentiality*; however, the apathy mentioned at the end of the vignette comes close to it. Longstanding passivity and avoidance will finally become part of the patient's habitus and essentially reflect the patient's second nature in dealing with the illness. The avoidance and passivity do not stand on their own; they belong to a conglomerate of illness characteristics, other personality factors, and contextual influences. The entire situation is characterized by a vicious circle of increasing helplessness, fear, and desperation. The description of the vignette suggests that Peter is largely aware of this (*self-awareness*) and that he thinks something like the following: "I am not the kind of person that is able to withstand these terrible and alarming symptoms," which represents a form of *self-interpretation*.

Paying attention to secondary and tertiary levels of self-referentiality is immensely important for clinical practice. Therapeutic success often depends on the subtle hand-ling of the implicit aspects of the way the patient relates to his or her illness. Under-standing secondary self-referentiality and weighing it against the direct influence of the disorder on the attitude of the patient toward the illness requires considerable clinical experience and empathy. This weighing of perspectives belongs to the heart of psy-chiatric practice and plays a crucial role in selecting the most promising and effective treatment options. In the case of Peter, the clinician must weigh the immediate impact of panic on avoidance behavior against the impact of Peter's personality on his avoid-ance behavior. The term "avoidance" refers here to Peter's unwillingness to face his condition and take appropriate measures. Similar considerations hold for the tertiary self-referential aspects of being ill, such as (possibly) Peter's apathy.

In summary, there is a complex dynamic among self-relatedness, self-referenti-ality, self-awareness, and self-interpretation. Self-referentiality is a fundamental layer in the understanding of the human psyche. Self-awareness helps one focus and prepare for action, whereas self-interpretation is meant to put one's emotions, gestures, attitudes, and interactional tendencies in a broader context.

Secondary reactions sometimes occur automatically. In other cases, they are the result of an act of will. Both intentional and unintentional secondary reactions may lead to alterations in the meaning of the original phenomenon (emotion, gesture, behavior, interaction), but usually not to the extent that the original meaning is wiped out. In the study of the psyche, it is sometimes difficult to disentangle the primary layer of affective, cognitive, and behavioral responses from later and more superficial layers.

The reader will note that I have been sticking to my original definition of self-referentiality, according to which the signifying (or referencing) occurs implicitly. Self-referring is a form of signaling inherent to emotions, gestures, attitudes, and interactions and independent of whether there is awareness of the emotions, gestures, attitudes, or interactions and their meaning. It is, of course, possible for one to become aware of complex forms of signaling. However, this fact usually does not stop the implicit signifying; it only makes it explicit and helps the sub-ject to recognize, categorize, interpret, and navigate through what he or she is feeling (or doing). A special case are psychopathological conditions in which the patient lacks or has lost self-referentiality. In these cases, secondary and tertiary forms of self-referentiality show that psychopathology, despite its apparent meaninglessness, might still say something about the patient as a person. We also saw that secondary and tertiary forms of self-referentiality may be relevant for the understanding of psychopathological phenomena. They add layers to the nuclear layer of primary self-referentiality.

2.4 Contexts

In this section, I briefly explore the impact of contextual influences on the way psy-chiatric illness is expressed. This is, of course, a huge subject. I limit my discussion to a conceptual outline, which will be developed somewhat further in Chapters 4 and 5.

The line of reasoning runs analogously to my argument in the previous section. It is hypothesized that, for the clinical manifestation of psychiatric disorder, the relationship between the patient and the context is *fundamental* and not *accidental*. Likewise, the relationship between psychiatric illness and the self is not accidental but fundamental. I will also show the need for some stratification of this relationship, as I did with respect to the relationship between psychiatric illness and the self.

Crucial for our understanding of clinical practice is that mental illness should be conceived as the product of an interaction, rather than the straightforward expression of an underlying dysfunction. This interaction involves the person, the context and, of course, the disordered mechanism, vulnerability, latent factor, dysfunction, or abnormality. In the previous section, I investigated the role of the person by addressing the self in different ways. These distinctions helped us to see that it is often not so much the dysfunction as such or its immediate expressions that are the main focus of clinical attention, but rather the overlay in the form of secondary reactions and consolidated forms of self-relatedness. These are implicit ways of interacting with oneself—under the influence of personality, context, or the illness itself—that in a secondary way refer to oneself (secondary self-referentiality) and that in consolidated form have become part of one's personality (tertiary self-referentiality).

By introducing these distinctions, I implicitly also imported a time dimension. What we see in clinical practice is not the "naked" disorder but the product of interactions that last for months, years, or even decades. Jeremy's indolence turned out to be a product of an internalized interaction between his personality, contextual factors, and the illness. It was not so much his depression "itself" but his passivity and demoralization that needed the therapist's attention. In fact, the interaction effects were so crucial that the idea of an underlying disorder became almost an abstraction—almost, but not entirely! Jeremy's symptoms could still be identified as belonging to the class of major depressive disorder. And, insofar as this class is established on scientific grounds, Jeremy's condition could also be addressed from a scientific point of view.

This also holds for the role of the context, as we will see. Contexts are not merely modifying factors on the road from dysfunction to symptom. They are not external to the process of symptom formation; on the contrary: They are constitutive. If mental illness is the product of an interaction, then the context is one of the producers of that interaction. Depending on the context, the expression of the disturbance will transform. This transformation may go so far that the "original" (or "naked", "nuclear") dysfunction, disturbance, or vulnerability nearly seems to disappear. In reality, however, the role of the original dysfunction simply changes within the web of interlocking dependencies. The situation is analogous to what I described with respect to the self-relational aspects of mental illness. There is an overlay of effects of interactions and relations between contexts, persons, and disturbances. By stratifying the role of the context, we will be able to disentangle this overlay.

This is enough to get an impression of the general plan. In Chapter 7, I develop a stratification with three types of context and interaction: individual, institutional, and societal. These distinctions are important because they allow us to see that each interactional layer produces its own conception of psychopathology, or, more precisely, of the object of psychiatry. In Diagram 2.1, "being ill" is the central focus. This diagram refers to individual interactions between the patient and the physician. We will see that in a wider institutional context, this definition of the object of psychiatry is too narrow. We will speak about *patient needs* in this institutional context. In the still larger societal context, the focus will be on the shaping, profiling, and cultural coding of *health problems*.

2.5 Conclusion

Let me summarize where we are. Chapter 1 sketched the need for a clinical approach to psychiatric illness, in addition to more scientific approaches. We saw that there is a tendency in current psychiatry to reverse the order of things, that is, to consider abstract, isolated, and reified concepts of mental disorder as the heart of the matter and as the starting point for a clinical practice that is ruled by guidelines and protocols, instead of viewing clinical practice as the heart of the matter and scientific concepts and explanations as tools that can elucidate what is going on.

According to one dominant view, psychiatric illness is the expression of the breakdown of a mechanism within a person's brain. Symptoms and signs that are not explicable in terms of disordered brain functioning are conceived as non-essential, derivative, and extrinsic. One other dominant paradigm is statistical and presupposes that psychiatric illness consists of clusters or patterns of co-varying items or symptoms. These clusters can be related to treatment algorithms according to the principles of evidence-based medicine.

The view I have been advocating in this chapter is complementary and entails that in clinical practice, we must think (and are, in fact, thinking!) reversely, that is, from the whole to the parts, from the full picture to the constituting elements and aspects. Disordered mechanisms should be put into perspective by relating them to the overall functioning of the individual and by weighing them against the adaptive capacities of the patient and against the roles of environmental resources and con-straints. What we have seen is that this holistic idea of overall functioning requires a concept of self-relatedness and explicit attention to the role of the context.

This chapter developed a conceptual framework for addressing the self in clinical psychopathology. A distinction was introduced between self-relatedness, self-referentiality, self-awareness, and self-interpretation. An additional distinc-tion was construed with respect to primary, secondary, and tertiary forms of self-referentiality. I emphasized the temporal dimension of the interactions and signifying relationships and suggested that the conceptual framework can help disentangle the intricate interwovenness between initial symptoms, secondary reactions, and their implicit and explicit meanings. The chapter ended with the suggestion that on the contextual side, we may suspect a similar interwovenness that can be disentangled by distinguishing among individual, institutional, and societal types of interaction. A further elaboration of this distinction will be given in Chapter 7.

3

SELF-RELATEDNESS, PSYCHOPATHOLOGY, AND THE CONTEXT: THE CONCEPT OF DISEASE

3.1 Introduction

This chapter and Chapter 4 provide the theoretical background and broader context for the distinctions made in the previous chapter. This chapter is devoted to the concept of disease, whereas the next chapter will deal with the concept of self. The conceptual stratification of contexts and their relevance for the clinical conception of psychopathology is dealt with in Chapters 6 and 7.

In the previous chapter, I suggested that mental illness, at a clinical level of understanding, is indissolubly intertwined with the self and with contextual influences. The question addressed in this chapter concerns the difference between this clinical conception and other conceptions of disorder, especially scientific conceptions. How is the clinical perspective on psychopathological conditions related to the scientific approach to these conditions? Are there models of mental illness that do justice to the self- and context-related aspects of psychopathology?

These questions are important in light of psychiatry's scientistic tendencies, particularly with respect to the concept of mental disorder. The reality of mental disorder is first a reality in the lives of people suffering from mental disorder. This seems a truism, but it is a truism that must be reconfirmed today. Scientific conceptions of mental illness are often conceived as representing a deeper and more "real" reality. This may culminate in a reversal in the order of knowing that was pointed out in Chapter 1. Then, the lived experience and concrete manifestations of mental illness are no longer seen as most "real" and comprehensive, but rather the scientific image of the illness. Science is considered to capture the reality of mental illness in a more essential and definitive way than clinical and everyday conceptions of mental illness. What is forgotten in this approach is that the theoretical attitude by definition presupposes some form of abstraction. Experimental design fixes reality so that confounding factors can be controlled for. It construes relationships between items that are artificially (i.e., experimentally) isolated from the phenomenon under study.

3.2 Transforming the story of the patient into a case

Let us begin again within clinical practice and ask how and when theoretical concepts of disease play a role in the mind of the clinician and in his or her interaction with the patient. How do these concepts mold what clinicians do and how they conceive of the patient's state? The most obvious answer to this question is that theoretical models are particularly influential in the phase of history taking and diagnostic assessment. Of course, concepts of disorder and explanatory models influence every phase of interaction between patient and clinician. One could even say that these concepts and models play a role before the patient enters the consulting room, in the patterns of thought that lie at the basis of the labeling of symptoms and signs by clinicians, administrators, and the general public, as well as in the patterns of thought that influence the proto-professionalization of the general public and that structure institutional practices and the organization of care. Important as these influences are, they are not our focus here. I begin in the middle of clinical practice, with interactions at an individual level and the role of concepts and models of mental disorder in these interactions.

It is by interviewing the patient (history taking) and by diagnostic reasoning that the story and the experiences of the patient are transformed into a "case." The clinician analyzes the patient's condition by interpreting it as an exemplar of a more general pattern or category. The clinician may subsequently develop a causal story that ideally explains what the problem is, how it came into existence, and how it can be solved. Identification aims at individual cases and is the cornerstone of clinical diagnosis. Identification is not the same as classification. Classifying is what taxonomists do when they define a new species or taxon. It consists of the delineation and definition of general characteristics of a class of entities (Blashfield 1986). Identification aims at individuals. Individuals are identified as belonging to a certain class (e.g., species, taxon).

The diagnostic process entails more than identification, however. Apart from identifying the illness with statements such as "You have X" or "This (entire set of symptoms) is what we call Y," a diagnosis typically involves a listing of environmental factors and of predisposing features within the patient. These predisposing features are referred to as "vulnerability factors" and are heterogeneous. They include genetic, biological, cognitive, behavioral, and personality-related factors. Clinical diagnosis finally highlights characteristics of the episode and/or the course of the disorder, for instance the number of episodes, the severity of the current episode, and the associated risks. A typical diagnostic formulation would sound like the following:

46-year-old lawyer, married, no children, with recurrent major depressive episodes, moderately severe, with a family history of mood disorder and personality traits that are sufficient to meet criteria for obsessive compulsive personality disorder; current episode presumably elicited by prolonged job-related stress; not suicidal at the time of diagnostic assessment.

The formulation combines the element of identification with a summary of the factors (intrapersonal and environmental) that are thought to be causally relevant to the genesis of the disorder. In the above case, the condition of the patient is identified as an exemplar of the category of major depressive episode, and it is also seen as the product of a network of interlocking, causally relevant factors, both internal (personality, genetic risk) and external (job-related stress).

Are diagnostic formulations such as these compatible with the self-relational and context-sensitive approach that I proposed in the previous chapter? I believe they are; however, this compatibility is not automatic or self-evident. Indeed, at first sight, the formulation suggests something different. It states that the patient "has" a certain condition, a disorder—a recurring disorder, even. This disorder is influenced by all kinds of factor that can be defined independently of the disorder itself. It is supposed that there are causal trajectories connecting these factors and the disorder. Taken together, this gives the impression that mental illness can be defined "as such," apart from its self- and context-related aspects.

We will see that diagnostic formulations such as the one above are usually based on the stress-diathesis model of psychopathology: the idea that psychopathology is the result of an interaction between stressful life events and vulnerability factors within the patient. We will discuss this model in more detail in Sections 3.4 and 3.5. For now, it is sufficient to note that diagnostic formulations of the sort that we are discussing do not necessitate essentialism or reification of the concept of disease. All one needs to do to prevent this is expand the scope of these formulations and pay attention to the self-relational and contextual dynamic. It is, after all, possible to include all five relationships that were discerned in Diagram 2.1 in such diagnostic formulations. Applied to the depressed lawyer, this could sound as follows (numbers refer to relationships described in Diagram 2.1):

46-year-old lawyer, married, no children, with recurrent major depressive episodes, moderately severe, with a family history of mood disorder [1]. The personality of the patient meets the criteria for obsessive compulsive personality disorder [1]. The patient is very worried about his condition [2]. His worry can partially be explained by the depression itself [1] and its influence on how the patient relates to his condition [4], partially by the patient's personality and its influence on how he deals with his illness [5], and partially by his self-image, which is colored by his preoccupation about being a member of a family with a predisposition for major depressive disorder [2; 5]. The current episode is presumably elicited by prolonged job-related stress [3]. The patient is not suicidal at the time of diagnostic assessment.

Therefore, the self- and context relatedness of clinical psychopathology should not be taken as precluding all forms of identification. The dynamic and many-faceted relationships among self, psychopathology, and context allow for interactions between discernable "identities," such as "being ill," "the patient as person," causal factors in the context, and predisposing factors within the patient. Moreover, nothing prevents the diagnostician from including in the diagnostic formulation the interactions with healthcare workers and with mental healthcare as a system. All these "identities" can be seen as nodes in a network. The network defines the nodes, but the nodes are themselves identifiable realities within the web. The interactions within the web are both constraining and enabling. The identities are conceptually diverse, i.e., the terms for them refer to conditions, persons, dispositions, and other causal factors.

3.3 Models of mental disorder: Rough contours

What role do models of mental disorder play in the identification of the patient's illness at a clinical level? Let us examine in more detail the formulations in the diagnostic statement and interrogate the imaginary diagnostician about the implicit assumptions of his formulations. As I have argued previously, these formulations are not necessarily reductionistic or essentialistic; although they may appear so initially, they can be adapted in a way that does not imply reductionism or essentialism. Nevertheless, most clinicians have some background assumptions when they use their diagnostic skills. Let us see how this works for the formulations that were given above.

The expression "46-year-old lawyer ... with recurrent major depressive episodes" refers to a state that lasts for some time (i.e., a syndrome). This syndrome is identified as major depressive disorder. This identification resembles the kind of identification we recognize from the classical disease model. This model views disorders as *categorically* distinct entities. Other parts of the diagnostic formulation, however, seem to fit better with other disease models, especially the dimensional and the (multifactorial) systems model. Dimensional approaches endorse the idea of a continuum between normality and abnormality, implying that mental illness is a matter of degree. They suggest that, in ideal circumstances, the space of psychopathological symptoms and signs should be subdivided into clusters of behavior and experience that are expressions of underlying psychobiological dimensions. Systems theorists interpret mental illnesses as complex and dynamic phenomena with expressions at multiple levels and with multifactorial causal histories. The diagnostic formulation of our vignette suggests a dimensional view when it says that the patient has "a family history of mood disorder" and that his personality traits "are sufficient to meet criteria for obsessive compulsive personality disorder." A positive family history for mood disorder suggests that genetic factors may play a role. Genetic and personality factors are usually conceptualized in dimensional terms. The systems approach emerges in the form of a bio-psychosocial formulation of causally relevant factors: There are biological (family history), psychological (personality traits), and social (job-related stress) factors contributing to the illness.

What stands out is the remarkable fact that even in short diagnostic statements such as the one given above, different models of disorder play a role. Despite its simplicity, the diagnostic formulation implicitly seems to refer to different concepts of disease. This is not something we must deplore. At the clinical level, diagnostic formulations tend to be so malleable that they may comply with virtually any model of disease. This corresponds with what so far has been found in research about implicit models of disease in clinical practice (Ralston 2019). Clinicians appear to be extremely pragmatic in their use of models of disease. They continuously mobilize the illness scripts that best fit their current understanding. The use of a particular term by the patient, psychomotor behavior, and general clinical impressions may activate these illness scripts, which are used with the aim to serve some practical goal.

That said, categorical, dimensional, and system models usually present a realist perspective on mental disorder that differs from nominalist and constructivist accounts. Realists view mental illnesses as things (entities, processes, systems, or even dimensions) that really exist "out there," (i.e., as essences). Nominalists think that mental illness only exists in the minds of psychiatrists. Constructivists hold the view that concepts of mental illness are only conceptual constructions that help to interpret, prescribe, and organize how we relate to people with mental illness.

3.4 The stress-diathesis approach

Diagnostic formulations like the one about the depressed lawyer are broadly compatible with a stress-diathesis (S-D) or stress-vulnerability (S-V) approach to mental illness. What is the stress-diathesis model? How does it work? Does it offer a clinical perspective on psychopathology? And what are its philosophical merits and implications?

The term "diathesis" refers to genetic, biological, psychological, or situational predispositions (or vulnerabilities) that put the individual at risk of developing a mental (or bodily) problem under a certain amount of psychosocial or biological stress (Monroe & Simons 1991). "Stress" refers to any burden that is put on the individual.

The S-D framework may be interpreted as a combination of a dimensional and a system approach to psychopathology. Diathesis refers then to dimensions, and the interactions between stress and diathesis fit best with a multi-aspectual systems approach. However, the S-D is also compatible with the classical categorical model of mental illness. The interactions between latent traits (or dispositions), on the one hand, and environmental and other causally relevant factors, on the other, may lead to disorders that can still be conceptualized in categorical terms. Disorders emerge at points where resistance has diminished. The general picture is that of an organism that is put under pressure and that manifests signs of illness at the weak spots, where the defenses fall short. The conditions that result from these interactions might well be conceivable in categorical terms.

Given this eclecticism, the framework appears suitable for clinical practice. As we will now see, however, there are still several terminological, empirical, and conceptual questions when the SD model is put to closer scrutiny.

Let us start with some terminological issues. It is not entirely clear whether the term "stress" refers to the burden itself or to the reaction of the organism to the burden. Selye, who coined the term "stress" in 1936, explicitly aims at the latter. Stress is "the non-specific reaction of the body to any demand placed on it" (Selye 1978). It is common today, however, to use the term "stress" to refer to these demands themselves and not to the (bodily) reactions they provoke. This is a bit confusing, of course. Another related issue concerns the valence of the stress factors: Are they by definition negative, or can they also be positive?

Selye introduced the concept of stress in his research on the so-called general adaptation syndrome. He was intrigued by the fact that there are many diseases that do not comply with the specificity typical of bacterial infections (i.e., the specificity of the relationship between microbes and organismic reactions). Selye recognized stress as the non-specific result of a range of factors, positive and negative. Thus, he focused on the non-specificity of stress reactions and not on their valence or on the specific nature of the factors causing them. Stress reactions show a large individual variability in terms of how they come about, how they are tolerated, and how they are dealt with. The stress-diathesis model is still as general as it was in Selye's days, with a tendency to focus on negative aspects. Koolhaas et al. (2011), for instance, refer to stress-related conditions as "conditions where an environmental demand exceeds the natural regulatory capacity of an organism." This definition ignores that stress may also have positive outcomes. So far, the terminological issues.

Since its inception before the Second World War, the stress-diathesis model has undergone many empirical improvements. What do these improvements mean for the conceptualization of psychopathology, especially for the self- and context-related approach to clinical phenomena? To answer this question, it is important to note that, almost from the beginning of the stress-diathesis model, scientists have distinguished between the natural, inborn capacities, weaknesses, and vulnerabilities of an organism and the defenses or coping mechanisms it uses when dealing with stress. About the developments with respect to both elements—the capacities/vulnerabilities and the mechanisms for dealing with stress—I will say a few words.

The *mechanisms* for dealing with stress are known as coping mechanisms or coping strategies. In the late 70s and 80s, the cognitive mediation of these coping strategies gained scientific attention. Lazarus and Folkman (1984) referred to these mediating structures as "mechanisms of appraisal." By using appraisal mechanisms, the subject was thought to be able to estimate the nature and possible impact of adverse events. Work in the field of stress and coping led subsequently to an interest in the subject of emotion regulation (Gross 1999). Emotion regulation refers to the ability to redirect the spontaneous flow of one's emotions by changing the direction of one's attention, by reinterpreting certain perceptions, or by actively influencing the action tendencies and physiological manifestations of emotions (Koole 2009). The introduction of the concept of self-regulation, which came in its wake, was the next conceptual improvement: It endowed organisms with the capacity to actively organize and shape their environments, including their own relations to it, in contrast to the concept of coping, which suggested an organism that—roughly speaking—merely defends itself against adversity.

The stress-diathesis model has also undergone improvements with respect to the conceptualization of *innate capacities* and *weaknesses* of the individual. The rise of attachment theory and emerging insights into the molecular basis of genetic and other traits has led to a much more dynamic view of vulnerability. Vulnerability factors are no longer conceived of as "static" causal factors that can be switched on and off depending on the level of stress. It appears that they can better be conceived of as products of the interaction between the organism and the environment. Vulnerability factors have also turned out to impact the development of one's coping repertoire. All these interactions were supposed to occur under the surface. The vulnerability factors themselves are usually latent; however, the factors that shape them and their influence on one's coping repertoire were also conceived of as being invisible to the clinician. Vulnerability factors, moreover, were construed as having subtle and differential effects at different points during one's lifetime, depending on the type of interactions that evolve with the environment. Moderating and mediating factors (or variables) completed the picture. Moderating factors are those that alter the strength of the relationship between independent (causal) and dependent variables (outcomes and illness manifestations). Mediating factors determine the kind of relationship that develops between independent and dependent factors.

Recently, the focus of research has shifted and expanded to "positive" rather than adverse events. Some people appear to have a disproportional susceptibility to the effects of enriching, supportive, and encouraging experiences and to be more predisposed than others to profit from such beneficial experiences. This is one of the reasons why Belsky and Pluess (2009) suggest using the term "plasticity factors" instead of "vulnerability factors."

So, where do all these empirical developments bring us? What stands out is the enormous variety and plasticity of both the vulnerability factors and the mechanisms for dealing with stress. The importance of the developmental dimension is also striking. Similar life events have a differential impact depending on the phase of one's lifecycle. Much of the developmental preparation for dealing with stress takes place subliminally. In short, the slightly mechanistic overtones of the early stress-diathesis model have been replaced by a much more dynamic, interactional, multilayered, and differentiated account.

3.5 Conceptual aspects of the stress-diathesis model

At this point, the reader may be inclined to believe that current versions of the stress-diathesis (S-D) model can only support the interactional, layered, and person-centered approach to clinical psychopathology that was proposed in the previous chapter. Some caution is warranted, however, when we focus on conceptual aspects of the S-D model. Current versions of the model are compatible with several models of disease. However, we must delve somewhat deeper at this stage of the argument. The point is that the current, more plastic and developmental versions of the S-D model still leave the conceptual structure of the old disease model intact. According to the traditional model symptoms at the clinical level result from underlying dysfunctions, disorders, mechanisms, or latent variables. The S-D model replaces these dysfunctions by vulnerability (or plasticity) factors. Recent developments have reshaped this slightly mechanistic view on genetic, developmental, and psychological susceptibilities by assigning a larger role to the organism's own activities and by emphasizing the developmentally determined, differential effects of certain susceptibilities. However, the more fundamental framework that undergirds and legitimizes the explanatory power of the model has remained intact.

Is this a problem? To a certain extent, yes. I will briefly discuss three issues. One issue is whether (and when) the underlying scientifically defined vulnerability factor, disposition, or latent variable can be considered identical with the vulnerability factor that is addressed by the clinician. When the clinician says that the patient is impulsive, is this impulsivity identical to what scientists mean by impulsivity? For the clinician, vulnerabilities are really "out there" and taking effect in relevant circumstances. But how are we to connect this with the statistical concept of traits (dispositions) and this, in turn, with the presumed biological or genetic basis of at least some of these traits (Strelau 2001)? These questions address the fact that scientific formulations of dispositions—whether they are statistical, genetic, or temperamental—tend to be abstract and bound to certain experimental designs. In addition, clinical operationalizations of these concepts (by questionnaires or sets of criteria) do not by definition coincide with what clinicians have in mind when they use identical terms.

The relation between *explanans* and *explanandum*, or, between theoretical concepts and what they explain at the clinical level, has been extensively handled in the literature (Allen & Potkay 1981; Chaplin, John & Goldberg 1988; Zuckerman 1983). In general, explanatory strategies operate somewhere between two extremes. One extreme selects for theoretical purity and attempts to separate definitions of explanatory constructs completely from descriptions of the *explanans*. At the other extreme, one finds approaches that are almost completely descriptive and clinical and of which the theoretical terms have hardly any explanatory value. Difficulties in the definition of the relationship between *explanans* and *explanandum* should make us aware that the distinction between clinical and scientific approaches to psychopathology might be more fundamental than we are inclined to think. Theories about causally relevant processes and factors move somewhere between clinical irrelevance and explanatory circularity. The bandwidth of explanatory power is limited and should be established on a case-by-case basis.

A second issue concerns the nature of the scientific construct of vulnerability as such. Is it a capacity, and, consequently, a concept with causal power? Or is it a conditional (and, therefore, logical) concept (i.e., a concept that refers to conditions necessary for the instantiation of certain events or properties of events)? Or does it have the status of a scientific hypothesis? These questions refer to the metaphysics and epistemology of dispositions (Kistler & Gnassounou 2016; Mumford 1998). The three options just mentioned (capacity, conditional construct, and scientific hypothesis) are distinct: The capacity interpretation refers to truly existing powers; it differs metaphysically from the two other approaches, which are not categorical but hypothetical. According to the capacity approach, the knowing subject is entitled to categorically say that someone has X or Y (X and Y being terms that refer to truly existing powers). By way of contrast, logicians and scientists tend to a hypothetical use of disposition terms; they refer to conditions under which a certain property becomes manifest (conditional) or to the possible explanatory power (statistical or otherwise) of a particular dispositional construct. So, what kind of explanatory relationship exists between the explanatory level and the *explanans* (clinical phenomena)? Clinicians are inclined to give realistic interpretations of explanatory relationships by considering them in terms of causal pathways. However, this may not be warranted given the conceptual structure of the factual explanatory relationship, which is frequently hypothetical in one of the two ways indicated above.

A third, related conundrum is whether dispositions as concepts can be defined independently from their possible realization. Can the conditions for which certain vulnerability factors are causally relevant be defined independently from these factors themselves? Circularity seems inevitable in cases in which the explanatory relationship is couched in dispositional terms. This is because dispositional terms (*explanans*) tend to be operationalized at the level of the *explanans*. Definitions of dispositions depend on descriptions of their possible instantiations, which implies that there exists no independence between *explanans* (the phenomena that are explained by the disposition) and the *explanandum* (the disposition). What was assumed to be an explanatory relationship turns out to be a relationship of logical entailment.

3.6 The gap between clinical and scientific conceptions of disorder

These questions and issues are rather technical. I nevertheless discuss them to make the reader aware of a compelling problem in medical epistemology: the epistemic gap between clinical and scientific knowledge. In a general sense, this gap has been widely recognized in the literature, and there have been numerous attempts to overcome it (Phillips et al. 2012). Researchers have pointed out, for instance, how scientific research can deal with clinical variation in the manifestation of disorders (Blashfield 1986). Other studies discuss how methods of clinical assessment can be made more objective and evidence based (First et al. 2004; Hunsley & Mash 2007). Some authors suggest how systems of classification can be improved (Kincaid and Sullivan 2014; Kupfer et al. 2002). On a more practical level, clinicians are instructed about how to use scientific knowledge in their practice. The very methodology of evidence-based medicine (EBM) offers a paradigm case of this kind of instruction (Sackett et al. 1997). Other practices have successfully integrated the use of Bayes' theorem (Gill et al. 2005; Wulff et al. 1986, Chapter 7; see also, however, Cooper 1992; McCrossin 2005).

However, most of these accounts don't make much work of the conceptual distinctions between clinical and scientific models of disease at a conceptual level. They not only fail to account for the clinical conception of disease as a phenomenon in its own right but also fail to directly address the question of what kind of explanatory relationships can exist between constructs at different levels of abstraction, especially between the clinical and the scientific level.

In our discussion of the dispositional type of explanation, we saw that at the most fundamental level, there is a gap that cannot easily be bridged between dispositional explanations that are developed in a scientific context—which are hypothetical (logical or statistical)—and the categorical interpretations of these explanations in a clinical context. Clinicians tend to transform hypothetical relationships into realistic and categorical ones. The depressed lawyer in our vignette may, for instance, have certain genes that predispose him to depression. The scientist will then speak in terms of statistical propensities. Contrariwise, the clinician will speak about the "real" influence of genes on the lawyer's condition (i.e., the relative strength of genetics within the context of other causally relevant factors). What prevails is a tendency to solve the conceptual problem with practical strategies and with an increase in psychiatry's level of methodological sophistication. I fear this will prove insufficient and will ultimately undermine psychiatry as a clinical discipline by urging the field toward an unattractive either/or: either to endorse "bridging strategies" that aim to bring clinical knowledge under the umbrella of science or to give up the entire project of a scientific psychiatry and fall back into eclecticism or an entirely social definition of the profession (or to go for yet a third way, allowing for "gut feelings"; see Stolper et al. 2011).

I hope most readers have now begun to sense that there is something important at issue in the distinction between clinical and scientific forms of knowing. I admit that we still do not have a full picture of what is at stake. What we have seen so far is that science makes use of abstractions (i.e., reductive measures that make the experimental field manageable) and that these abstractions cannot easily be corrected for when scientific insight is "applied" to clinical problems (Chapter 1). We have emphasized the context dependence and self-relatedness of psychopathology in a clinical context (Chapter 2). We saw that there are conceptual challenges in the use of dispositional explanations (this chapter). However, what we need is a conception of disease that escapes from the either/or mentioned above—a conception of disease that does justice to the self- and context-related nature of clinical psychopathology and gives scientific insight its due place in clinical practice.

To see whether such conceptions of disease exist and how they could work, I broaden my perspective by discussing some other disease models and explanatory strategies. I investigate how the science/practice distinction is dealt with in these models and strategies. It will appear that the classical philosophical debate about concepts of disorder has stalled. It is my hypothesis that this lack of progress is related to difficulties in adequately dealing with the fundamental differences between clinical and scientific knowing. I plead for an account that not only makes a firm distinction between clinical and scientific knowing but also acknowledges that we need a plurality of disease concepts. Arguments for a fully clinical disease concept are quite rare, but suggestions toward plural conceptions of disorder are less rare. What we need is an account that has the resources to conceptually locate and typify the different practices—scientific, clinical, institutional, and societal—in which different concepts of disorder operate.

Leading scholars in the field do acknowledge the different roles disease concepts play (Kincaid 2014; Zachar 2014). We will see, however, that the question of how contexts shape concepts of disease has still not been fully addressed at a conceptual level. We will see that other scholars still tend to attribute the differences among concepts of disorder to different levels of scientific sophistication. Kendler et al. (2011), for instance, plead for a move from an instrumentalist approach, in which disorders are viewed as practical instead of natural kinds (see Zachar 2014; and Section 3.7), to a "more ambitious" and "bolder" commitment to research that again focuses on the objective causal structure of psychopathology, this time along the lines of the mechanistic property cluster approach (see also Kendler 2008a; 2009). I suspect that this strategy will not work; it still insufficiently distinguishes between scientific and clinical ways of understanding psychopathology and has no clear answer as to how this distinction should be dealt with.

So, what we are investigating is whether there is a concept of disorder that can do justice to the difference between scientific and clinical ways of understanding and to construe explanatory relationships that meaningfully bridge the distance between the two. If such approaches don't exist, we must ask whether there is a viable plural disease concept.

3.7 Natural kinds and the science/practice distinction

One important approach to the concept of disorder that is relevant in this context has become known as the natural kind approach. This approach is usually taken as a form of scientific realism. As I am going to show, however, this is not necessarily so. I discuss the natural kind approach first, because it has been paradigmatic for the disease concept of medicine as a whole and an important ideal behind the reform in psychiatric classification expressed in the third edition of the Diagnostic and Statistical Manual of Mental Disorders (DSM III; APA 1980). It was the explicit aim of this reform to describe classes of disorder such that their definition could fulfill two roles: that of providing an intersubjectively reliable nomenclature of psychiatric disorders and that of defining the *explanans* for explanatory theories about mental disorder. DSM-III and its successors largely succeeded in fulfilling the first aim, but they did not succeed in fulfilling the second.

The natural kind approach holds that mental disorders are "natural kinds" or families of properties. Famously, these families of properties are meant to "carve nature at its joints." They refer to an underlying reality that lacks the messiness of the everyday clinical experience of psychopathology. In an ideal world, systems of diagnosis and classification would describe these underlying clusters of properties insofar as they are relevant to diagnosis, treatment, and scientific research.

Natural kinds are natural in the sense that the properties occur naturally (i.e., independently of human interference). And they are kinds in the sense that it is possible to group the properties based on some sort of similarity. One traditional and more technical definition runs as follows:

> Natural kinds are sets of intrinsic natural properties that are individually necessary and jointly sufficient for a particular to be a member of the kind. (Bird & Tobin 2015)

The intrinsicality of the properties is traditionally associated with what philosophers call "essentialism." Natural kinds denote essences, things of which the properties are intrinsic in the sense that they belong to the very nature or essence of the thing.

There is a tendency in the philosophy of psychopathology to restrict the term "natural kind" to the categorical disease concept. However, as the above definition shows, this restriction does not necessarily follow from the concept of natural kind itself. Dimensions and systems can equally be considered as representing "sets of intrinsic natural properties."

There are intriguing metaphysical discussions about the concept of natural kind. For the purposes of this chapter, it is sufficient to briefly address two areas of discussion. First, some scholars hold the view that a commitment to natural kinds does not necessarily imply that one endorses scientific realism. According to them, it is possible to hold a pragmatic, conventionalist, or even nominalist view on natural kinds (Kincaid & Sullivan 2014). One need only drop the criterion of intrinsicality of the properties that are clustered in the natural kind. Natural kinds will then only serve as conceptual tools to make scientifically or clinically relevant distinctions, without the pretention of referring to truly extant sets of properties or entities in the world. Peter Zachar (2000), who discusses this option, calls this the practical kind approach. In my opinion, for the sake of clarity, it is better to use this expression and to reserve the term "natural kind" for the clustering of intrinsic natural properties (Zachar 2014; Zachar & Kendler 2007).

The second main topic of discussion is whether the concept of natural kind is bound to properties that are fixed. The idea that properties need to be fixed would rule out the species concept in biology as a candidate for natural kindness. Species evolve over time, and their properties change. Ruling out the species concept would also have consequences for the concept of disease, which is traditionally oriented around the species concept. This seems not only highly unattractive but also unnecessary. It is possible to allow for some changes in the sets of natural properties and maintain that they remain intrinsic (or essential). It is not clear beforehand, however, where to draw the line between intrinsic-but-changing and changing-and-no-longer-intrinsic. Instead of stretching the boundaries of the concept of natural kind, it is preferable to follow the suggestion of Haslam (2002; 2014) and to group the different forms of kindness under the umbrella of a "kinds of kinds" model. Haslam distinguishes a series of five different kinds that satisfy increasingly stringent criteria. These kinds of kinds are as follows: dimensional, practical, fuzzy, discrete, and natural. Each successive kind of kind meets one more requirement than the kind below it (Haslam 2014, p. 13).

Within a scientific context, natural kinds are interesting for their explanatory rather than their metaphysical or descriptive merits. The groupings of properties serve explanatory purposes, either in and of themselves or because these groupings represent a causal relationships. Philosophers of science have called these causal relationships, or patterns of causal relations, "mechanisms" (Bechtel 2008; Craver 2007; Woodward 2003). Mechanisms lie at the basis of the clustering of properties. They are "patterns (or systems) of causal activity" or "entities and activities organized such that they are productive of regular changes from start or set-up to finish or termination conditions" (Craver & Darden 2013, p. 15). The *mechanistic property cluster* (MPC) approach, mentioned earlier, is one of the variants of this view.

From the MPC perspective, the kindness of disorders "is not ... produced by a defining essence but rather from more or less stable patterns of complex interactions between behavior, environment and physiology that have arisen through development, evolution and interaction with an environment," according to Kendler et al. (2011, pp. 1146–1147). These patterns of interaction find their origin in and are maintained by causal mechanisms. Kendler et al. suggest that the MPC approach goes back and forth between the natural kind and the practical kind approach (ibidem). The quotation identifies contextual factors as potential elements belonging to the causal patterns underlying mental disorder and as contributing to explanatory relevant forms of kindness. In spite of this flexibility and inclusiveness, it is still not clear how the MPC perspective could include the self-relational aspects of psychopathology at a level of abstraction that is also clinically relevant.

The natural kind approach has always been attractive as a strategy to connect explanatory and clinical-descriptive approaches to psychopathology. The approach has, in fact, been highly influential. It formed the basis for the conceptual renewal that took shape in the third edition of the Diagnostic and Statistical Manual of Mental Disorders (DSM–III; APA 1980). In the classification system, the criteria for each disorder were assumed to offer an intersubjectively reliable basis for clinical practice, as well as a valid point of departure for scientific hypothesis building and theorizing. The history of psychiatric classification since 1980 is well-known and has been extensively documented. The message of this history is clear: Even today, after almost 40 years of intense scientific research, clinicians and scientists are not in a position to formulate sets of criteria for disorders that are both valid from a scientific point of view and capable of serving as a starting point for the scientific study of the causal mechanisms underlying mental disorder. All we have are piecemeal artificial constructions, knowledge of causally relevant factors and of statistical probabilities, validators of disorder, endophenotypes with predictive power but often little clinical specificity, and mixtures of scientific insight and clinical prototypes. We have no clear-cut descriptions that define disease in a clinically reliable way that can also serve as anchoring points for scientific research. From a scientific point of view the expectations have simply been too high and based on simplistic and old-fashioned positivist ideas surrounding the role of explanations, causal mechanisms and statistics in biology and medicine (Kincaid 2014). Philosopher of science Nancy Cartwright (1999) says that scientists should learn to live in a "dappled" world instead of a unified world of universal order (see also Kendler 2012, who adopts the term "dappled"). Laws form at best a patchwork. The world of science is so heterogeneous and the *ceteris paribus* conditions (under which laws and law-like relations hold) are so strict that scientists are always working in largely artificial contexts and within constraints that by definition limit, or at least should limit, their more practical aspirations.

3.8 Dysfunctions and the science/practice distinction

We focus our attention now on another important notion in discussions about the concept of disorder: the concept of dysfunction. Much has been written about the concept of disorder in psychiatry, and much of it relies in one way or another on an account of the notion of dysfunction (Boorse 1975; 1976; 1977; Fulford 1999; 2000; Glas 2008b; Hempel 1961; Kendell 1975; 1988; Kendler et al. 2011; Sadler 2005; Wakefield 1992a; 1992b; 2000). The discussion about dysfunction runs largely parallel to the previous discussion on (natural) kinds. I will, therefore, be brief in this section. The question is, again, how does the concept of dysfunction play out in the context of the science/practice gap?

Dysfunctions ideally connect determinants of disease with their clinical manifestations. Terms for dysfunctions sometimes belong to the *explanandum* and sometimes to the *explanans*. In other words, they sometimes describe what is going wrong at a clinical level and in other cases why there is something going wrong at all. In still other cases, it seems ambiguous as to whether the terms for dysfunctions refer to explanatory processes or to clinical events and processes. Having a "dysfunction in the brain's serotonin metabolism" is an example of the explanatory (scientific) use of the term dysfunction. "Having a sleep dysfunction" (as in insomnia disorder, one of the sleep disorders in the DSM-V) is an example of a descriptive use of the term. An example of an ambiguous use of the term dysfunction could be "having a disturbance in your working memory."

Delving deeper into the semantics of dysfunction leads to some confusion. For one, terms for dysfunction and disorder are often used interchangeably in an inconsistent way. Terms for dysfunctions usually refer to explanations of disorder. Sometimes, however, dysfunctions *are* disorders, instead of their explanation. In other, rarer cases, disorders are conceived of as explanations of dysfunction. This especially occurs when diagnostic terms or categories in classification manuals are reified. Terms for disorders are then taken as if they denote processes that explain what is going on. This might lead to skewed formulations such as: "Your insomnia is caused by your insomnia disorder." The dysfunction and the disorder denote identical phenomena; nevertheless, the one is spoken about as if it is an explanation for the other. Ironically, the sexual disorders in the new DSM-V are taken together under the heading "sexual dysfunctions." So, we have erectile dysfunction, of which clinicians are asked to say that it is "an expression of" or even "caused by" an erectile disorder which, in turn, belongs to the general category of sexual dysfunctions.

This is not a plea for semantic rigidity, however. The history of science has taught us that the meaning of terms is malleable and their use changes over time. Blurring of the distinction between explanation and description is not necessarily catastrophic. Atherosclerosis offers an example. The term originally referred to a broad range of molecular and cellular processes that explain several somatic conditions. Today, however, nobody would be surprised if a physician said, "You suffer from atherosclerosis," or ""Mind you, you have atherosclerosis!" The explanatory term is so common that it has become part of our lay vocabulary, which is (mainly) descriptive. In the context of psychiatry, the term alarm system offers a similar example of semi-reification of a metaphor. The alarm system has become a common-sense term for the neural substrate of stress and anxiety. The term was invented in a scientific context and explicitly introduced by neuroscientist Joseph LeDoux in his book on the neural underpinnings of pathological forms of anxiety (LeDoux 1996). Alarming the organism is a function of what he calls the "hippo-campal-amygdala system." What happens with this term in a clinical setting is intriguing and subtle. The clinician who says "Your anxiety is caused by a dysfunction in your alarm system" identifies and explains what is going on in lay terms and suggests at the same time something deeper and more "real" at the explanatory level. The deeper reality is that "there is something wrong with circuits in the brain that function as an alarm system." The suggestion of an explanation is, in other words, based on a shared assumption that ultimately the patient's condition should be couched in the language of disturbed brain functioning. The physician adapts his or her language to what the average layperson can understand; however, at a deeper level, this same language refers to a reality that is presumed to be more fundamental, the reality of malfunctioning neural circuits.

Metaphors play a very important and underestimated role in bridging the science/practice distinction, but this is no place to go deeper into the issue. The suggestion above is that these metaphors enlighten, obscure, and lead to new myths. They illuminate how brain processes are related to clinical phenomena. However, they obscure too, for instance, by simplifying the complexity of the underlying brain processes and by ruling out other relevant points of view. This may lead to myths about, for instance, brain functioning, as if the alarm system is a kind of device that can be turned on and off and functions as a more or less separate module within the brain. Nothing is less true, of course, given what neuroscience has taught us about the spatial distribution and the stochastic nature of neural information processing.

3.9 Network approaches and the science/practice distinction

One final approach that can also be grouped under the heading of realist theories of disease is the network approach to psychopathology (Borsboom 2008; Borsboom & Cramer 2013; Borsboom et al. 2011). Borsboom et al. criticize the traditional psychometric approach to psychopathology, which considers symptoms of disorder as expressions of variation on underlying latent variables. This approach is no longer plausible. The promise that findings in genetics or cognitive neuroscience will solve the problem of comorbidity or the lack of specificity of causally relevant factors is not convincing anymore. What we see, 15 years after the "decade of the brain," is an increase in complexity, not a reduction to clinically manageable causal relations. Borsboom et al. state that this means that there is something wrong with the underlying model. The psychometric approach mimics the traditional "medical" approach to disease; latent variables have simply taken the place of dysfunctions or "causes" in the traditional disease model. Hence, all the problems of traditional models return. The network analysis approach Borsboom et al. suggest is based on the idea that from a psychometric point of view, symptoms are themselves causally interacting elements that form clusters instead of expressions of underlying latent variables.

The conceptual renewal Borsboom et al. propose is daring and revolutionary. Borsboom and his group belong to the first who really bite the bullet by giving up the idea that symptoms should be explained by "underlying" variables and by advocating instead for symptoms as causally interacting nodes in a network. They refer to Ryle's famous comparison between a scientist searching for essences ("the disorder") and the visitor to Cambridge who, after being shown the colleges, libraries, scientific departments and administrative offices, asks where the university is (Borsboom & Cramer 2013, p. 116; Ryle 1949, p. 16). According to Borsboom et al., diseases are not essences; they are collections of symptoms, i.e., patterns of interacting elements (e.g., symptoms, predispositions, environmental influences, and developments).

The proposal does not imply that genetic and neural abnormalities have no place in the explanation of mental disorder—on the contrary! Their role should be conceptualized differently, however, "instead of searching for 'genes that cause MD' [major depression] we are searching for 'genes that cause certain risky network structures in individuals'" (ibidem). Genetic abnormalities, neural and cognitive dysfunctions, and environmental factors are usually seen as operating on different levels that are intrinsically ordered. According to the network approach, "it is extremely likely that once researchers start taking the dynamics of symptomatology seriously, they will find feedback loops that cross the border of traditional thinking." Genetic, neural, and environmental factors can themselves be conceived of as nodes in the network or—at one level of abstraction higher—as patterns of relative strength within the relationships between certain nodes. The authors refer to the experience sampling method as one that is amenable for the advanced statistical modeling techniques that are now used in behavioral genetics. Experience sampling refers to a research method that asks patients to systematically register symptoms and other experiences and activities during the day. The iterative nature of the process makes it possible to detect time series of patterns of symptoms, activities, and other experiences and observations. It may appear, for instance, that there are strong reciprocal connections between symptoms of negative affect (e.g., worry) and daily hassles. The strength of these connections can then be viewed as a "risky part of a person's network structure" and as putting the individual at risk for the development of major depression. Endophenotypes can be conceived of in a similar vein (i.e., as representing patterns of relative strength of connections between certain nodes).

In one sample of 9000 individuals, the architecture of the connections conformed to a "small world structure." The sample consisted of participants in the National Comorbidity Survey Replication (Kessler and Merikangas 2004; Kessler et al. 2005), which registered all 522 symptoms of the DSM-IV. The degree of clustering between the nodes was high, with a short average path length and with distances between the clusters that reliably predict comorbidity rates (Borsboom et al. 2011). (Path length is the length of the causal paths between nodes.)

The causal network modeling approach seems very attractive, because it is clinically highly plausible to suppose that symptoms themselves causally interact. Sleep deprivation, for instance, may lead to fatigue, fatigue to concentration problems, and concentration problems to irritability. Network analysis is also attractive in that it can be "personalized"—for instance with the experience sampling (ES) method—and be used to tailor make individual treatments. With the help of this ES method it is, in fact, possible to give the kind of "personalized" feedback that was suggested by the person-centered model presented in Diagram 2.1 (van Os et al. 2017). However, it is also possible to study patterns of interactions at a group level. Scientific, generalizing research on networks does not exclude the personalized approach. The direction of causality may, moreover, be two way; genetic factors, for instance, may predispose to the development of mental disorder, but "persistent symptomatology (e.g., insomnia or loss of appetite) may cause differential gene expression just as well" (idem, p. 117). This may have effects on brain maturation and cognitive development, which in turn may feed back into the environment. Network analysis is, henceforth, helpful for the study of the interactions among phenotype, neural development, environmental input, and behavior. Borsboom et al. suggest in this context that causal network analysis comes close to Kendler's MPC approach and might be compatible with it. The MPC approach conceives properties as mechanistically connected, which is a different way of saying that symptoms can be seen as causally interacting nodes in a network.

At this stage of development, it is difficult to determine whether the conceptual problem that we are discussing—that of bridging scientific and clinical approaches to mental disorder—will be solved by causal network analysis. Clinical and scientific analysis both make use of a research methodology that aims at the unraveling of causal trajectories between nodes, although in different directions (the clinical approach in the direction of "personalized" networks and the scientific approach in the direction of general patterns). This suggests that the two approaches are at least complementary.

However, some caution is warranted: The analysis of more general patterns in their applications to subgroups might lead to problems similar to those generated by the more traditional statistical or causal-modelling approaches. The relevance of general patterns for these subgroups will always prove to be a matter of numbers and of interpretation, and there are worries about both. The numbers are still insufficient. For instance, findings in the field of genomics suggest that the human genome simply does not explain much of the variance of common human diseases and that the variance it explains is rarely susceptible to direct medical or public health action (Joyner & Paneth 2015). This also holds for interpretation, especially the interpretation of the associations that are found with data-mining techniques on large numbers of parameters in different domains. How are investigators to responsibly and adequately make sense of all the information?

However, these worries are not relevant to the individualizing strand of network analysis, only to the generalizing approach in its application to individual cases. The idea of personalized network analyses still seems highly attractive, important, and challenging (see de Haan 2015 for a similar appreciation).

3.10 Conclusion

How does the clinical concept of psychopathology outlined in the previous chapter relate to models of mental disorder? This has been the topic of the previous sections. We began with clinical diagnosis and saw that it conforms to the stress-diathesis (S-D) approach to mental disorder. The S-D approach itself appeared to be a mixed bag, with elements of dimensional and systems models in the explanatory parts of the diagnostic formulation and elements of the categorical model in the identification of disorder. Considering the S-D model more closely, we focused on its dimensional constituent (the diathesis or vulnerability). We saw that the structure of the dimensional model did not differ from that of the classical (or categorical) disease model. I briefly addressed three conceptual problems with the dimensional (dispositional) account of explanation in psychiatry: differences in the definition (and operationalization) of dispositions (clinical vs. scientific), the nature of the concept of disposition, and the circularity and explanatory vacuity of dispositional terms.

Next, we focused on natural kinds and dysfunctions. They appeared to be the kind of concepts that were originally designed to connect the scientific-explanatory and the clinical-descriptive perspective on psychopathology. In the discussion about natural kinds and dysfunctions, we saw that the prospects for both concepts, in their most strict interpretations, were dim. There is little reason to expect that psychiatric illness behaves like somatic disease and that clinical syndromes can be reduced to essences (natural kinds) or to dysfunctions on a 1:1 basis. We should also be skeptical of the hope that joined efforts in genetics, brain imaging, and epidemiology will lead to new demarcations of disorder. This hope has recently taken shape in the Research Domain Criteria (RDoC) approach to mental illness, briefly mentioned in Chapter 1 (Insel 2013).

However, developments in the most advanced parts of the sciences that inform psychiatry point in a different direction: to a plurality of kinds (kinds of kinds), to mechanistic property clusters representing "patchy" causal patterns, and to networks of causally related symptoms and context-related factors. It is uncertain which of these approaches will fully do justice to the self-relational and context-sensitive aspects of psychopathology, although so far, the idea of personalized network analysis promises a truly person-centered approach to psychopathology and psychiatry.

4

SELF-RELATEDNESS, PSYCHOPATHOLOGY, AND THE CONTEXT: THE CONCEPT OF SELF

4.1 Introduction

In our search for a clinical concept of psychopathology that is both self-relational and context sensitive, we now focus on the notion of the self. Further elaboration of the context sensitivity of psychopathology will be discussed in a later chapter.

So, what is a "self" in the context of psychopathology? What kind of self are self-relatedness, self-referentiality, and self-awareness referring to? Recently, extensive literature has been published about the concept of self in psychology, philosophy, cognitive neuroscience, and psychotherapy (Bermudez et al. 1995; Christoff et al. 2011; Damasio 1999; 2010; Fonagy et al. 2002; Gallagher 2000; 2013; Gallagher & Shear 1999; Glas 2006; Hobson 2010; Hood 2012; Immordino-Yang 2011; Kircher & David 2003; Lambie 2009; Leary & Tangney 2003; Legrand 2007; 2011; Northoff et al. 2011; Schechtman 1996; Strawson 2009; Taylor 1989; Zahavi 2005). This is not the place to review the various debates, not even those on terminology. In the next sections, I focus on the concepts of self-relatedness (3.2.2) and self-referentiality (3.2.3) and unpack them a bit more, especially as far as their philosophical background is concerned. I do this to further substantiate my claim that clinical psychopathology needs a self-relational approach. I also answer many questions and objections to the framework developed in the previous chapter. Let us begin first, however, with a brief terminological exposition about the term "self."

4.2 "The" self as term

To begin with, I adopt a pragmatic stance with respect to the definition of the self. When I use the term "self," I mostly refer to persons (i.e., to myself or oneself) and not to a component or quality of a person, such as character, personality, self-concept, or a particular form of self-experience. When I use the term "self-relatedness," I am referring to the fact that persons relate to themselves as persons. When I am relating to myself, I am usually relating to myself as a person seen-from-a-particular-perspective or in my capacity of being-such-and-such or doing/experiencing-this-or-that. When I say, "I don't like what I did," I am referring to myself in my capacity of having done something. I am relating to this "myself"—not to myself as a whole, including my past and all possible things that can be said about me. I am, by the same token, also not referring to a part of myself, my character, for instance, or my conscience or self-image. If I were, I would have to say something like "I don't like my character" (or conscience or self-image). Of course, my character, conscience, and self-image influence how I feel and what I say about what I did. But that is something different. The object of the expression "I don't like what I did" is something I did, an activity, not an aspect of my personality or self-concept. These terms come conceptually later; they are the objects of a second-order form of reflection. When I refer to "aspects of the self" I mean something similar; they are not components of a person, but rather a person viewed from a certain perspective, for instance a person in his or her capacity of doing/experiencing this or that.

I emphasize this—that the term refers to persons and not to parts of persons—because there is a tendency in the literature to abstract from this broader background and to associate the concept of self with more specific capacities and roles. Phenomenological philosophers and neuroscientists such as Damasio (1999; 2010) tend to conceive of the self as either a particular form of self-experience (i.e., as "core [sense of] self") or as a narrative construction (i.e., as the story one can tell about oneself (the "narrative" or "autobiographical self"). Psychologists are inclined to view the self as a processing unit or integrating *device* (a "psycho-social dynamic processing system," cf. Mischel & Morf 2003). I do not say that these concepts are invalid. Instead, I suggest that these more specified conceptions presuppose and build on broader, less specified, and more common-sense notions of selfhood that refer to persons and to who they are (not to "parts" of them).

It is obvious why it is so tempting to use the term "self" in these more specific ways. This is because the word "self" is not only used as a reflexive pronoun but also as a noun in ordinary language. We are not only speaking about ourselves—or oneself, or myself—but also about someone's self, my "self" and even "the" self. In these last cases, one's being-oneself has become quasi-objectified. Expressions that refer to parts of oneself—one's self-concept, for instance—should be conceived in a similar vein, as quasi-objectifying statements that pick out one aspect of one's functioning and consider it as if it exists in itself, more or less dissected from myriad interactions and relations of one's functioning.

Languages do this in different ways. The French *soi* refers to both (the) self and oneself, independent of whether the term *même* is added (as in *soi-même*) (Ricoeur 1990, p. 2). In English, German, and Dutch this is different. The reflexivity (i.e., the self-referring quality) of the term oneself (*sich-Selbst, zichzelf*) is lost in the noun "self" (*Selbst, zelf*). It is legitimate, therefore, to speak about one's self-esteem or self-concept, thereby implying that there is something, a "self," that is involved in the activity of esteeming or conceiving. These concepts assume a certain independence of the self in its capacity of esteeming or conceiving (i.e., independence from other capacities, activities, experiences, and/or roles of the same person). They also presuppose that the exertion of the capacity (to esteem what one does or to conceive of oneself) ideally leads to an achievement. Selfhood has, on this account, something to do with achievements (Evans 2006, p. 265). These achievements acquire their status of achievement often based on recognition by others. Being a self is then regarded as a status that is granted by being attributed by others, often based on certain criteria (related to rationality, language, human rights, and communicative and/or interpretative capacities).

Terms such as "self-esteem" and "self-concept"—although often attributed by others—may acquire a self-relational denotation in expressions in which the person who speaks is talking about him- or herself, such as, for instance, in: "My self-esteem has improved the last month." The expression refers to the speaker explicitly (i.e., self-relationally). It is a statement about oneself as a speaker that presupposes the capacity to assess one aspect of one's functioning, namely one's self-esteem. The "self" in self-esteem is again referred to in an objectifying way. And it is the objectifying —together with the linguistic structure—that eradicates the reflexivity of the term.

I can refer to my "self" in contexts in which I am speaking about myself as an agent or as a subject of experience. We saw that the agential use of the term "self" does not imply reflexivity. It is compatible with a self-relational type of expression, however, e.g., when the speaker is referring to him- or herself while speaking. This also holds for talk about ourselves in a receptive, experiential sense. We speak about ourselves as subjects of experience. This may occur in many forms: in explicit statements—about what certain events have meant to me, how I was affected, or why I myself felt such-and-such—but also, more subtly, in the form of implicit references to oneself as a person who feels, perceives, and appreciates. The sentence: "This is painful" may refer to feelings of the subject, but it may also refer to feelings that are shared by others. Facial expression, bodily posture, and context are usually sufficient to understand what the speaker means. Sometimes, verbal clarification is needed, as in: "This is painful for me" (reference to oneself) or "We feel very sorry for you; this is so painful" (reference to a larger group).

In the most elementary form, this subject of experience is not so much spoken *about* as it is *announced in* the experience of mineness. "Mineness" refers to a particular quality of one's conscious states (feelings, thoughts, and desires) whereby one knows that it is oneself who has the feeling or thought or desire. It is an immediate, non-thematic, implicit, and immersed awareness that it is me who is experiencing. More technically, mineness refers to the "first personal mode of givenness of experience"; it is a "primitive experiential self-referentiality," according to Zahavi (2005, pp. 119, 122, respectively). It is a non-objectifying experience within one's stream of consciousness, to use the terminology of William James (1890). Or, as Harry Frankfurt puts it, it is an awareness of me being aware, which reveals an "immanent reflexivity" (Frankfurt 1998, p. 162). Experiential self-referentiality is part of one's awareness of the situation; it forms the background and embedding of object-directed experiences and acts.

As the reader may have noticed, in the last paragraph I have begun to broaden the focus. I first analyzed how terms referring to the self are used and what they mean. In the last paragraph, I focused on varieties of experience instead of language. This broadening of perspective is needed in order to answer the next question: Are there different forms of self-referring?

In the second chapter, I restricted the use of the term "self-referentiality" mostly to implicit references to the self in emotions, gestures, activities, attitudes, and interactions. Self-referentiality was conceptualized as a non-verbal and sometimes also non-conscious form of self-signification. I said that awareness of self-signification usually does not put an end to self-signification. I suggested that implicit self-referring and explicit awareness of oneself may co-occur and that they usually coincide with respect to their content, although they also may diverge. For instance, persons may for feel disempowered (self-awareness), but their face and bodily posture may (self-referentially) express anger. However, I did not restrict the use of the term "self-reference" to implicit forms of signification only. I used the term "self-reference" in the context of self-awareness by saying that self-awareness is a form of referring to oneself. The experience refers to the person having the experience.

The question we must address now is how these different types of referring relate to one another. So far, I have maintained a distinction between implicit self-referring in emotions and gestures and consciously referring to oneself in self-awareness. I have not addressed the question of whether and in which way the two vary. This question becomes more urgent in the context of the discussion about mineness. Mineness is an experience at the border of awareness. One can be aware of the mineness of one's experience, but this not necessarily the case. Mineness may reside at the background of one's experience, like street noises we do not notice. So, if mineness may adopt the form of an "implicit" or "dormant" sense of self within one's self-awareness, what kind of self-referentiality does this implicit self-referring then represent? Is it a signifying one, as in emotion, or is it a different, "presentational" one, as in self-awareness? I answer this question in two stages. I give an initial response in this section and a more detailed exposition in the section on self-referentiality (4.2.3).

My initial response is pragmatic. Self-referentiality was defined in the previous chapter as an implicit form of referring to oneself; however, I also emphasized that self-referentiality does not rule out self-awareness and self-interpretation. Emotions and gestures may implicitly signify something about the self and, at the same time, also involve a conscious experience of oneself. As conscious experiences of oneself, they refer to oneself-seen-from-a-certain-perspective or oneself-in-one's-capacity-of-doing-or-experiencing-this-or-that. So, both are forms of self-referring, but emotions, gestures, and the like are forms of signification (or sense making), whereas self-awareness can better be described as a form of (inner) "presentation." I use the term presentation instead of re-presentation to emphasize the pre-reflective, immediate, and non-thematic content of self-awareness. Body sensations play an important role in this non-thematic self-awareness. They help to anchor one's thoughts, images, and associations in a spatio-temporally bounded "me," so that the sense of mineness of pre-reflective self-awareness is not something that freely floats around.

There are two elements in this pre-reflective self-awareness that can be distinguished and conceived as being present to oneself. One element is that one is present to oneself in the experience. The other is that one is present to or for oneself. Sartre, who extensively deals with the subject, speaks of non-thematic (non-positional) consciousness as being *pour soi* (for oneself). Self-consciousness, even in its most primitive forms, is different; it is being oneself for oneself. In pre-reflective consciousness, there is no self outside consciousness; there is only the consciousness of one's own being conscious, which can be conceived as a "presence for oneself" (Sartre 1943, p. 115). The process of signification is, seen from this perspective, something completely different. It can best be seen as a form of sense making that is generated by one's emotions, gestures, attitudes, and actions in their relation to a context and to a subject with a biography and all sorts of preoccupations and concerns. However, again, both forms of self-referring can co-exist, beyond a doubt. This is the pragmatic and first part of the answer.

What does this distinction mean for the mineness of one's experiences? Is mineness a form of self-presentation or of intrinsic signification? Surely, we can refer to mineness as a quality of one's experience. But this is not what is meant here. Referring to mineness as a quality of one's experience is to consider it as a quality that can be addressed in a third-personal way. Mineness as experiential reality, however, refers to itself. It is first personal and refers to oneself in one's capacity of being an experiencing creature. I will attempt to elucidate this in my second response in 4.4, when I return to the nature of mineness.

4.3 Self-relatedness

Let us first focus on the concept of self-relatedness. One of the first explicit accounts of this concept can be found in the work of Sören Kierkegaard, who coined the term and made it a central aspect of his anthropology. The idea of self-relatedness was, of course, not invented by Kierkegaard. It was already emerging in the work of Augustin. It is also important in the philosophies of René Descartes, Blaise Pascal, Jean-Paul Sartre, Helmuth Plessner, and Charles Taylor (1989), to mention only some of the great masters.

Kierkegaard views the self as a relational category. Anti-Climacus, the pseudonymous author under whose name Kierkegaard published his *Sickness unto Death*, defines the self as "a relation which relates to itself, or, that in the relation which is its relating to itself. The self is not the relation but the relation's relating to itself" (Kierkegaard 1848/1980, SKS IV, p. 129). These somewhat puzzling formulations reveal that the self is not a thing (an "entity" or substance), or an illusion, or the "passive" result of an interaction, but a kind of activity, or, as Anti-Climacus puts it, that which, in the relation, consists of "its relating to itself." When the (I–self) relation relates to itself, it "is" or becomes a self.

This self-relating, as Kierkegaard elsewhere suggests, co-occurs with other acts and interactions. It is by speaking and interacting with others that I am (also) relating to myself. And it is by this relating to myself that I show who I am and who it is that I call my "self."

Self-relatedness lies at the basis of Kierkegaard's famous doctrine of indirect communication, which he develops in his treatment of the topic of truth (Kierkegaard 1846/1992; SKS VII, pp. 55–62). The term "indirect" should be read as in contrast with "direct," which, in the case of Climacus—the pseudonymous author who voices the position of the skeptical humorist—means "objective, factual, as a state of affairs one can be informed about." What Climacus means is that truth is no report about objective facts, no chunk of information isolated from the context, but something more. Truth deserves its name only when it is also an expression of a way of self-relating that is truthful, trustworthy, and appropriate with respect to the context. People may lie with truths; their messages may factually be true, but existentially be distortions of truth, and their direct communication may refer to factual truths, but their indirection communication may be at odds with it. Climacus calls the objective concept of truth "abstract." These abstract truths turn into falsehood when they are not brought into perspective with other truths and the appropriate context and when they are not an expression of the way one lives. Truth, in short, presupposes soundness in one's way of self-relating; it implies truthfulness, and truthfulness can only be communicated when the manner of communication is consonant with that which is communicated. The how (the form) and the what (the substance or content) of the truth cannot be viewed separately. The message and the medium should be in tune.

Kierkegaard is very much aware that the desired consistency between content and form is often illusory, and not only with respect to the subject of truth. His work is packed with descriptions of distorted characters and with analyses of the seeming inevitability of imperfection, imbalance, and ambiguity. This makes his work interesting for psychiatry. I already mentioned that psychotherapy often thrives on the inconsistencies between psychomotor expression and verbal content. But the notion of self-relatedness shows its relevance in a much broader way: in the struggle between different forms of relatedness to oneself. I am referring to situations in which the patient is longing for inner peace (discrepancy between the current and the desired state) or is struggling for acceptance by others or for self-acceptance.

In this book, I consider self-relatedness a broad and general category indicating that persons relate to themselves. They do this in part by adopting a stance toward what they are doing or undergoing. This may occur implicitly (non-consciously and non-deliberately) or explicitly (consciously and deliberately). It is the person him- or herself that is relating to him- or herself. Stance taking, as one of the most obvious forms of self-relating, presupposes a temporal dimension: I relate to who I was in the past, to who I am in the present, and to who I wish to be in the future.

But there are many other forms of self-relatedness. I can relate to an aspect of my present "self," i.e., myself seen-from-the-perspective-of A or B or in-my capacity-of X or Y. I can relate to myself as a physical, psychological, social, or political being. And I can relate to myself in my capacity as an agent or a subject of experiences. None of these forms of self-relating exists in isolation; they are fundamentally shaped by one's relationships with others and with the conditions in which one lives.

Self-relatedness is conceptually closely related to the concept of personal identity. The self-relational perspective I am endorsing is considered—by Paul Ricoeur among others—as offering an alternative for both bundle theories and essentialist conceptions of personal identity. I see self-relatedness as structurally given and as fundamentally encompassed and opened up within relations with important others. A focus on self-relatedness is, therefore, fully compatible with a position that emphasizes a second-person perspective; that is, the primacy of one's connectedness with others as a precondition for one's becoming oneself. From a developmental psychological perspective, this conceptual move makes sense given the fundamental role of caretakers in early infancy (Hobson 2004). However, it is not a widely accepted position in philosophical circles (Hermans & Kempen 1993).

One of the reasons I find this approach attractive is because it circumvents some of the longstanding problems with the concept of the self in approaches that take a Cartesian-style philosophy of consciousness as a point of departure. These approaches tend to result in a forced choice between first-personal and third-personal accounts of the notion of the self. By "Cartesian-style philosophies of consciousness" I mean theories of consciousness that see consciousness as a "glassy essence" and an "inner theatre," in which the world outside consciousness is in some way reproduced. Such philosophies construe knowledge as the inner reproduction (i.e., the representation within one's consciousness) of the relationship between a subject and an object. The subject is the theorist's mind, and the object is the inner representation of an object in the world. In a Cartesian universe, the self can be taken on the one hand in a first-personal sense, as a subject of experience, in which case it either becomes an abstraction or a disengaged experience, torn loose from its roots, bodily and otherwise. By way of contrast, it can be viewed from a third-personal point of view, in which case the self becomes an object, a thing.

Descartes' famous dictum "I think, therefore I am" is a good starting point to illustrate these problems briefly. Who is the "I" who thinks? The subject of thinking is, in the Cartesian approach, a consciousness of oneself, a consciousness of me as thinker. In order to know this thinking me, we need to make it the object of a new act of thinking. But this new act of thinking requires—again—a subject, a thinking "I," which, in order to become known, must become an object for a next thinking subject, and so on. This is the well-known problem of infinite regress. Infinite regress leads to volatilization of the self, the self disappears in an endless series of more and more abstract "I"s. Philosophers after Descartes tried to solve this problem by making the "I" a transcendental idea (or precondition). The "I" thus becomes that which necessarily should be presupposed in order to make sense of our knowledge and experiencing. In this approach, the "I" becomes a formal category, the logical and, in fact, anonymous subject pole of our acts of thinking.

The abstractness of this concept of the "I" of the subject is at odds with the concreteness of the experience of being an "I" or me. For the clinical approach to psychopathology, we need more mundane versions of self-relatedness than the transcendental one. We need versions that do more justice to the ambiguity and contradictions within the patient's everyday existence. In short, both the Cartesian and the transcendental self are abstractions, the first as a result of endless backward questioning (infinite regress) and the second as a result of formalization of epistemic conditions.

The other problem with a purely first-personal account of the self is that it may lead to a view in which the self is no more than a disengaged experience torn loose from its bodily anchoring and broader embedding in the life world. I referred to this already above when I suggested that the self is anchored in bodily sensations and in body memory, which prevents it from becoming a "freely floating" and isolated entity. In Descartes' philosophy, the threat of such separation and isolation is obvious, given his views on mind–body dualism and solipsism (for nuance, see Glas 1989). But we saw also how a similar concern might arise with respect to, for instance, Sartre's account of consciousness as *pour soi*, especially the idea of pre-reflective consciousness as a consciousness of one's own being conscious, which is conceived as a "presence" or "being present" for oneself. Presence differs from re-presentation. For Sartre, the most primitive forms of self-awareness do not represent something else (e.g., a self outside consciousness). The awareness is not the manifestation of something else. Minimal self-awareness *is* the presence of a self. It is the way the self *is* present, "for itself." And there is nothing outside this awareness.

This is no place to go into all the intricacies of the discussion on minimal (pre-reflective) self-awareness. We should take phenomenology as it presents itself: as a method to investigate experience from a first-person perspective. It is without a doubt too simplistic to suggest that this method leads to an idealistic metaphysics. The point I want to raise is not about metaphysics, or about the methods of phenomenology as such, but about the interpretation of the results of phenomenological investigation of the self and of self-experience. What kind of consciousness is left after the phenomenological reduction, when self-awareness has been stripped of all its references to all identifiable aspects of who one is, whether psychologically or bodily? What is the self of self-consciousness when it is abstracted from all thematic content? Does this "self" still embody a kind of personhood? Can it in a meaningful way be connected with who one is? Or is this self-awareness so minimal that it only refers to itself *as* mere awareness, disconnected from everything else? Is it, in other words, an awareness of *itself* or of *oneself*? This is not the place to answer this question. It is a well-known question within the phenomenological movement itself: Jean-Paul Sartre once admitted that pre-reflective self-awareness—in its most elementary form—is no longer an awareness of a self, but awareness of a subject-less awareness. Michel Henry (1973, p. 467) and Dan Zahavi (2005, p. 124ff) resist this egoless concept of subjectivity. Henry argues that in minimal self-awareness we are dealing with a real self, a self that is touched ("affected") by itself. This auto-affection testifies to both the concreteness and the individual selfhood of the minimal self. Zahavi distinguishes between the pure and formal subject of experience and the personalized subject that appears in the social sphere. The individuality that is inherent to the first-personal givenness of experience represents "a purely formal kind of individuation" (2005, p. 129). This experiential self should be kept distinct from the narrative self with its concrete individuality, its "personal history" and its "abilities, dispositions, habits, interests, character traits, and convictions" (ibidem).

We do not need to adopt a position in this discussion, so long as we—like Fuchs (2000), Gallagher (2005), Legrand (2007), and others—put sufficient emphasis on the role of the body and of body awareness in minimal self-awareness. Pre-reflective self-awareness "presents" a self because it refers, inter alia, to a body. Pre-reflective self-awareness is minimally body awareness (i.e., awareness of the immediate presence of one's body). I am not referring here to isolated body feelings, but to all one's bodily feelings at a particular point in time, including the feelings that represent one's general condition. The ensemble of these bodily feelings forms a background experience and, thereby, provides a sense of self in the here and now. They locate my awareness in a spatio-temporal and bodily felt "me." The personhood of this "me" does not depend, in my view, on some difficult to define core-experiences or on the "mineness" of one's experiences. It depends first on the wholeness of one's experiences (i.e., on their coherence and their reference to a felt body that is located, mine, and bounded by the not-me). This suggestion does not contradict my earlier statement about the (non-) self-referentiality of body feelings. This statement aimed at more or less isolated body feelings: twinges of pain, pressure in one's chest, waves of nausea. Such feelings refer to parts of one's body. At best, one can say that they refer to oneself-seen-from-the-perspective-of-one's-physical-body. But self-referring does not necessarily imply self-awareness. The "oneself'" in the expression "oneself-seen-from-the-perspective-of" is experientially not necessarily "present" in these cases (i.e., at least not in the experiential reference to the body part). The issue is tricky, I admit. Body sensations are still my sensations; one can, in other words, attribute mineness to these sensations. But mineness is an attribute; it is not the sensation itself. Mineness refers to a self, but we still have to decide (in the next section) whether this means that it "presents" a self. Apart from this, it seems wise to assume that there is a broad divide between sensations that refer to body parts and experiences that refer to selves.

These last paragraphs suggest that phenomenological accounts that put exclusive emphasis on the notion of minimal (or pre-reflective) self-awareness (as in Sartre's thinking) indeed may claim to have successfully withstood the threat of infinite regress and to have overcome the formalism of transcendental approaches. However, such accounts still run the risk of cleaving the self from its anchoring in the body and its broader anchoring in the lifeworld. I am not saying that this risk cannot be undone, or that there is an irreparable deficiency in this type of phenomenological thinking. But there is a risk, a tendency, a threat that is more difficult to overcome the more self-awareness is stripped of its thematic referents. The threat is that it becomes impossible to connect the self of minimal self-awareness with the concrete, everyday experience of selfhood. This everyday experience is bodily anchored and socially embedded, even when we are not aware of it.

So far, the vicissitudes of the Cartesian perspective on the self, when the self is seen from the perspective of its first-personal mode of givenness, i.e., as subject. I can give a much shorter treatment of the other horn of the dilemma, which focuses on the self as an object. Earlier, I questioned who it is who thinks in the "I think, therefore I am." We investigated this question by reasoning backwards and immersing ourselves in the thinking subject. We can also reason forward by viewing the self as an object, as a being with attributes instead of a subject of experience. By viewing the self as an object, we adopt a third-personal point of view. The thinking "I" appears as an object, as something in the world that can be described and analyzed. There is one obvious problem with this approach, which is that it divorces from the self qualities that seem to be vital to it. Our existence is marked by self-concern, by expectations, valuations, and ideals that we deem important. The concept of self is connected with what matters to us. Our identity, says Taylor, is:

> [D]efined by commitments and identifications which provide the frame or horizon within which I can try to determine from case to case what is good, or valuable, or what ought to be done, or what I endorse or oppose. (1989, p. 27)

Being a self means being connected with a more encompassing framework (i.e., a set of assumptions) within the background of one's life, assumptions that are pre-existent and, nevertheless, open for revision. These assumptions are essentially conceptions of the good, according to Taylor, who strongly objects to the "disengaged," "naked," "punctual" self of Enlightenment philosophers like René Descartes and John Locke (idem, p. 143ff, p. 159ff). It also means that we are bound to a web of interrogation, a "space of interlocutors," a horizon of implicit and explicit expectations and strongly valued goods that function as quasi-transcendental conditions of one's language and identity. Being a self means orienting oneself with respect to this horizon of meaning. The fundamental move Taylor makes consists of a shift from the third-personal approach to selfhood to a second-personal perspective. According to this perspective, I become a self by orienting myself against a horizon of shared expectations, values, ideals, and hopes. Selfhood depends on recognition by a wider community.

4.4 Self-referentiality

"Self-referentiality" is a term with a wide use in logic, linguistics, computer science, mathematics, robotics, and philosophical linguistics (Hofstadter 2007; Perlis 1999; Shoemaker 1968). In this book, I use the term to mean something quite limited and specific: that certain behaviors—most notably emotions, gestures, acts, attitudes, and interactions—refer to a "self," i.e., to the person displaying that behavior. To refer means to point at, to signal, to signify, to implicitly address or focus on or intend. I have borrowed the concept initially from Paul Ricoeur (1990, p. 48ff), who considers self-referentiality as key feature of "ipseity" (selfhood). The term ipseity was not invented by Ricoeur; it can also be found in the work of Jean-Paul Sartre (1943, p. 142 ff.) and Michel Henry (1973, p. 459ff). Among contemporary philosophers, the term is little used, except by Zahavi, who gives it due attention in his book on the first-person perspective (2005, pp. 108, 115ff; see also Slaby & Stephan 2008; Stephan 2012).

In his account of personal identity, Ricoeur distinguishes between identity in terms of *idem* (sameness) and *ipse* (oneself, self-reference). *Idem* refers to the features by which an entity, event or person can be identified, either as an individual or as an exemplar of a more general category. This first (individual) kind of identification refers to what has been called numerical identity, whereas the second (general) kind of identification has become known as qualitative identity. The *ipse* (or *soi* in French) is something else. It refers to who I am. Who I am is not what I think of myself, as a form of self-consciousness, or as the ego that posits itself rationally, as in the work of Descartes. It is a self that "finds itself" in its own acts, narratives, and social interactions.

In other words, the self is always "implied" and mediated; it needs a detour via its manifestation in the world to find itself (Ricoeur 1990, pp. 2–3, 16–19). One can compare this with what Kierkegaard meant by "indirect communication." The self is, again (as in Kierkegaard's view), not a substance or entity (idem, p. 118ff); not a predicate (idem, p. 34), or an objectifiable event (idem, p. 48). It is "who I am" while speaking, acting, and interacting. Ricoeur uses the term self-referentiality (or *sui*-reference) to indicate what this means: the implicit referencing of a speech act, or act, or narrative to the "I" or self of the person who is speaking, acting, or narrating (idem, pp. 48–53, 57, 118–125). This referencing is implicit, which means that the references to aspects of who one is are implied in the act or narration.

In the previous chapter, I took self-referentiality as a concept that refers to the implicit signifying aspect of emotions and moods, whether pathological or not. This use of the concept is clearly narrower than Ricoeur's, which includes forms of explicit (Kierkegaardian or Sartrean) self-relatedness. We saw in 2.3.1 that it is possible to say that experience refers to a self or to aspects of it, but this referring appears to be a result of inner presentation, not as signification by the act—or gesture, emotion, attitude, interaction—itself. So, I am restricting the term self-referentiality to the implicit signifying aspects of these behaviors themselves. It is the emotion itself that refers and not the person, as is the case with acts in which I am relating to myself. Self-referentiality is not adopting a stance toward one's emotions. It refers to what emotions by themselves "say" (signify, indicate, or reveal) about the person having them.

Self-referential signifying does not exclude self-awareness or self-interpretation. Emotions don't lose their self-referential qualities when one becomes aware of them. This may change when emotions and their meanings become the explicit target of reflection, as in psychotherapy. Mentalization, explicit reflection, and "working through" may change what emotions signify, but this only occurs after extended elaboration. I do not further pursue this intriguing subject here. What is needed is that one keeps in mind that (a) self-referentiality and self-awareness may go together and that it nevertheless makes sense to distinguish them conceptually, and (b) we need to distinguish the self-referentiality of self-signifying behaviors from the self-referentiality of some experiences. We mainly focus on the first in this book.

We must now return to an issue that was raised in the previous, in which I discussed the notion of mineness and asked what kind of self-referentiality it represents. I described mineness as the immediate, implicit, non-thematic awareness of oneself when one is immersed in one's activities and experiences. I suggested that the experience of mineness, qua experience, may reside at the background and adopt the form of an "implicit" or "dormant" sense of self within one's self-awareness. I also said that self-awareness can best be described as a form of inner "presentation." Pre-reflective self-awareness is, accordingly, the awareness of a self that is literally present to itself in the act of awareness. But what of cases of self-awareness in which the mineness of the awareness is not felt, cases with a dormant sense of mineness? Do such cases still have the resources to signify something about the self (oneself)? And, if so, how does this signifying occur? Does the self-referential potential adopt the form of self-presentation or of intrinsic signification?

The initial answer in the previous section was pragmatic: Presentation of the self and implicit signification of the self can be conceived as complementary manners of involvement of the self in one's behavior and experiences. But the issue we are discussing is more complicated. What should we think of situations in which self-awareness is robbed of all thematic content and in which mineness as a felt quality keeps itself dormant, at least temporarily?

Perhaps there is no answer to this question apart from the practical one. It is, after all, very hard to imagine situations of minimal awareness in which there is no immediate, implicit, non-thematic self-awareness at all; that is, states of pure consciousness that are stripped of any reference to an experiencing, spatio-temporal me, even mineness as the most elementary awareness of selfhood. Maybe there are some rare neurological conditions or cases of intensive Buddhist meditation that come close. But it is much easier to imagine that even in such cases, not all traces of self-awareness—understood as the most elementary experience of being present to oneself—have been wiped out. Let us assume, however, that such cases nevertheless exist, cases in which no immediate, non-thematic self-awareness whatsoever has been left. Even in such situations, we would still think about them as deviations of a standard situation, as somewhat artificial conditions that under certain circumstances could be restored to their default position, which is one of primordial self-awareness. Lack of a sense of mineness is then reinterpreted as a condition with potential self-awareness. This potentiality can then be accounted for in different, overlapping ways: phenomenologically, in terms of a theory about the structure of consciousness (i.e., as inherently self- [and object-] directed); in terms of philosophy of mind, by giving a dispositional account of consciousness; or even in terms of a cognitive neuroscience or psychology of consciousness, referring to particular subpersonal processes.

I have distinguished between three forms of inner presentation: (a) a classic form that is usually referred to with the term "intentionality" and in which presentation adopts the form of being directed at an intentional object; (b) a primordial form in which the "presentation" occurs immediately, implicitly, and non-thematically (this is what I called pre-reflective self-awareness), and (c) a form of presentation with no awareness at all of a self or any aspect of the self. This last form of presentation appeared to be tentative and somewhat theoretical. The question of whether references to a self in awareness [c] are possible and if so, whether they are of the implicit signifying or the inner presenting kind is very difficult to answer. It seems impossible to "present" a self if there is nothing left to present. However, self-signification by experiences like [c] are of a different order; such self-signification is not bound to the first-person perspective (others signify too), it lacks the immediacy of [a] and [b], and the signification is the expression of something with which it does not coincide: an act, a behavioral expression, an attitude, and/or an interaction. I am nevertheless inclined to suggest that insofar as awareness [c] can be construed as an act, expression, or attitude, there is nothing that withstands the attribution of self-referentiality to this act, expression, or attitude of awareness. The meaning of such referencing would then be of a different order compared to the "primitive experience of self-referentiality" of awareness with its idea of presence of the self [b]. So, I am inclined to deny that [c] presents a self, and I am ready to admit that experience [c] may have self-referential qualities, provided that it can be construed as a (self-referring) act, expression, or attitude.

There remains an important conceptual distinction between implicit self-signification and conscious self-presentation. Self-referentiality is a form of sense making or meaning generation. It needs time to evolve, as we saw in the previous chapter. It is the temporal dimension that explains the layeredness of self-referential sense-making; initial self-referential expressions and (inter)actions are valued in light of one's own hopes and desires related to the expectations of others. They are shaped against the background of one's personal history and of a socioculturally established horizon of meaning. Self-referring is, in other words, a process of signification that presupposes and builds on networks of relations that themselves are imbued with meaning. Signification can be seen as an emergent phenomenon of interactions in these networks; it is an expression of one's being-in-the-world (to borrow from Heidegger) that reveals one's stance with respect to the inherent meaning of these relations.

Being-aware-of—whether explicitly, implicitly or dormantly—is something else. Self-awareness is a state of mind with a certain directedness that takes shape against the background of an implicit understanding of the self (and the situation). Most of all, it should be seen as a form of "being present" to myself, a presence in the mode of the first-personal givenness of the self. Questions about dormant forms of mineness lose their urgency once one has understood the fundamental difference between self-signifying and being conscious-of-oneself.

Before I conclude this section, there is still one point that I need to mention to locate my account of self-referentiality, this time in relation to philosophers who conceive of self-referentiality in terms of character. Some of these philosophers deny the need for a concept such as self-referentiality. They claim that the conceptual work that self-referentiality is thought to do can already be done by the notion of character. Their argument runs as follows: Character is a concept that implies that people adopt a stance toward what occurs in their lives. They particularly adopt a stance toward occurrences that matter to them. This stance reveals who they are. Who one is, one's identity, is consolidated in one's character or personality. In so far as one's experiences and acts are an expression of one's character, they reveal one's identity.

I don't think this argument is conclusive, but it needs a response, which focuses mainly on emotion. Throughout this and the previous chapters, I have said that emotions are about what matters to us. This fact has not remained unnoticed in academic psychology (Frijda 1986) and philosophy (Baier 2004; Goldie 2000; 2002; Kenny 1984; Nussbaum 2001). What I have been aiming at is more specific, however. It is the idea that emotions implicitly and intrinsically refer to (aspects of the) persons having them. Emotions are not merely expressions of *what* one is, they say something about *who* one is. They are not merely indicating in what state one is or expressions of what kind of person one is (i.e., of one's character and habits). They are (also) expressions of who one is in a more immediate and personal way. Emotions show who I am or relevant aspects of who I am, as the person having the emotion in this specific situation and at this point in time. These statements make a distinction between references to general features (such as character traits) and to individual and actual features of the person. At first sight, the distinction seems gradual. There is a deeper dimension to it, however, which is elucidated by Ricoeur in his narrative account of character, (i.e., conceived as the character in a plot [a narrative, a play, a life history]) (Ricoeur 1990, pp. 119–123).

The concept of character is important in that it shows that *idem* (identification by general features) and *ipse* (answering to the question of who one is) may overlap and, in fact, often complete one another. Character refers initially to the constant features (the "what") of a person's personality. These features enable us to identify the person (i.e., by pointing out what type of personality he or she has). Character also addresses a normative dimension of personhood, however. References to a person's character are also an answer to the question of who one wants to be, for others, for oneself, and in the world. Both elements—the constancy of certain traits and the normative dimension of who one strives to be—presuppose one another. The self (*ipse*) is inscribed in the *idem*, according to Ricoeur. The self is not a free floating ipseity but is anchored in the *idem*. The self-referential aspects of my feelings and doings are anchored in identifiable features of my behavior and speech. Rather than viewing general and individual forms of self-referring as extremes of a continuum, it is better to view them as intertwined layers. Self-referring to the individual and actual "me" should be seen as a specification and revelation of the normative dimension of personhood. This normative dimension is anchored in references to general and identifiable traits, which enable us to locate, specify, and direct the normative dimension of personhood.

4.5 Application to psychotherapy

The relevance of the distinctions I have made can easily be shown with respect to the practice of psychotherapy. Helping the patient understand what he or she is going through forms a substantial part of the therapist's job (Gabbard 2010; Hobson 1985). Frequently, feelings and emotions are initially distorted, suppressed, or simply not noticed by a patient. In this initial phase, the therapist tries to point out, in collaboration with the patient, (a), that he or she is feeling something and, (b), what this feeling means. Step (a) concerns the transition from unnoticed (but self-referential) emotions to emotions of which the patient is aware. Step (b) concerns the transition from self-awareness to self-interpretation: The patient gradually gains an understanding of what the emotion says about him- or herself. He or she will then be able to interpret the emotions.

The distinction between self-referentiality and self-awareness is useful because emotions may signify something about the patient even when the patient is not aware of this signifying (Solomon 1983, p. 188ff; Stephan 2012). The distinction between self-awareness and self-interpretation (or self-understanding) does justice to the fact that self-awareness does not automatically imply that one knows what one's emotions or feelings mean. Interpretation goes a step further than mere awareness: It requires a fuller picture of the situation, an ability to reflect on what is going on, and above all recognition of the fact that the emotion signifies something about oneself.

Let me give a brief example.

> Judy, a 30-year-old woman, employed, with no husband and no children, is depressive and sad after the loss of her mother. Judy's sadness can be seen as a physiological and psychological state. As a psychological state, it involves an appraisal of how the world looks after the loss of her mother. The kind (and intensity) of her feelings and mood expresses what kind (and strength) of attachment she had with her mother (I consider deep attachments like Judy's attachment to her mother as part of her character). However, Judy's sadness also refers to something more individual and actual. It indicates implicitly why her mother's death has struck her in this particular way and not in some other way, why it seems so senseless to her, and why she feels so alone, numb, hopeless, ambivalent, and full of bitterness. In other words, the emotion not only refers to what matters to people like Judy in general, or merely to what kind of person she is in general, but also to what matters to Judy in her specific situation. This specificity is indicated and implied by the phenomenon itself: Judy's emotion of sadness. The emotion refers to what matters to Judy in her particular situation. Judy is not only sad (general category); there is a story in her feeling, something deeply personal in the way she experiences what has happened to her (see, in a similar spirit, Hobson 1985; Ratcliffe 2008; 2010; Sadler 2007).

To fully understand this, we must further discuss not only the embodied but also the embedded nature of emotions. Emotions do not exist in isolation. They are, in fact, part of one's life. In daily life and in psychiatric and psychotherapeutic practice, they make sense when and in so far as the contextual and temporal specificity of this embeddedness is taken into account (Stern 2004). Following a suggestion by Ratcliffe (2010), I indeed think that it makes sense to view the double-sidedness of emotions/moods (as both situational and self-directed) as overarched and integrated into a (Heideggerian) concept of the world.

4.6 Conclusion

In this chapter, we investigated the concepts of self, self-relatedness, and self-referentiality, and applied them to the clinical practice of psychiatry. I endorsed a broad and common-sense notion of selfhood that refers to persons and who they are, and not to parts of persons or aspects of how they function, such as one's self-image, the autobiographical self, or the "core" (or minimal) self (how valuable these concepts as such are). I next focused on the so-called "mineness" of one's experiences, that is, the immediate, non-thematic, implicit, and immersed awareness that it is me who is experiencing. This mineness is also described as "first personal mode of givenness of one's experience." I investigated the distinction between implicit self-referring in emotions and gestures and implicit referring to a self in self-awareness. This distinction was subsequently applied to pre-reflective self-awareness, especially the mineness of this self-awareness. There appeared to be (some) cases in which the mineness of one's self- awareness is "dormant" or implicit.

I subsequently developed the notion of self-relatedness, starting with Sören Kierkegaard's seminal phrases on the subject in *Sickness unto Death*. I argued why this notion is helpful in the conceptualization of emotions and psychopathology. In the traditional Cartesian-style interpretation of mental phenomena emotions and psychopathological experiences are interpreted either from a first-personal or a third-personal perspective. The first-person approach leads to a view in which feelings are torn loose from their bodily anchoring. The third-person approach is inextricably bound to the problems of objectivism. With respect to emotions and psychopathological experiences the objectivist approach implies that these are merely psychobiological states: they don't have a meaning and do not say something about the person having them. We saw that in a self-relational view body sensations are important, also for the understanding of mineness. They help to anchor one's thoughts, images, and associations in a spatio-temporally bounded "me," so that the sense of being a me in pre-reflective forms of self-awareness is not something that freely floats around.

Next we discussed self-referentiality. Emotions, gestures, attitudes, and interactions refer to a self, that is, to the person displaying that behavior. I traced the roots of this concept and introduced Ricoeur's distinction between *idem* and *ipse*. I argued (again) that self-referentiality and self-awareness may go together and that it nevertheless makes sense to distinguish them conceptually. I related self-referentiality to the notion of character and, broader, the ideas of embodiment and embeddedness. I warned that the self should not be viewed as a free floating ipseity, but as anchored in the *idem*. Self-referential aspects of my feelings and doings are rooted in identifiable features of my behavior and speech. In the final section, I illustrated the layeredness and complexity of these self-relational and self-referential aspects of one's psychic functioning with a clinical vignette.

Our discussion so far suggests that self-referring to an individual and actual "me" can be seen as a specification and revelation of a normative dimension of personhood. It is about this normativity that more will be said in the second part of this book—normativity with respect to both patients in the relationship with their illnesses and professionals in their relationship with their professional roles.

PART 2

Psychiatry as normative practice

5

BEING A PROFESSIONAL: SELF-RELATEDNESS AND NORMATIVITY

5.1 Introduction

In this second part of the book, I focus on what it is to be a professional. I do this by analyzing the relationships within which professional practices evolve. I also show how philosophy can contribute to the development of a normative approach to the practice of psychiatry. The result of these reflections is what I call a "normative practice approach" (NPA) of psychiatric practice. This approach proves relevant to contemporary debates on the role of the psychiatrist in individual, institutional, and societal contexts.

The current chapter argues that professionalism is inherently normative because of the inherent normativity of the relationships that support and guide professional activities. I build on the self-relational approach to psychopathology that was described in Part I. Just as patients don't coincide with their disorder but relate to their illness roles, professionals don't coincide with their professional roles; they relate to them (see Diagram 5.1). We will see that these relationships are also intrinsically normative.

Professional roles can themselves be seen as embodying certain values, which are transmitted by role modelling, supervision, training, and education. Different forms of self-relating, when put in temporal, narrative, and social contexts, give depth and perspective to professional role fulfilment. Professionalism, in fact, appears to be a complex concept. Attitudes toward one's professional role will over time be appropriated and internalized. These internalized attitudes become part of one's professional identity. I use the dynamic self-relational and (threefold) self-referential framework of the second chapter to illustrate and analyze this complexity.

5.2 Being a professional: The diagram updated

Diagram 5.1 provides an expanded version of the diagram that we discussed in Chapter 2. One of its main functions is to show that professionalism does not solely

The professional relates in different ways to his/er own professional role fulfilment [A] – [E]

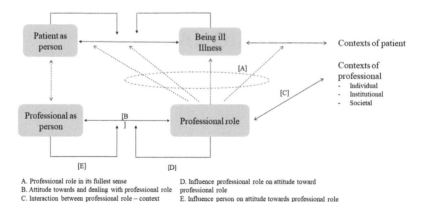

A. Professional role in its fullest sense
B. Attitude towards and dealing with professional role
C. Interaction between professional role – context
D. Influence professional role on attitude toward professional role
E. Influence person on attitude towards professional role

DIAGRAM 5.1 The professional relates in different ways to his/er own professional fulfilment [A] – [E]

consist of a set of skills plus a sufficient level of knowledge but is embedded in a network of relationships.

5.2.1 The relationships

Relationship [A] concerns the professional role with the full spectrum of issues that can be the focus of clinical attention. This full spectrum entails all relations [1] to [5], discussed in Chapter 2: the clinician's attention to the illness, to the patient's relation to the fact of being ill, to interactions between illness and context, to the influence of the illness on one's relating to the illness, and to the person of the patient, i.e., the influence of the patient's personality, her values, expectations, and interests on her being ill.

The next interaction, [B], concerns the relationship between the professional as person and his/her professional role. How do professionals as persons relate to their own role fulfilment? Are they capable of monitoring their own behavior? Can they reflect on their role fulfilment?

The Canadian Medical Educational Directives for Medical Specialists (CanMEDS) mention professionalism as one of the seven core competencies of any physician (Frank et al. 1996). These directives describe a framework for competency-based medical specialist's training. Professionalism is the ability to deal professionally with one's role as a psychiatrist. This includes having insight into one's own role, awareness of and ability to deal with role conflicts, and maintenance of professional and ethical boundaries with respect to value-sensitive matters, privacy, and informed consent. Traditional medical virtues return in the conceptualization of professionalism: honesty, altruism, compassion, integrity, trustworthiness, beneficence, accountability, and humanism (Gabbard et al. 2012).

Professionalism can be seen as a second order competence that helps to maintain the right balance between the other six competencies (Birden et al. 2014).

Relation [C] focuses on the interaction between professional behavior and all sorts of contextual influences. Today, these influences are so dominant that they affect and, some would say, threaten the professional identity of the psychiatrist. The institutional settings of psychiatric practice have significantly changed in the last 20 years. The administrative burden has sharply increased in most Western European countries and in North America. The economic context in which professionals operate puts its stamp on how individual professionals organize their practices.

Relation [D] refers to the shaping of one's attitude toward one's professional role by the execution of this role in various contexts and in the course of time. Think of a young colleague, who has recently begun her residency training and, after having been on call the entire night with a succession of problems that were difficult to handle, asks herself: "Is this what I want to do for the rest of my life?" Much of the emotional energy of being in training as a professional must be put into the process of becoming acquainted with one's role. Later in their career, professionals may feel that their professional self-image no longer fits with what their healthcare organization, professional association, or patients require them to be. Professionals may also simply outgrow their roles.

Professionals describe their professional identity sometimes in terms of the context in which they flourish optimally, as in: "I am typically a community psychiatrist," or "I am most at ease in my private practice, where I can organize my time better and be there entirely for my patients." In still other cases, it is the professional context itself that has changed, such that it leads to a redefinition of professional roles. An example of this is new occupations in healthcare. Nurse practitioners and physician assistants have taken over tasks that traditionally belonged to the domain of the physician, and this has led to a reshuffling of roles. The basis for the reshuffling may be legal: new laws and/or state regulations that redefine the jurisdictions of different professions. But this legal basis is usually the endpoint of long discussions between stakeholders with diverging interests: health economists, patient groups, professional organizations, the public health sector, and representatives of the state.

Relation [E], finally, focuses on the professional as person, on who one is as a professional and who one was and wishes to be. One's learning history is of course of great importance for the development of professional identity. It is the basis on which one's current role fulfilling builds and is given shape. Personal values are an important source for the development of one's professional identity.

5.2.2 Tensions and ambiguities

I began this chapter by suggesting that the professional role involves more than a collection of competences and executive functions. The question is what this "more" is. I answer this question in two stages: first, by describing the tensions and ambiguities typically inherent to professional role fulfilment, and, second, by giving a brief analysis of the values and normative principles that belong to each of the five different aspects of being a professional. To make this more vivid, I begin with an example:

> George is a psychiatrist in a regional mental hospital and, for over ten years, chief of a clinical ward for the treatment of people with severe mental disorders. The patients he and his team are treating have complex problems: schizophrenia or autism with severe behavioral problems; chronic, severe depression with comorbid personality disorder, suicidality, self-mutilation and/or substance use; and severe personality disorders with externalizing tendencies (acting out, impulsivity, reckless behavior). Most of George's patients have illness histories of more than 15 years and have been treated according to the relevant, evidence-based guidelines and treatment protocols without much success. Most patients know they will not get better and have no prospect of ever living a life outside the clinic. Their next destinations will be either forensic settings or high-security settings with short-term intensive treatment.
>
> George loves his work, despite all the misery he is dealing with. He is dedicated and inventive. George has quite unconventional ways of approaching his patients. He counters their unruliness with sometimes even more unruly verbal means. He is direct and at times authoritarian. But he has a nicer side too: If there is time, he takes patients out for a walk; he listens to music with them; once a month he prepares a dinner for his patients. George is a skillful clinician and has done his work energetically. In the past couple of years, however, the administrative burden has increased tremendously. He has difficulty finishing his administrative work. The electronic patient records are very inconvenient to work with; it is unclear where to write what and navigating through the system is a time-consuming job. The coupling of the records with the financial administration has, moreover, become a nightmare. Every bit of treatment must be registered. Many of the treatments George gives are difficult to specify in terms of the modules and treatment algorithms the hospital has introduced to serve as the basis for reimbursement by insurance companies. The problems of his patients don't fit with the categorizations that are used to describe the treatment modules. George says that the work he does simply cannot be translated into the linear language of modules and algorithms.
>
> Even more important is the insidious change in the attitudes of some of his patients and their relatives. They are behaving differently and have become more distant and demanding. George has less and less time to speak with the patients. There have been a couple of incidents with lots of aggression on his ward. The turmoil has led to unrest and feelings of unsafety among the patients and to burnout of some staff members. In response to these incidents, the Inspectorate for Mental Health has asked for clarification and a plan of action. It has also announced a visit to the ward. Apart from writing an

extensive report for the Inspectorate, George is also asked to report to the Executive Board of the hospital. He feels aggrieved by the attitude of suspicion of the member of the Board who questions him about the incidents. In the last few months, he has had doubts about whether to continue in this job. To make matters worse, the Executive Board has announced new budget cuts. This time, these will also impact George's department. George is worried; his attention is more and more focused on issues that have little to do with patient care; collegial relationships are under pressure.

The above case gives an impression of the complexity of the psychiatric profession today. This complexity is not only a reflection of the complexity of patient problems, but increasingly of changes in the administrative, economic-financial, legal, institutional, and sociocultural context of mental healthcare and the effects these factors have on the social psychology of larger organizations. In the first decade in his career, George could honestly say "I am there for my patients"" Now, he has the feeling that his professional existence is mostly absorbed by the "system," i.e., by all the institutionalized ways of accounting for and giving legitimacy to what he and his team are doing. It feels for George as if he is living in a different world. His previous world was based on respect and trust. The world he now inhabits is based on distrust and plagued by a hypertrophy of measures of control. The change is not local or accidental; it is a change in the system. At a personal level, he still has a grasp on what is going on, at least to a certain extent. Colleagues respect him, and he is supported by most of the members of his team. But at an institutional level, he doesn't have a grasp on or sufficient insight into the changes in the bureaucratic landscape.

The case—based on a mix of real-life cases in the Netherlands—illustrates how the professional role is influenced by a variety of factors. It shows abundantly the impact of changes in the reimbursement of psychiatric treatment and of the increased emphasis on efficiency and transparency. It highlights the duty to account for the nature, duration, and efficacy of treatments and shows how this leads to a shift in the focus of the clinician's attention. It describes how all these changes affect the self-image of the clinician and, in fact, reorganize the landscape of values in which clinicians such as George are working. In sum, and plotted against our diagram, contextual factors at an institutional and societal level [C] affect not only the definition of the professional role [A] but also the way in which the professional relates to this role [B]. George's working style has developed in an unconventional direction [D]. For a long time, this was no problem, since he was always fully committed to the well-being of the patient. But the administrative changes and the subtle changes they bring about in the definition of what a good professional is gnaw on George's professional identity (influence of [C] on [B] and [D]). This in turn leads to self-examination about what kind of professional George wants to be and about whether the current context allows him to strive for his ideals [E]. Does "the system" allow George to fulfil the role he needs to have given his commitments and ideals?

5.2.3 The normative dimension of these relations

From this, it is not a large step to a first qualification of the value domains and the types of norm that belong to the five aspects ([A]–[E]) of professionalism. I call it a first qualification because we are only dealing here with the individual professional–patient relationship and not with the larger context of professional relationships. Diagram 5.2 gives an overview of the different aspects of the professional role, the relevant value domains, and the qualities and virtues that are associated with these value domains. The overview is not meant to be complete; it gives only an impression of the broadness of the topic and of what a stratification of the different value domains could look like.

Aspect [A] of professionalism concerns the professional role proper with—in terms of the CanMEDS competencies—emphasis on the roles of medical expert, scholar, collaborator, organizer, and communicator. This role, moreover, requires sensitivity toward moral issues that are related to clinical performance. With respect to the latter, one might think of adherence to the codes of conduct of a certain profession, including rules with respect to confidentiality and informed consent, accountability, commitment to excellence, and subordination of one's interests to the interests of patients and their families. Professionalism can be seen as a second-order competence that enables the professional to navigate properly among different roles and interests.

With respect to relation [B], psychological competencies, such as insight and openness to peer review, appear to be important. Associated with these competencies are general self-directed virtues such as honesty, integrity, and trustworthiness.

The interaction between the professional and context [C] is characterized by qualities, values, and norms in at least three domains: collaboration and organization, the social context, and moral notions that are implicated in the social contract. The social contract involves the idea that physicians are worthy of trust bestowed on them by their patients and the public because they are working for the patients' and the public's good (Swick 2000). Health advocacy, one of the CanMEDS competencies, also belongs to this sphere. Responding to societal needs is an even broader category that draws the public sphere almost literally within the consulting room.

Relation [D] is about the influence of the professional role on one's dealing with that role. One important topic in this context was addressed in our description of George's career. George has felt gradually alienated from his original commitments and his professional role. Keeping a balance between one's own ambitions and those of the organization with respect to one's role is one of the important qualities of the professional. Integrity is another important value.

Relation [E], which addresses the impact of one's personality on one's task fulfilment, requires psychological capacities (self-reflection, insight) and is based on more general and overarching virtues such as the one's mentioned above (honesty, integrity, and trustworthiness), but also compassion, altruism, and respect.

Aspects of professional role	Domains	Qualities, values, and norms
A. Professional role in *sensu stricto*	Medical expertise	Clinical skills, craftsmanship Diagnostic skills Dealing with complexity and uncertainty
	Scholarship	Expert knowledge, medical expertise Scientific orientation
	Social	Competence in organization and collaboration Communicative skills, empathy
	Moral	Commitment to excellence Accountability Subordination of one's own interests to interests of others Adherence to codes of conduct
B. Professional relates to professional role	Psychological	Insight Openness for peer review
	Moral	Self-related values: honesty, integrity, compassion, altruism, respect, trustworthiness
C. Interaction between context and professional role fulfilment	Collaboration and organization	Attuning to meso- and macrolevel contextual changes/influences
	Social	Responding to societal needs Awareness of social contract between society and profession Health advocacy
	Moral	Trust by the public
D. Influence of professional role fulfilling on how one relates to professional role [B]	Psychological	Ability to balance needs of the organization with fulfilment of one's professional role
	Moral	Integrity
E. Influence of person-related factors on how one relates to professional role [B]	Psychological	Self-reflection and critical attitude Insight
	Moral	Other directed "humanistic" values: honesty, integrity, compassion, altruism, respect, trustworthiness

DIAGRAM 5.2 Aspects of the professional role, domains, and competencies

5.3 Professionalism

5.3.1 Definitions

There have been extensive discussions of professionalism in medicine and other occupational domains (Abbott 1988; Freidson 2001; Larson 1997; Parsons 1963; Schon 1983; Wear & Aultman 2006). Definitions of professionalism vary. Most definitions mention expert knowledge and skills as one of its core features, together with certain jurisdictions or privileges of the professional. These jurisdictions and privileges are granted by society and/or patients based on the professional's commitment, accountability, and competence. Among these privileges (and their related requirements) are self-regulation with respect to standards of excellence, membership in the professional subgroup, training requirements, and criteria for licensing and quality control. Rueschemeyer describes the traditional (functionalist) conception of professionals as follows:

> Individually and, in association, collectively, the professions "strike a bargain with society" in which they exchange competence and integrity against the trust of client and community, relative freedom from lay supervision and interference, protection against unqualified competition as well as substantial remuneration and higher social status. (Rueschemeyer 1983, p. 41)

He also emphasizes that the way we think about expert occupations transcends the confines of occupational sociology and comes close to a central theme in classical sociology: the emergence of modern society and culture as such:

> How expert knowledge is deployed in different institutional forms, how it is controlled, how it is used as a resource of power and a basis of privilege, and how in turn different institutional forms of deployment, social control as well as individual and collective advantage, are affected by other and wider social structures and processes—inquiries into these questions tell us much about the structure and the dynamics of society as a whole. (Rueschemeyer 1983, p. 38)

Moore gives a practical overview and defines the professional as having a full-time occupation, which sets his efforts apart from amateurism. The professional has a commitment to a calling; the fulfilment of the profession's requirements is a response to a set of normative and behavioral expectations. Professions are set apart from other forms of occupation by various signs and symbols and are identified by their peers via membership in formalized organizations. Usually the possession of skills and knowledge requires intensive and prolonged training. Professionals need to exhibit an orientation to service; they proceed by their own judgment and authority and are, therefore, professionally autonomous (Moore 1970, pp. 5–6). Freidson's more recent account enumerates similar criteria. He states that professionals have:

1. "Specialized work in the officially recognized economy that is believed to be grounded in a body of theoretically based, discretionary knowledge and skill and that is accordingly given special status in the labor force;
2. Exclusive jurisdiction in a particular division of labor created and controlled by occupational negotiation;
3. A sheltered position in both external and internal labor markets that is based on qualifying credentials created by the occupation;
4. A formal training program lying outside the labor market that produces the qualifying credentials, which is controlled by the occupation and associated with higher education; and
5. An ideology that asserts greater commitment to doing good work than to economic gain and to the quality rather than the economic efficiency of work." (Freidson 2001, p. 127)

An important and more recent impetus for the study of professionalism is the educational reform in residency training programs. This reform has occasioned an upsurge in writings on professionalism as clinical competence and on the assessment of this competence (Birden et al. 2014; Gabbard et al. 2012). This body of literature focuses on the appropriate attitudes and behaviors of the physician, given his or her unique privilege of being a professional. It also investigates how these attitudes and behaviors can be operationalized in a way that makes them suitable for clinical assessment. The new CanMEDS framework combines the two broader perspectives—the profession's responsibility for defining its own standards of excellence and the societal legitimation for the profession's doing this independently—in its definition of professionalism as a core clinical competence (see also Diagram 5.2):

> Physicians have a unique societal role as professionals who are dedicated to the health and caring of others. Their work requires the mastery of a complex body of knowledge and skills, as well as the art of medicine. As such, the Professional Role is guided by codes of ethics and a commitment to clinical competence, the embracing of appropriate attitudes and behaviors, integrity, altruism, personal well-being, and to the promotion of the public good within their domain. These commitments form the basis of a social contract between a physician and society. Society, in return, grants physicians the privilege of profession-led regulation with the understanding that they are accountable to those served.

Being a professional consists of a unique combination of roles, excellence, and commitment, which includes personal dedication to the welfare of others, mastery at a high level of certain skills and knowledge, sensitivity to the art of medicine, and a wide range of other commitments. Note that in the quotation, these commitments are positioned as the "basis" for the social contract. It is not unusual to see the social contract described as legitimizing the exertion of certain skills and to see commitments narrowed down to the duty to keep the contract (i.e., to use these skills appropriately). The CanMEDS framework recognizes a broader embedding of responsibilities and commitments within the professional's role. This is, of course, in line with one of the meanings of the word "profession," which not only refers to a paid occupation but also to the vows people make (i.e., what they "profess") on entering a certain group. The Hippocratic Oath qualifies as a declaration of this dedication on entering the medical profession.

In this and the next section, I briefly discuss the history of professionalism as a social phenomenon. I outline how professionalism has come under attack and what this means for professional autonomy. I also say a few words about the rise of the service user movement. In Chapter 7, I will complete the analysis of professionalism by providing more detail about the broader (meso- and macro-) contexts of psychiatry. There, I will also introduce a distinction between the levels and contexts of professionalism and begin with a short analysis of the meaning and relevance of contextual variation for the idea of professionalism

5.3.2 Professionalism from a sociological perspective

Professionalism is a big topic in sociology. The history of the concept is complicated, a fact partially reflected by the lack of a single definition of it, not even within the field of medicine. It is nevertheless not uncommon to see the sociology of professions described as having gone through at least three stages (Evetts 2003; Kanes 2010; Sciulli 2005). The division into three parts is somewhat artificial, but it may well serve for our purpose, which is to give an impression of the kind of discussions there have been on the professions from a broader societal and social perspective. I think it is important to give this broader background. It is remarkable how little of the extensive sociological studies on professional competence has resonated in the medical educational literature (exceptions are, for example, Cruess & Cruess 1997). In order to see that professionalism is more than an ability to use a set of skills, we need this broader background.

The first *functionalist* or *structural-functionalist* phase started in the 1930s. The early studies give descriptions of the development of the professions and give a rationale for their emergence. Professionalism is generally seen as representing an outspoken, institutionalized form of division of labor. The term "division of labor" was not new at that time. It was, for instance, an important topic in the works of both Karl Marx and Max Weber, although obviously for different reasons. Marx considered the division of labor as an evil because it lies at the basis of class differences and of man's alienation from the products of his hands. Max Weber, by way of contrast, saw the division as the inevitable counterpart of the processes of modernization and rationalization of Western society. These processes are characterized by the institutionalization of purposive-rational economic and administrative activities. These activities crystallize in two broad domains: the market (the capitalist enterprise) and the bureaucracy (public administration). Examples of bureaucratic control are activities of supervisory bodies, of authorities that are occupied with the enforcement of legislation, and of institutes that control whether certain standards are met.

Characteristic for both domains are the functional and specific relations between providers and consumers and between representatives of the bureaucracy and those who make use of its services. Other resemblances are the existence of a restricted domain of competence and/or power and the application of universalistic, impersonal standards.

This first phase in the development of professions is usually seen as the expression of this rational and functional division of labor. Leading sociologists like Talcott Parsons (1964) emphasize not only the rationality of this process but also its integrating function and uplifting potential. Professions have an integrative function because their members are not only experts but bound to certain norms and codes of conduct. These norms and codes embody goods that never would have been realized when professional–client relationships would have been defined in terms of the market. Freidson suggests in his later work that the professional–client relationship conforms to a "third logic" (Freidson 2001), apart from the logic of the market (consumerism) *and* of the bureaucracy (managerialism). Most significant for professions is that they are permitted to regulate and control their own practices. Professions would lose all resemblance to their current manifestations if they became, on the one hand, "mere casual labor in a spot market controlled by consumers" or, on the other, "mere job-holders in firms controlled by managers" (Freidson 2001, p. 7; see also Chapter 8). The third logic consists therefore in the specific form of giving-and-taking within the social contract that underlies the professions.

The second, critical (or revisionist, ideological, or postmodern) phase in the sociological analysis of the professions puts emphasis on the negative effects of professionalism. The way these negative effects are described sometimes seems a far cry from Karl Marx's objections against the division of labor. The professional is now seen as someone who exploits his or her position of power to sustain a privileged, self-interested monopoly (Evetts 2003). Larson, for instance, one of the major voices in the critical camp, states that the medical profession in the US has not shown enough integrity to safeguard its public mandate. Doctors have been more interested in their own private interests than in pursuing the collective value of health. She deplores the lack of benefit the medical profession has yielded for the public good (Kanes 2010; Larson 1977; 2003, p. 460). Illich (1976) goes one step further in his influential book *Limits to Medicine* by suggesting that the system of healthcare produces its own illness (iatrogenesis). Modern medicine disempowers people and expropriates their health. Such criticisms are not restricted to the medical field, however.

Freidson mentions three general issues in what he calls the assault on professionalism: criticism on the monopoly of professions, on social closure, and on credentialism. These three issues are complementary. The monopoly concerns the privileged position of professions in the market, i.e., their jurisdiction and exclusive command about how expert knowledge and technical means are used. Social closure refers to the claim that professions have the right to determine their own criteria for membership. And credentialism denotes the profession's right to establish its own credentials, i.e., its standards of excellence and systems of accreditation.

Focusing specifically on medicine, Marmor and Gordon (2014) discuss several themes in the critical literature. Critics complain that the inherent inequality in terms of knowledge and skills has turned into misplaced superiority and display of authority (paternalism). Another issue is self-regulation. This has become a protective shield, instead of a way to strike a balance among the competing priorities of self-interest, service to the public good, and striving for the appropriate level of competence. This is the mild version of Larson's criticism. Another issue is the traditional disdain of doctors for any form of competition and competitive commercialism. This disdain has sometimes turned into detrimental indifference to medical costs and the problem of controlling them. Finally, the individual patient–doctor relationship has become so central that it has led to a relative neglect of medicine's role with respect to larger societal problems and public health concerns.

Such criticisms have brought some scholars to predict the decline and even the end of professions (Broadbent et al. 1997; see also Tallis 2004). According to Kaul (1986), professional elites are becoming "proletarian," and this will dramatically change the medical landscape. The term "proletarianism" refers in this context to the envisioned process of deprofessionalization. The idea is that, as the proletarian has been alienated from his labor, so the professional is being alienated from his work. Krause (1996) states that professions behave like guilds and that, because they keep doing so, they will die out. However, with the exception of some radical proponents of the free market, like Milton Friedman (1962), few scholars really believe that patient will behave like consumers. They will never be able to independently gain all the relevant information and use it in their own interests. The information that is available in the media and on the Internet is often incomplete or distorted by the framing of interest groups. The transaction costs of deprofessionalization will, moreover, be enormous. Transaction costs are costs that are made in order to make the exchange of goods a transaction. Inexperienced service users need to reach the point at which they can assess the risks and benefits of the different options realistically and adequately. Many users will never reach this position or will simply not be willing to deliver the amount of effort that is needed (Freidson 2001, p. 205).

The third phase in the sociological study of the professions began in the late 1980s and early 1990s. This phase is characterized by a cautious reappraisal of the role of professions and by a search for balance and a more empirical orientation (Irvine 2001). Abbott (1988), for instance, puts more emphasis on the internal dynamics within and between professions. Professions are not only interacting with governments and other bureaucratic agencies and financial partners but also with each other; there are constant negotiations between professions about their jurisdictions. Abbott also draws attention to the relationship between kinds of professional work and the way the respective professions safeguard their credibility, accountability, and level of expertise. Different types of work require different credentials and different forms of education, quality control, and organization.

Other studies point to the different ways of organizing work and how this has led to a plurality of professional styles, also in medicine. Castellani and Hafferty

(2006) mention seven of these styles for medicine: nostalgic, unreflective, academic, entrepreneurial, empirical, lifestyle, and activist. Bloom et al. (2008) see this plurality in the creation of new partnerships between states, market players, and civil society organizations. Given the larger role of formal and informal markets in the system of healthcare, the information asymmetry between experts and clients has become increasingly important. This asymmetry requires additional regulatory arrangements to protect vulnerable consumers against exploitation, misinformation, and insufficient care. These new arrangements require new and targeted negotiations on specific aspects of the social contract. Today, these negotiations are more than ever mediated by non-market institutions, such as public health bureaucracies, non-profit organizations, advocacy groups, and regulatory bodies.

5.4 Philosophical reflections

Let us move on to a philosophical reflection on the concept of professionalism, including its history and its future. I briefly focus on two issues: the role of (expert) knowledge and the impact of differences in context on the definition of the object and purpose of professional activity.

5.4.1 Professionalism and the role of expert knowledge and skills

We have seen that the expert role is contested today. It is criticized by the service user movement. It is threatened by ongoing specialization and concomitant fragmentation of the field of (mental) healthcare. Introduction of market incentives have eroded trust in the unselfish beneficence of the professional. Inter- and intra-disciplinary competition have made things even worse.

At a more fundamental level, there are other issues that influence the very notion of expert knowledge and skills. The fortunes of professionalism are part of a more general and subtle change in society's relationship to knowledge and expertise (Beck & Young 2005). In a postmodern world, citizens relate differently to knowledge and skills. Competence is no longer seen as owned by scholars, and professions are no longer conceived as embedded in contexts and traditions. Knowledge has been reduced to bits of information that are freely available wherever one lives, and skills are seen as more or less isolated abilities that can be appropriated where and when one wants. The relationship between subject and knowledge and between practitioner and competence has become instrumentalist (or functionalistic). Knowledge and skills do not mean anything in themselves. They acquire meaning depending on their use. Ideally, competences should effortlessly be transferrable from one context to another. This is similar for knowledge: It should be "generic," or suitable for use in as many contexts as possible. As a result, education and professionalism are no longer seen as embedded in practices with different styles, cultures, and implicit understandings of the world.

This issue is especially topical in discussions about the reform of medical specialists' training. According to the functionalist paradigm, it would be ideal for residency training programs to uncouple contexts from the acquisition of skills. In the Netherlands, there even appeared a policy document in which—based on similar ideas—a plea was made for marketizing of medical specialists' training. Competences and knowledge, the document stated, are after all products of an educational system that, to optimize efficiency and cost effectiveness, must be dealt with as if it were a market.

The ideology behind these suggestions and proposals is questionable, however. There are at least two major drawbacks: First, the instrumentalist approach to specialists' knowledge and skills is too abstract. It is simply not true that the possession of competences can be operationalized apart from contexts. The competence of communication, for instance, involves various abilities that largely depend on the context. Talking with a severely psychotic and violent patient in a police station requires communicative skills that differ from those that are needed in psychodynamic psychotherapy. Negotiating with a patient about the level of restraint that is needed to keep the situation safe at a closed ward requires different collaborative skills than those necessitated by negotiating about treatment options with a fully competent anxiety disorder patient. Therefore, competences like communication and collaboration refer to a wide variety of skills that are highly context sensitive.

Another drawback is the abstractness of the idea that skills can be separated from the persons who use them. As discussed in Section 5.3.2, the professional role is more than a set of loosely coupled skills. Professionals relate to their role, and the manner in which they do this becomes part of their professional identity. Residents need to grow into their future roles. This growing requires one to be embedded in the relevant environments. These environments should, ideally, allow residents to discover their own personal fit—the fit between who they are and who they are required to be in terms of knowledge, skills and attitudes. We will revisit this issue in the final chapter.

The relationship between the postmodern professional and his or her knowledge and skills is changing, indeed. These changes are not new, however; they are even not postmodern. In fact, they are predictable in the light of Weber's idea of an ongoing division of labor and Dooyeweerd's notion of increasing interlacements between different spheres of life. These changes do not go so far that they offer arguments for a fundamental revision of the notion of professionalism. On the contrary, they ask for a concept of competence in which transferability (of skills) is reinterpreted as requiring context sensitivity. The increasing complexity of current mental healthcare, contextually and qua the expert role, should not be addressed with a decontextualized concept of competence but with a notion of competence that is even more radically contextually sensitive than it used to be. Transferability of skills should indeed be put high on the priority list of educational programs, but transferability does not necessarily imply isolation and decontextualization. It should be conceived as compatible with increased context sensitivity.

5.4.2 Contexts and their role in the legitimation of the professional role

The dominant role of the context in the shaping of knowledge and skills brings us to a related subject: the conceptualization of expert knowledge in view of the dominance of contextual factors on its nature and legitimacy. What is it in expert knowledge that justifies its special role? How should the relationship between knowledge (or the expert role) and contexts be conceptualized in order to do justice to its special status in mental healthcare?

To orient ourselves, let me discuss two extremes in the conceptualization of expert knowledge: absolutization and devaluation. We discussed already examples of both. I addressed absolutization of knowledge in the first chapter of this book, where I associated it with scientism. Scientism is the conviction that science and science alone is epistemically justified in its claims about truth and about what exists. I interpreted scientism as being based on neglect and even denial of the abstractness of scientific knowledge. Due to this neglect, the boundary between scientific knowledge and worldviews (paradigms) becomes blurred, and science adopts the role of a worldview by functioning as an ultimate horizon and touchstone for truth.

Openly confessed statements of scientism are rare in psychiatry, but we saw that subtler variants are the order of the day, especially when viewed from the perspective of clinical practice. For instance, the much criticized paternalism of medical professionalism cannot be separated from the hidden scientistic views of its defenders. The doctor knows best. Why? Because science tells him what the facts are and how the patient's problems can be solved. The relationship between scientism and paternalism is not so much logical as it is motivational and attitudinal. If it is science that determines what exists, then it is the professional, as a representative of science and guardian of truth, who understands the patient's situation. It is the professional who speaks with authority. Patients can only offer opinion. Technology plays of course an important mediating role in this context. It strongly enhances the expectation that the professional is in control and that the object of investigation can be manipulated and made transparent.

It is from this perspective not so much the expert role itself that lies at the basis of the absolutist attitude but rather the improper valuation of science's limitations—limitations that follow from the abstract mode of observing and thinking of the scientist. It is superfluous to say that scientists may speak with authority when they do respect the limitations of their methods and say no more than can be justified based on their proper use.

The other extreme, devaluation of the expert role, not surprisingly, comes as a reaction to this self-acclaimed authority of the profession. This reaction is based on exactly the same neglect of the distinction between science and worldview as the paternalistic absolutization of the scientific basis of psychiatry. Expert knowledge is regarded as belonging to a system with totalitarian traits. This system is by definition oppressive and disempowering, according to the critics. Professional knowledge is instrumental to this oppressive role because it identifies the abnormal and provides the conceptual tools for its correction.

So, here we are. The professional claims to have authority. This authority is primarily based on the expert role. But this role is limited, like the knowledge behind it. Professional authority, therefore, cannot be solely based on this role. As Gorovitz and MacIntyre (1976) rightly remark, medical knowledge is characterized by an intrinsic and necessary fallibility. Even in the ideal case of a complete knowledge of all the relevant causes and mechanisms, doctors are never able to predict with 100% certainty what will happen in the individual case. There are, therefore, epistemic reasons to argue for a broader than epistemic basis for medicine's legitimacy. Expert knowledge is important; it is even crucial, and without it there is no medical professionalism. But it cannot be the only or the ultimate ground for what doctors do. In the next chapter, I will argue that science and expert knowledge are foundational to a normative account of professionalism. They offer the basis (or foundation) for what doctors do, but they do not qualify medicine as the (moral) practice that it is. In a framework that distinguishes between qualifying, conditioning, and foundational norms, scientific insights and expert knowledge are foundational. What qualifies the relationship between the (medical) professional and the patient is trust and the doctor's commitment to the well-being of the patient (beneficence). This trust and commitment are morally qualified. This point will be further developed in the next chapter, where we will see how mental healthcare can be conceived as a normative practice. So, my answer, so far, to the question of how the relationship between knowledge and contexts should be conceptualized in order to do justice to the special status of expert knowledge is as follows:

- expert knowledge and skills deserve a special status because they are foundational to the practice of medicine
- the expert role functions in a broader framework of normative relations
- contexts are part of and delimit this framework of normative relations
- the doctor–patient relationship should be conceived of as a moral relationship because it relies on trust by the patient and a commitment to beneficence by the doctor
- this trust cannot solely be based on epistemic grounds.

To conclude this subsection, we must take one additional step. There is still one characteristic of professional practices that has not been addressed so far: the fact that they are practices. Professional knowledge is never merely knowledge but always part of a practice. This is an element that is easily overlooked in discussions about the justification of the special role of expert knowledge. The term practice refers in this context to a whole range of practices: the practice of knowing something (as in science), the practice of construing and reconstruing (as in technology and engineering), and the practice of predicting (for instance, in policymaking or treatment planning). These practices have, as we have seen, normative dimensions. These normative dimensions give (scientific) knowledge and the practices to which it contributes a certain specificity and direction. In the next chapter, I will specify this practical side of medical knowing by introducing the notion of disclosure or "opening up." A normative account of expert knowledge requires a careful analysis of how the different normative (contextual) dimensions open up (shape, specify, and guide) knowledge and expertise in a way that contributes to the ultimate goals of the practice.

In summary, expert knowledge by itself cannot fully justify the authority of doctors and undergird the legitimacy of what they do. I nevertheless emphasize that expert knowledge and skills are a *sine qua non* for medical professionalism. I suggest that the legitimacy of expert knowledge and skills should be found in what doctors do with their knowledge and skills. Medicine and psychiatry are practices, after all, and they are meant to contribute to the patient's good. Knowledge and skills should lead to the opening up of one's understanding; they should attune clinical understanding to the specific features of the situation and pave the road to the right choices with respect to treatment, rehabilitation, and support. Meeting these needs requires a view on mental healthcare that also takes its broader contexts into account.

5.5 Conclusion

This chapter began with an analysis of the relationship between the professional and his or her role in five dimensions (5.2). This analysis showed that the relationship between professionals as persons and their roles is much more intrinsic than an instrumentalist and merely functionalist view on professionalism tends to concede. Professionalism is more than a collection of skills and techniques that can be put to use at will. Professionals are inclined to identify themselves with the roles they play in the various settings in which they work. They identify, both individually and as a group, with broader and more fundamental commitments with respect to the good of the patient and of healthcare as a practice. This good is, of course, related to—but cannot completely be accounted for in terms of—competences and measurable performance (Hafferty 2006b; Sullivan 2004).

Practices are organized in ways that ideally correspond with what professions consider to be meaningful and valuable. Professionals internalize these meanings and values. The more and the longer the professional is embedded in a certain practice and becomes used to it, the more his or her professional identity will tend to coincide with the values that are inherent to these practices. Contrariwise, personal inspiration and sensitivity for meaning will also flow back to professional practices and codetermine how they evolve.

The developments we have discussed are ambiguous, pluralistic, and somewhat ironic. We saw this in the second part of the chapter, which focused on the sociological concept of professionalism (5.3). In the last few decades, more and more emphasis has been put on the validity of clinical knowledge and the transparency of treatment protocols. The managerial translations of these epistemic requirements have contributed to a technical and instrumentalist view on the professional role. At first glance, this instrumentalist view on professionalism fits well with a functionalist interpretation of professionalism, such as that described in the first phase of the sociology of professions. Important elements of this functionalist approach have remained in the current, more pragmatic views on professionalism. Today's (mental) healthcare requires flexibility, employability, interchangeability, and accountability. Knowledge and skills are dealt with as if they are "functions" that can be employed wherever needed. The professional has become a "bearer" of functions, which derive their meaning from the rational framework of which they form a part. This framework also needs to partially conform to the logic of the market and to the logic of bureaucracy.

From a theoretical point of view, changes at the level of the system of (mental) healthcare form a perfect match with this technical and instrumentalist conception of the professional role. However, as we have seen, what seems perfect in theory does not always work in practice. The irony of the process appears to be that the very logic behind the triad of functionalism, managerialism, and consumerism also led to an erosion of trust between physicians and patients and between the medical profession and society. This crisis of trust was counteracted by additional bureaucratic measures meant to improve the transparency of patient–physician interactions and the accountability of the profession. However, these measures were taken without prior re-establishment of the kind of good that is embodied by the practice of (mental) healthcare. What was seen as an inseparable part of the concept of professionalism in the early sociology of professions, especially by Parsons—that its norms and codes integrate and embody a greater societal and moral good—no longer appears to be self-evident in contemporary Western societies. The result is—and this is the irony—that instead of promoting trust, the new managerialism has led to preoccupation with control and to avoidance of risk, together with an even more reduced concept of professionalism. In other words, instead of integrating common interests, the new bureaucratic arrangements led to collisions between managerial approaches and professional ideals. Instead of enhancing trust, they brought a paradox of control, with a diminishment of trust because of ever increasing measures of control.

Normativity still appears to be the forgotten dimension in the renewed negotiations about the social contract between medicine and society (Wynia et al. 1999). It is interesting to see how this has been recognized in the most recent debates, for instance in Margolis' plea for "fiduciary duty" instead of market-driven interests as a central concept for administrators and directors of healthcare facilities (Margolis 2015). Normativity will be the topic of the next chapter.

6

TOWARD A NORMATIVE PRACTICE APPROACH FOR MENTAL HEALTHCARE

6.1 Why a normative account of practices?

The previous chapter outlined the ideas, tensions, and ambiguities behind today's concept of professionalism. I attempted to sketch out a perspective that offers an alternative to both scientistic absolutization and critical devaluation of the expert role. We saw how a self-relational/self-referential approach can provide the bare bones of a new concept of professional identity. We analyzed how professional responsibilities at individual, institutional, and societal levels overlap but do not coincide. We reviewed how today, institutional and societal aspects of (mental) healthcare play a more dominating role than they used to in terms of how professionalism is viewed and shaped. We also considered the rise and impact of service user movements and their influence on the definition of what it is to be a professional. We concluded that normativity and responsibility form the forgotten dimension in recent discussions between stakeholders about their rights and duties.

With this, we have already given a general answer to the question in the heading of this section (i.e., why is a normative account of practices needed?). We need this account because normative issues have been insufficiently addressed in recent debates about the social contract between mental healthcare and society. We now focus more specifically on this normative dimension and develop a heuristic framework for psychiatry as a normative practice. The first sections explore what terms like "normative" and "normative practice" mean and enumerate the requirements for the framework, i.e., for psychiatry as a normative practice. The second part develops this normative practice approach. It outlines its background, explains its constituents, and defines some of the roles it might play in various discussions.

6.1.1 Normative is broader than ethical

In this chapter, I make a distinction between ethical and normative aspects of a practice. I prefer to speak of the normative aspects of psychiatric practice. Ethics is a science and a branch of both philosophy and theology. Ethicists refer to moral theories, but not all ethics is normative. There are also descriptive ethics and meta-ethics. However, the main reason for my preference of the term normative is that it spans a broader domain than the domain of (normative) ethics per se. Like medicine, psychiatry needs a broader than strictly moral analysis of its "normative structure." This is because there are other kinds of normativity than ethical normativity alone, such as socially, economically, legally, and politically qualified normativity. The kind of normative analysis I am aiming at is an attempt to intuitively probe the inherent normative principles (rules, maxims, and values) of a certain practice. This attempt begins from within, i.e., in the form of a phenomenological and/or ethnographic descriptive analysis of mental healthcare as a practice. This kind of analysis ideally provides a substantive account of the practices under study, with glimpses of an implicit normativity, which is subsequently unearthed by conceptual analysis as thoroughly as possible. My contribution mainly consists of the second part: the conceptual analysis. With respect to the first part, the descriptive analysis, I mainly refer to the work of others.

This method—the bottom-up unraveling of normative constituents of practices—does not imply that values can be derived from facts. The phenomenological and/or ethnographic type of description does not suffer from a naturalist fallacy. It is the other way around: It is precisely this kind of investigation that elucidates how abstract the idea of value-neutral description is. We have already seen that psychiatric practice is inherently and in every respect value laden. This also holds for descriptions of this practice and the analysis of these descriptions. The kind of normative analysis I am aiming at begins *in medias res*, not as a purely theoretical endeavor, but within practice, as an attempt to make the implicit explicit.

As a result of this bottom-up approach, a certain degree of circularity in the design of this chapter cannot be avoided. To introduce the normative practice approach, I briefly compare it with other approaches, which also need some introduction. When the discussion becomes more focused, more detailed arguments and more fine-grained analyses are needed, for instance in the fields of medical ethics, philosophy, and meta-ethics. In other words, the normative practice approach will be developed as an extension (or variant) of clinical understanding. Competing approaches will initially be described at this level. Later, the normative practice model will be placed in a philosophical and meta-ethical context and again be compared with these other approaches.

Although we start at the clinical level of understanding psychiatric problems, it would be shortsighted and naïve to think that the kind of clinical-normative reflection that I am proposing can be performed without references to broader philosophical and meta-ethical discussions. Many issues in clinical-normative reflection have an important conceptual and metaphysical core, and many conceptual issues can be addressed much more precisely at a philosophical than at a practical-clinical level. I nevertheless insist on the bottom-up approach, because I am convinced that most normative discussions in clinical practice are settled based on grounds that express one's sense of appropriateness, proportionality and holism and not on more refined philosophical grounds. It is at this level that the normative practice approach should be of help, as a relatively coarse-grained systematic heuristic device that helps to bring some order to the discussion.

6.1.2 Normative practices: What are they?

The term normative usually refers to behavior that is "established by, relates to, or is derived from a standard or norm" (Oxford Dictionary). In the context of psychiatry, this means that activities are constituted by, relate to and are derived from standards, norms and principles, which are typical and specific for medicine/mental healthcare. The normative aspects of a practice become manifest in the legitimate expectations people tend to have about that practice. These expectations concern issues people deem important, valuable, and/or indispensable for that practice. The normative practice approach that will be developed in this chapter limits the use of the term normative still further and aims only at *constitutive* characteristics of practices. When I am referring to norms, I am therefore not aiming at external standards or at criteria with a merely descriptive status or at averages. Norms and normative principles are, in the normative practice approach, the kind of things practices must realize and embody in order for those practices to be what they are. Norms and normative principles are, in other words, inherent, or intrinsic, to practices.

I derive the idea that what holds for a practice is inherent to that practice from the classical virtue-ethical approach. In Book I of the *Nichomachean Ethics*, Aristotle suggests that the excellence of a practice is not some abstract ideal. It is, instead, intrinsic to that practice (1097a15–1098b8). There is not lyre playing and then, apart from this, good lyre playing as a distant ideal. Paraphrasing Aristotle, one could say that if lyre playing is not good enough, it is no longer lyre playing but making noise. Goods are not abstract ideals, but inextricably connected with the excellence, or perfection, of a practice. They are, to say it in a more Kantian than Aristotelian way, constitutive for that practice, which means that the practice cannot be conceived apart from its perfection, its perfect realization, or excellence.

Alasdair MacIntyre, whose *After Virtue* heralded the return of virtue ethics in moral theory, refers to these norms as "goods that are internal to practices":

> By a "practice" I am going to mean any coherent and complex form of socially established cooperative human activity through which goods internal to that form of activity are realized in the course of trying to achieve those standards of excellence which are appropriate to, and partially definitive of, that form of activity, with the result that human powers to achieve excellence, and human conceptions of the ends and goods involved, are systematically extended. (MacIntyre 1984, p. 187)

I quote this well-known definition not only because it offers a succinct statement of what a practice is but primarily because of its reference to implicit notions of appropriateness. These notions are similar to what I referred to above when I spoke about "glimpses of implicit normativity" and of "a sense of appropriateness, of proportionality, and of holism." The reference to inherent norms appeals to normative intuitions, most of all a sense of what is appropriate in a given case. The question is, of course, whether we can trust this sense of appropriateness. How much common ground do we have? How far does the appeal of our intuitions reach? And how much weight can they bear in terms of content? More about this later. For now, it is sufficient to note that MacIntyre's definition connects goods (norms) with the definition of a practice, and it connects dispositions (virtues) with human conceptions of the end (or *telos*) of a practice. The definition recognizes, moreover, that the realization of the excellence of a practice takes time. I will return to MacIntyre in Chapter 8.

6.1.3 Requirements for a normative practice approach

Let us now turn to the requirements for the approach of normative practices we envision. It is clear by now that the analysis of psychiatry as a normative practice should result in more than a list of desiderata or a professional code. The analysis should ideally deliver a coherent view on psychiatry, a view that gives a proper justification of the psychiatrist's job, for instance, by providing a coherent account of the role of (scientific) knowledge in clinical knowing (i.e., an account that avoids both absolutizing and relativizing of the role of scientific knowledge). The approach should outline a plausible view on the various responsibilities of psychiatrists and how these responsibilities relate to those of other stakeholders. It should also provide a perspective on how micro-, meso-, and macro-contexts of professionalism intersect.

Some readers might be inclined to interpret the normative practice approach as an answer to a cry for "more ethics." This cry has been heard in medical circles for a long time. What we require from the normative practice approach is more specific, however. The model should provide an organizing idea, a principle, or set of principles or ideas to get a grasp on the bewildering multitude of normative issues, contexts, insights, and points of view with respect to psychiatry as a profession. What psychiatry needs is not only recognition of the significance of normative analysis but also and more specifically recognition of the importance of a coherent account of how the different normative aspects and points of view cohere. What is needed is insight into the normative structure of psychiatric practice. This insight should be sufficiently deep by showing how professional competence is anchored in existential and moral attitudes (i.e., in the ethos of the profession). Competence should no longer be one-sidedly defined in terms of outcome and performance. Instead, it should be conceived of as an expression of inner conviction and dedication (Brint 2015; Hafferty 2006a; Levinson et al. 2014, Chapter 5; Sullivan 2004). The normative practice approach should do justice to the complexity of psychiatric practice, by paying attention to how different types of norm cohere and interact in the different (micro-, meso-, and macro-) social contexts of psychiatric practice. It should finally offer a convincing account of the role of scientific knowledge in psychiatric practice.

In short, the normative practice approach should:

- do justice to the differences and the coherence between types of norms that shape professional practices
- properly locate and define the role of expert knowledge and skills amid the many different roles and responsibilities doctors and patients have
- avoid both scientistic absolutizing and critical relativizing of professional knowledge
- give a coherent and plausible outline of norms, duties, and responsibilities other than the epistemic ones
- give a social and moral justification of the professional role
- bear relevance for other than merely the micro-context of individual caregiver and caretakers
- provide a convincing approach to solve the legitimacy crisis in (mental) healthcare and, in general, the public's distrust of professionalism.

6.2 A normative practice approach for psychiatry

6.2.1 Background of the approach

The normative practice approach (NPA) as it will be presented here was initially developed by Jochemsen, Hoogland, and this author for medical practice in general (Glas 2019; Jochemsen 2006; Jochemsen & Glas 1997). The approach has also been applied in the fields of education (Hegeman et al. 2011), developmental studies, journalism (van der Stoep 2011), and healthcare economics (Polder et al. 1997) (for an overview, see De Muynck et al. 2011).

The approach was born as a result of reflection on four issues. Three of these issues have already been addressed in previous chapters. The fourth issue has so far not been discussed, so I mention it, but I will postpone its full explanation until the next chapter.

The *first* and most general consideration found its origin in the unease with principlist approaches in medical ethics, philosophy, and theology, which pre-suppose that moral deliberation should be conceived as a form of reflection by which general moral principles are applied to individual cases. One problem of this approach has become known as the manipulability worry (Alexander & Moore 2016; MacIntyre 1967, p. 198). General moral rules and principles are simply too general to be applicable unambiguously and straightforwardly. An analogy can be drawn between the application of moral rules and the application of scientific insights. There are strong arguments to deny that clinical knowledge consists of the application of general scientific knowledge to individual cases. There are, analogically, equally strong reasons to deny that moral deliberation consists of the application of general moral rules and principles to the problems of individuals. The application approach sees clinical diagnostic reasoning as a form of subsumption: Individual problems are subsumed under general categories. We called the application approach therefore the subsumption view (subsume = to include under a more general heading or category) (see also Gremmen 1993).

The subsumption view disregards fundamental differences between types of reasoning. The clinician is not aiming at the confirmation of general knowledge, neither is the practical ethicist interested in establishing the truth of moral theories. The clinician is primarily interested in solving a specific problem of this individual patient. Likewise, the ethicist—in his or her role as counselor—is first and foremost interested in helping this person with his or her specific moral problem. Science aims at the discovery of lawful generalizations, whereas clinical practice focuses on individual cases. Ethics as a philosophical discipline is interested in moral theory (aiming at general relations), whereas the counselor focuses on the peculiarities of the individual case.

The subsumption view not only disregards epistemic differences between theory and clinical practice but also overlooks the strong interdependence between practices and knowledge. How knowledge is used in clinical contexts depends on specific features of the case and on the context. This holds also for ethics. The crucial conceptual point is that the method of applying itself is highly informed by case-based estimates of context-related factors. What a particular theory—whether pathophysiological or moral—says in concrete situations depends not only on the theory itself, or on some meta-theory, but also on specific features of the situation. The application of general points of view requires, in other words, a special capacity, indicated with terms like insight, wisdom, and sense of proportionality. This capacity is not based on theory (scientific or moral); it is a second-order type of competence. It is an ability to weigh the evidence and determine its relevance for the explanation of a specific phenomenon. This capacity has been associated with the Aristotelian notion of *phronèsis*, both in medical ethics and in the literature on clinical knowledge (*Ethica Nicomachea* 1106b36–1107a2, 1140a24 ff). *Phronèsis* means literally practical (or moral) wisdom, prudence, the ability to find the mean between two extremes. This meaning is not a numerical, spatial, or logical category but a practical one. It is an experience-based capacity to adapt general insights to specific situations. It is the ability to estimate the appropriateness of a certain action. Aristotle mentions courage as an example: The same behavior is courageous in one situation and reckless in another. *Phronèsis* is an important notion in Gadamer's conception of philosophical hermeneutics, which, in turn, has gained some influence in the hermeneutical approach to clinical knowledge (Gadamer 1960, pp. 297–307).

The *second* issue is in fact an extension of the first: norms (or goods) are not abstract and general principles, far removed from everyday practices. They are, instead, embedded within these practices. Fundamental for the NPA is the idea that normativity is inherent to professional practices. Medical practice does not become ethical because of the application of ethical principles to that practice. It is ethical because of its inherent normativity. This normativity is not an add-on; it is no arbitrary addition to a practice that is conceived of as neutral by itself. It is precisely the opposite: It is because of norms that practices exist. Norms belong to the very heart of the medical profession; without them, the profession would not be what it is. This was, in fact, one of the messages of the overview of sociological literature on professionalism in the previous chapter.

Brought back to its most elementary form, the practice of medicine consists of the meeting between two individuals, one with an illness and the other with expert knowledge and skills with respect to the illness and its treatment. The key conceptual question behind the normative practice approach is the following: Is it possible to spell out the norms that hold for and are inherent to this relationship? This question is especially important for the identification of what it is that qualifies the doctor–patient relationship. What is it that qualifies the doctor as a doctor and the patient as a patient? Of course, the doctor–patient dyad is part of more extensive relational networks. The organization of (mental) healthcare has become so intricate that there are many other normative relationships that bear relevance for the interaction between doctor and patient. But we begin by focusing on the most elementary forms of medical practice: doctors and nurses who take care of patients and ask what it is that qualifies their relationships with patients.

A *third* consideration finds its origin in the rediscovery of the Aristotelan–Thomist account of virtues and the substantive view on practices that came in its wake. Virtue ethics holds the view that practices, like the practice of professionalism, by themselves embody certain goods. These goods are thus intrinsic; they belong to the heart of the practice and function as *sine qua non*. Without their realization, the practice would no longer be the practice it is supposed to be. We discuss the theoretical contribution of virtue ethics to the development of the normative practice approach more extensively in chapter 8.

The *fourth* consideration was based on recognition of the relevance of the work of the Dutch philosopher Herman Dooyeweerd (Chaplin 2011; Dooyeweerd 1953–1958, Volume III). In Dooyeweerd's social philosophy, one finds many examples of the type of analysis of social practices we envisioned for medicine. Dooyeweerd develops a systematic philosophical framework that gives an account of how different types of norm and principle are related and cohere within the functioning of institutions and practices, such as the state, the family, churches, industrial companies, and volunteer associations. Apart from this "constitutive" side of social practices, he also discerns a "direction" or directedness in the process of "opening up" or "disclosure" of practices.

Professional and other practices not only have a structure (the constitutive side); they also develop in a certain direction. This directedness can be conceptualized in terms of concrete targets or objectives, but it also entails and represents a broader, regulative dimension. Virtue ethicists call this regulative dimension "telos." The telos is the overarching purpose of a practice; it indicates its internal destination. Dooyeweerd himself would hesitate about the term *telos*. He would consider it as too much bound to a natural law approach to practices and to a metaphysics of substances with their necessary inner teleology. Dooyeweerd and the virtue ethicists concur, however, that practices are determined, both in their existence and in their development, by an internal destination.

Dooyeweerd puts much emphasis on the crucial role of cultural development in the emergence and growth of scientific, technological, and other practices. His concept of opening up of practices—under the influence of cultural shifts, new scientific insights, technological progress, or changing worldviews—acknowledges the dynamic and adaptive nature of developing social practices. It is by developing in a direction that conforms with their inner destination that practices flourish and express their purpose and richness. This purposiveness is not some abstract ideal; it is anchored in the structure of a practice (i.e., its constitutive side). It is also embodied in the ethos of the participants in that practice.

6.2.2 An outline of the normative practice approach

Diagram 6.1 gives an outline of the most essential components of the NPA. The approach is meant to serve as a heuristic conceptual framework for discussions on the work floor. It is not a blueprint, neither does it describe the essence of psychiatric practice. The approach provides an ideal typical description. It does not so much prescribe how to look at psychiatry as invite one to adopt the point of view the approach proposes and investigate whether this elucidates and solves the problems we have discussed so far.

The diagram contains two boxes: one listing different types of rule and one indicating a regulative dimension. What stands out initially is the distinction between constitutive rules and a regulative direction. In this subsection, I discuss this distinction; the next subsection is then devoted to how they interrelate.

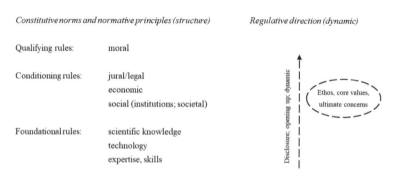

Psychiatry as normative practice

Constitutive norms and normative principles (structure)   *Regulative direction (dynamic)*

Qualifying rules:	moral
Conditioning rules:	jural/legal
	economic
	social (institutions; societal)
Foundational rules:	scientific knowledge
	technology
	expertise, skills

Disclosure; opening up; dynamic

Ethos, core values, ultimate concerns

DIAGRAM 6.1 Psychiatry as normative practice

I call constitutive those aspects or dimensions of professional practices without which there cannot be such a thing as a professional practice. Constitutive rules or principles define psychiatry as the practice it is. To use the well-known analogy with chess, the rules for chess playing define which moves are allowed and which are not. These rules constitute chess as the game it is. If the player performs a move that is not allowed according to the rules of the game, the player is not playing chess differently; he or she is not playing chess *at all*. It is only possible to play chess on the basis of and within the confines of its rules. This also holds for the rules and principles that are constitutive for practices, in our case, the practice of psychiatry.

With respect to rules, often a distinction is made between knowing that and knowing how. The rules that hold for the practice of psychiatry refer to both. Among them are rules with a clearly prescriptive meaning ("do not harm," for instance), but there are also rules that refer to implicit capacities. Based on these capacities, we know how to do things. Principles are foundations that form the basis of a practice and at the same time serve as integrating normative ideals or maxims that guide practices. The principle of beneficence is a well-known example: It is the basis and foundation for all helping relationships in medicine and functions at the same time as an integrative norm and ideal that guides professionals when they are dealing with ambiguous or otherwise difficult situations.

The other box refers to the regulative dimension of psychiatric practice. Regulative means in this context that practices are determined by their inner, intrinsic directedness, which—ideally—is reflected by the commitment, motivation, and dedication of those who execute and shape such practices. Regulative ideals provide a general idea about the inner destination of a practice. These ideals are embodied in the motivation and dedication of practitioners. This motivation and dedication can be conceptualized in terms of ultimate concerns, core values, or meaningfulness.

The regulative ideal or purpose of a practice is not some distant or abstract goal that stands apart from that practice. It is, instead, the perfect realization (or excellence) of that practice. The regulative dimension of a normative practice embodies the attitudes, motivations, and ideals in virtue of which the practice becomes the practice it is meant to be. We will elaborate later on the expression "it is meant to be." For now, it suffices to see that the purposiveness of a practice is embodied by the practice itself, as a fundamental motivation, commitment, or ethos that helps psychiatrists and other stakeholders fulfill their proper roles.

I will add a few words about the term "regulative." Many readers will associate this term with Immanuel Kant, who ascribed a regulative role to what he referred to as "transcendental ideas." These ideas regulate theoretical thinking and guide it to a dimension of understanding beyond what can be known by the senses and by logic, the dimension of the *Ding-an-sich*, which is unknowable in itself. In my use of the term regulative, the term refers to practices instead of to knowledge. It has more to do with the ethos of practices themselves than with what is beyond them. By ethos I mean the sum of a practice's most fundamental motivations, attitudes, and guiding ideas. The regulative side of practices refers to their dynamic, to the way they evolve over time, to their tendency to integrate or disintegrate, to develop into one direction or into another, to flourish or to fall into decay. The analogy between the transcendental and the practical use of the term is that both refer to the guiding role of a more fundamental dimension. But unlike Kant, I use the term "regulative" in an affective, motivational, moral, and spiritual, instead of transcendental, sense. The term "ethos" comes close to what is meant here. It is what the Greeks meant by character. It is the spirit that motivates the fundamental attitudes, ideas, and values of a practice. Dooyeweerd used the term ground motive for similarly deep and motivating driving forces in the cultural history of our civilization.

Diagram 6.1 outlines three types of such constitutive rule: qualifying rules, conditioning rules, and foundational rules (or principles). These three types of rule or principle refer to different roles of the rules and principles in the normative structure of a practice. There are rules and principles that qualify psychiatry (and medicine) as a professional practice. There are rules and principles that function as conditions or as conditioning factors for professional practice. And there are rules and principles that function as a foundation for professional practice. These different types of constitutive norm hold simultaneously.

6.2.3 How do the constitutive and the regulative sides of a practice work together?

The most difficult aspect of the NPA is imagining how the constitutive and regulative sides of psychiatric practice work together. Neither can exist without the other, and thus the schematic presentation in Diagram 6.1 is off the mark because it essentially locks the two sides into two separate boxes. In reality, however, the constitutive side is opened up under the guidance of regulative notions (ideas and overarching values), whereas the regulative side can only be brought to life via the existence and holding of different sorts of constitutive principles and norms.

One can simplify the image still somewhat and call the entire constitutive side of a practice "structure" and the regulative side "direction." The question then becomes how structure and direction interact. The easiest way to understand the interplay between structural features and the direction of a practice is to focus on the historical development of a practice. Practices evolve over time and develop into a direction that corresponds with or deviates from their destination. Practices may flourish or fall into decay. Their directedness may be conceived of as a kind of dynamic that pervades the practice as a whole. This still may sound a bit vague, and, indeed, it remains vague if one thinks of this dynamic as if it were a component or aspect or otherwise objectifiable element of a practice. The dynamic I am aiming at is more fundamental, however. It precedes every form of objectifying or purposeful action. It is that which gives perspective and meaning to one's practice, not as a mission statement or ideology, but in a more embodied and embedded form. What precedes it is a set of attitudes, aspirations, and ideals driving a motivating force that operates from within.

Contexts again play an important in role in the way this dynamic unfolds. It is in the interplay between contexts and practices that certain aspects of a practice become more important than others. Small-scale practices are often part of larger networks with their own dynamic. One of the advantages of the term dynamic is that it allows us to see practices as subject to heterogeneous dynamic forces. This corresponds with the experience that practices are usually somewhat mixed and that participation in a practice often leads to a certain measure of ambivalence. It is not uncommon for practices to fall under the influence of more than one dynamic. Different motives guide them in different directions, and this may lead to ambivalence, alienation, and conflict.

We have analyzed several such ambivalences and conflicts in the previous chapters. We saw, for instance, the deep divide between the patient movement and the medical establishment that arose in the 1960s. Patients longed for autonomy and struggled against the paternalism of doctors, who in the name of science claimed to know what was best for them. The collision was the expression of an opposition—or as Dooyeweerd would call it, "dialectical antithesis"—within the ground motive of medicine. This opposition consisted of the inner contradiction between a technology-driven desire for control (by doctors) and a longing for freedom and autonomy by patients. We saw how medical professionalism itself more recently has come under the spell of managerialism, i.e., the urge to keep medical practice under control, not only economically, but also in terms of efficiency, accountability, and transparency. At the basis of this managerialism lies the almost uncontrollable growth of medicine and its lack of self-regulation—economically and qua expansion of technology—as well as the distrust of the public about whether the sector really puts all its efforts into the service of others instead of into its own interests. We have discussed these tensions and analyzed the irony of bureaucratic control. The massive increase of control—administrative, economic, and in terms of accountability, patient safety, and access of care—paradoxically led to an increase in discomfort and distrust, both in the service user, who is confronted with an increasingly complex system of care, and in the professional, who feels more and more alienated from his or her proper role.

With the help of the normative practice approach, we can understand these tensions as the product of interactions between structure and direction, i.e., between anomalies in the interpretation and development of the structural side of medical practice and ambiguities and contradictions in the motives guiding those who take part in medical practice. Tensions in the basic motives of medical practice may lead to overemphasis on one type of norm and end in unsurmountable disharmony and conflict. The unbounded urge for technocratic control (as a ground motive or direction), for instance, may lead to one-sided emphasis on the foundational side of medicine, that is, on science, technology, and professional specialization as prerequisites for technocratic control. This urge may subsequently jeopardize norms that qualify medical practice, for instance the norm of beneficence. What is good for the patient does not necessarily coincide with what is possible technologically.

Structure and directedness always interact and cannot be analyzed apart from one another. In the analysis, one can begin at either side. One can start with an analysis of the structure of practice and argue toward underlying tensions in the direction. Or one can begin, like we did above, with the identification of an underlying tension within medicine's ground motive(s) and then reconstruct how this tension affects the opening up of the structural side of a practice, the constellation of its constitutive norms.

6.2.4 Two examples

Let us move now to mental healthcare and briefly review two examples of the interaction between "structure" and "direction," the first starting off with a structural analysis and the other with a tension in the fundamental motivations for psychiatric professionalism.

An example of the first approach is given in the analysis of the managerialism that is so prominently present in today's mental healthcare in some Western countries and that I have begun to analyze at the end of the previous chapter (5.4). Managerialism can be interpreted as the consequence of a distorted view on the structure of psychiatric practice, a view which is determined by a role reversal between conditioning and qualifying norms. The conditioning, economic norm of efficiency is dealt with as if it were a qualifying norm. This role reversal leads, for instance, to a different definition of professionalism. In healthcare systems in which efficiency norms prevail above other values, a good doctor is an efficient doctor, not primarily a caring doctor. Efficiency, instead of beneficence, becomes the overarching and qualifying norm for a sound and sustainable practice. Of course, advocates of efficiency in medicine claim that there need be no contradiction between efficiency and caring for suffering people; indeed, they argue that these aims are complementary. But that is not the issue. The issue is the specific role that is ascribed to the norm of efficiency and the place it takes in the hierarchy of values of medical practice. Efficiency is no longer an auxiliary quality, together with the other necessary conditions for healthcare as a practice. It becomes the most defining (or qualifying) characteristic of good practice, with, as we have seen in the previous chapter, deleterious effects on the ethos of medical professionalism (see also Tallis 2004). Managerialism is an example of a distorted view of the structure of mental healthcare. This view has a strong, eroding effect on the ethos of psychiatrists and other mental healthcare workers. It ultimately leads to antinomies in the direction of psychiatric practice.

Analyses of how the spirit of scientism affects the practice of psychiatry offer an example of the other way of analyzing the structure - direction interaction. Here it is the dynamic that is brought about by fundamental convictions that makes role reversal between structural norms understandable. One example of a fundamental conviction is scientism, the belief that it is science and science alone that leads humanity to true knowledge. One variant of this spirit of scientism can be found in some branches of neuroscience and neuroscientifically informed psychiatry. It is a

way of conceiving and interpreting that may be indicated with terms like neuroessentialism (O'Connor et al. 2012; see also Farah 2012) or neurocentrism (Satel
& Lilienfeld 2013). Neuroessentialism means that the essence of what can be said
about human behavior, whether pathological or not, can be found in the brain.
Neurocentrism means that in explanations of behavior, brain mechanisms are central. This one-sided highlighting of the brain and of brain mechanisms leads to
negligence of the importance of psychological explanations and of the role of the
environment in the genesis of abnormal behavior. The patient is seen as the
extension of a brain problem, instead of the other way around.

The consequences for the practice of mental healthcare are potentially large.
Neuroessentialism not only implies one-sided emphasis on the foundational (i.e.,
scientific and technical) side of psychiatric practice—and this moreover in a restricted,
biological sense—at the expense of its moral, juridical, social, and economic aspects.
It also inevitably leads to changes in the governance of mental healthcare facilities
and in the distribution of financial and other resources. On the basis of a neu-
roessentialist view of mental problems, it could be argued, for instance, that patients
should receive care only insofar as their problem can be translated into a brain problem. If not, their problem falls outside the scope of psychiatry because it is merely a
problem of living. One-sided emphasis on the foundational aspect of psychiatric
practice has consequences for the definition of disease and, consequently, for the
boundaries of the profession. This might imply exclusion from care of all those who
are ill without evident brain dysfunction.

The NPA acknowledges the important role of knowledge of the brain and of
techniques that influence brain functioning. Both are necessary for, even foundational to, the understanding and treatment of psychiatric patients. However, they
don't qualify what psychiatrists do. Psychiatrists, like other physicians, are called to
heal and to provide comfort to patients and their families. The NPA does not deny
that science plays a role in the demarcation of the boundaries of the profession, but it
emphasizes the role of other—moral, legal, and practical—points of view as well.
Deciding about the boundaries of the profession is a collaborative endeavor; it
requires the voices of all stakeholders, not only the voice of science; it admits that the
answers will be different, depending on the nature and complexity of the context;
and it insists that the ultimate destination of psychiatry, like all of medicine, is a
moral one. This is the topic of the next subsection.

6.2.5 Qualifying norms and principles

The term "qualifying" refers to those aspects, modes of functioning, or functions of
psychiatric practice that give this practice its own, distinctive quality. The term
aspect, or mode, is an abstract expression for a particular way of functioning
(operating, working, or fulfilling a role) of a thing, event, or activity.

For instance, one can say that one of the modes of functioning of a tree is the biotic
(or biological) mode. The tree is a biotic subject. Trees, when they are alive and
growing, have this biotic quality in and of themselves. By human interference, trees

may also acquire other qualities, for instance, economic or aesthetic qualities. This is the case when they are sold (economic) or put in an ornamental garden (aesthetic). They then function as economic and aesthetic objects, respectively. Qualifying modes or aspects are those aspects (modes of functioning) that qualify the thing (event, activity) as the kind of thing (event, activity) it is. The sentence: "Trees are qualified by their biotic aspect" means only that trees are the kind of things we identify by their biotic qualities (i.e., that they are alive and grow). A tree can also be qualified by the economic or the aesthetic aspect. These aspects qualify, characterize, or determine the tree as merchandise and as an aesthetic object. Merchandise is a kind of thing we identify as economical. Aesthetic objects are the kinds of thing we identify with aesthetical principles. Aspects or modes determine an entity, event, or act. Determination means in this context that the entity "obeys" or behaves in accordance with the laws or lawful norms or principles for that particular mode (i.e., biotic laws or economic or aesthetic norms and normative principles, respectively). I will say more about the background and meaning of the concept of mode (mode of functioning, aspect, or modal aspect) in Chapter 8.

As has been said earlier, we are primarily interested in norms, rules, and principles that are intrinsic. The question we focus on now is which norms, rules, and principles are intrinsic to the practice of mental healthcare, and, more specifically, what the subset of qualifying norms looks like. In my answer, I take the physician (or nurse)–patient relationship as a paradigm case. This is not undisputed, given the advanced stage of the division of labor in medicine and the dominant role of organizations. However, given the analysis of professionalism in the previous chapter, it still seems reasonable to take the individual relationship as a starting point. I see the default position of medical professionalism as existing in the relationship between a person who offers help to another person who suffers from an illness. The helping person is legitimized to use his or her knowledge and skills to that end. I see the role of other, allied professionals as codetermined by this ground situation. As we have seen in the previous chapter, the professional relationship is determined by expert knowledge and skills and sustained by a social contract that presupposes certain moral obligations. These obligations require a form of character formation and, ideally, lead to virtues such as beneficence, unselfishness, dedication, and commitment.

On a deeper level, the obligations and virtues are an answer to a fundamental drive to solidarity with others. The helper helps because he or she recognizes that under different circumstances, it could have been him or her who is sick and needs help. This fundamental reality is not different for allied professions, including nursing or psychotherapy. This solidarity is, of course, not permanently felt. At the basis of the professional relationship is not feeling, but the social contract, which, in turn, should be seen as the collective answer to a fundamental reality, i.e., the reality of the contingency of our existence, physically, emotionally, and socially. We are all in the same position; something wrong and beyond our control might happen to each of us. Physicians from Hippocrates to well into the 21st century (cf. the *Physician's Charter*) have recognized this and have indicated that beneficence and benevolence belong to the key virtues that qualify the interaction between the doctor (or nurse) and the patient. Both terms have a primarily moral meaning. It is for this reason that I think the moral aspect or mode of functioning should be identified as the one that qualifies medical (psychiatric) practice. Medicine and psychiatry deserve their moral status because the patient–physician (nurse) relationship is characterized by a distinctively moral kind of dedication (i.e., by benevolence and beneficence, by the drive of doing good to the patient).

Of course, there are specialties in medicine in which the technology so much interferes with normal communication that it sounds a bit improper to speak of a doctor–patient relationship. And, of course, the experience of being ill has significantly changed. Laypeople know much more. The level of technological sophistication has strongly increased. The modern patient is proto-professionalized. Medical knowledge and expectations about what medicine can bring about influence how we view our bodies and minds. We seem much less vulnerable than previous generations with respect to what can happen to our bodies and minds.

Nevertheless, I think that all these changes have not fundamentally altered the medical ground situation, one in which the sick individual has become dependent and is seeking help from someone who has the qualifications and the jurisdiction to do so. Illnesses still disturb our lives. We still suffer from conditions we haven't chosen and that limit our opportunities. We, as patients, still entrust ourselves to physicians because of their status as experts and because of their professional morale, which prevents their activities from being determined by self-interest instead of our well-being. I see, in short, the professional relationship as a fundamentally moral relationship, and I am inclined to adopt this view also with respect to non-medics, such as technicians and administrators. These professions too refer to—and ultimately find their basis in— the medical ground situation. It is the moral core of the medical relationship that qualifies the (medical) professional relationship.

The qualifying aspect of professional practices is sometimes called the leading aspect, indicating that among the different properties, aspects, or modes of functioning of a practice, the qualifying aspect fulfills a leading role. The term leading implies that other aspects or modes of functioning ideally open up to this aspect. They should, in other words, function such that they optimally support and sustain the practice in its ultimately moral meaning.

The relationship between the different types of norm is reciprocal, intrinsic, and determined by their specific roles in a practice. The opening up of the foundational and conditioning norms occurs under the guidance of qualifying properties (i.e., the qualifying aspect or mode of functioning). This guidance can best be seen as a form of enrichment and specification of the guided modes of functioning by the leading function. Dooyeweerd speaks of anticipation of lower functions on the higher (moral) mode of functioning.

Here is an example of this enrichment and specification: Over the ages, the legal principle of justice has differentiated from an egalitarian intuition into a more refined and deepened sense of duty. If medicine were based on egalitarian principles, people would simply get back what they invest in healthcare as a collective service. However, medicine is based on a more nuanced view of justice, informed by principles such as solidarity and benevolence. According to this more specific and richer view, some weak and sick people deserve solidarity in the form of medical care, even if they are never able to pay for the benefits granted to them. The (higher) moral mode of functioning enriches and specifies the juridical mode of functioning within medical practice.

With respect to the core of these modes of functioning, especially the moral one, there has been some discussion about characteristic features, both in general and in relation to medicine and psychiatry. Dooyeweerd saw love as the core of the moral mode of functioning. He carefully distinguishes the moral sphere of existence from the sphere of religion, the sphere of justice (law), and the sphere of feeling (psychology) (NC II, pp. 140–163). Love in a moral sense is associated with altruism, care, self-acceptance, and recognition (of the other), not with romantic love (psychology), or with religious self-surrender. Puolimatka (1989) prefers the term benevolence above the term beneficence for the moral mode of human functioning. Benevolence refers to the sphere of volition and beneficence to making and doing. For him, the first seems more appropriate than the latter as a qualification of what it is to behave morally. Dooyeweerd would have problems with this suggestion, however. He thinks that the will (i.e., willing the good) is too unspecified to shed light on the proper sense of the moral sphere. There are many goods, but not all of them are moral. Others have put emphasis on care as central qualifying principle of healthcare (Cusveller 2004). The problem with the term care, however, is also that it also has so many meanings. Care may refer to a psychological disposition ("this is a caring person"), to activities ("he is caring for …"), to taking responsibility for someone ("I will take care of him"), but also to the practice of healthcare itself.

My take on the issue is that in the context of medicine, terms such as beneficence and benevolence are sufficiently specific to elucidate why medical practice is determined by a morally qualified relationship between caregivers and caretakers. It indicates that there is something irreducible in the functioning of professional relationships in the context of healthcare. This irreducible, altruistic element in healthcare relationships does not function on its own, however. It is part of a whole range of other, equally irreducible elements, properties, aspects, and modes of functioning. These other elements support, color, and codetermine the medical-professional relationship as a moral relationship. One may compare this with the facets of a crystal. Professional relationships can be moral because of the role of all different aspects, for instance legal, social, and psychological aspects. In order to behave morally appropriately, a sufficiently stable and specific legal context is required. Institutions, hospitals, and professional organizations should function properly. Stakeholders (including local government, patient representatives, insurance companies, the pharmaceutical industry) should cooperate in a constructive way. Professionals need to possess certain psychological qualities, such as empathy.

Their altruism presupposes a sense of proportion and of justice, which refers to the economic and legal aspects of healthcare, respectively. All these aspects are needed, irreducible, and co-constitutive for medical practice. In the way they intersect, they give medical practice a certain splendor, like the facets of a crystal. All facets are important, albeit in different ways and in different constellations. Similarly, it is in the interactions among all the different aspects of medical practice (psychological, social/institutional, economic, legal, and technical/scientific) that medicine as an ultimately moral endeavor is realized.

6.2.6 Foundational norms and principles

Let us now turn to what it means to say that medical practice has its foundation in science and in expert skills. Earlier, in subsection 6.2.3 and 6.2.4, I spoke about science and technology as foundations for mental healthcare. I referred to neuroessentialism and neurocentrism as examples of how one-sided motives (i.e., a spirit of scientism) may lead to a distorted view of the structure of mental healthcare (i.e., to absolutization of the foundational norms for the practice of psychiatry). The NPA resists role reversal between qualifying and foundational norms. The guiding role of certain moral principles should not be substituted by a view in which science and technology dictate what good practices are. Scientific knowledge and technology are crucial for modern healthcare, but only in a foundational and not in a qualifying sense.

But how exactly should we conceive this? What does it mean that science and technology represent the foundation of medical practice? Does it mean that the practice of mental healthcare and the practices of science and technology overlap, or that parts of science and technology are part of medicine? Well, in a certain sense, yes. The two do indeed overlap. Science and technology are also practices, and they partially overlap within the practice of mental healthcare. But this is not what is meant here. Throughout this book, I have described the clinical practice of psychiatry as a practice in its own right, not as merely the field of application of scientific insights, or solely as a blend of different practices. So, we are talking about those elements of science and technology that are factually present in the practice of mental healthcare: cognitive (or logical) artefacts in the form of (parts of) theories and hypotheses, derivatives of scientific knowledge in the form of treatment algorithms, technical devices and the practices of their use, and, indeed, elements of scientific practices, for instance in various forms of data collection.

What the NPA says is that this scientific and technical input is enormously important, but that it does not qualify medical practice and mental healthcare. The gathering of knowledge and the formulation of new hypotheses and ideas are a *sine qua non* for contemporary mental healthcare, but they are not ends in themselves and do not make psychiatric practice what it is. In short, they offer the foundation, but not the destination of psychiatry.

If we go one step further and adopt a modal point of view, as Dooyeweerd did in his analysis of the functioning of social practices, we must locate the role of science in the cognitive (or logical) sphere (or mode of functioning). Scientific insights come to expression in the logical-analytical ("cognitive") aspect of psychiatric practice. Theories function in professional practices as cognitive artefacts. These artefacts are "opened up" toward and point at the mode of functioning that qualifies a practice. Cognitive artefacts, such as theories and hypotheses, are thus molded so that they contribute to the optimal functioning of mental healthcare as a moral practice.

This ideally occurs in the formulation and application of guidelines, protocols, and treatment algorithms. Under ideal conditions, such guidelines are phrased such that they optimally contribute to the well-being of the patient, for instance, by specifying as precisely as possible the conditions of their application and/or by giving suggestions about how to discuss guideline-based treatment advice with the individual patient. How this occurs depends on how professional associations, scientific journals, and representatives of these associations in boards and committees frame the role of guidelines and protocols. Much depends on how diagnostic and treatment practices themselves develop. Some professionals conceive of the guidelines and protocols as blueprints; other professionals see them as recommendations. Local contexts determine to a large extent how guidelines and protocols are dealt with and spoken about. There emerges, in other words, a new practice: the practice of dealing with guidelines and protocols. This practice defines itself in relation to all kinds of practical, legal, professional, and ethical norm and standard.

This also holds for technology, which is more difficult to "locate" in the list of modal aspects or functions. Technical devices are, as such, physically qualified. However, they don't exist for themselves; it is their role to function in various practices in medicine, for instance, in diagnostic procedures (imaging techniques, radiology, EEG, laboratory measures) and in treatment (robotics). In such practices, these devices themselves acquire a function that is derived from and intrinsically related to the nature and qualitative distinctness of that particular practice. It is their function to make these practices possible and to open them up such that they can become beneficial for the larger practice of mental healthcare.

This is another way of saying that technology plays a formative role. The term "formative" combines the two elements just mentioned: the aspect of making a (sub-) practice possible and the aspect of opening up a new field of medical practice. In Dooyeweerd's systematics, these functions would be called "historical"; they are expected to function according to the proper role of the historical aspect. Dooyeweerd associates this proper role with the (legitimate) exertion of power. This power contributes to the differentiation and opening up of a field of human activity. The civilization process itself is one large historical process in the sense that it successively unleashes powers that over time lead to the successive opening up of new spheres of existence. Which fields are opened and how this occurs depends on the stage of the development of a certain civilization. Dooyeweerd argues, for instance, that the emergence of science as we know it never would have been possible in the ancient Greek world. The kind of openness that was characteristic of the late Renaissance and early Reformation view on reality—an openness that led to experiments and to the mathematization of physical relationships—was unthinkable in the scholastic world with its metaphysics of substances guided by their *causae formales* and *finales*. With respect to the formative role of technology, I am inclined to emphasize not only the role of power and control but also the importance of imagination and creativity. The opening up of new fields of practice and the innovative potential of new techniques and devices presupposes imagination, creativity, and the capacity to design.

I allow myself this digression to give an impression of how the Dooyeweerdian approach to the interaction between scientism, technology, and utopian longings can be conceptualized. The opening up of new fields of practice is not something neutral and detached. New developments and technical advances in medicine always raise expectations about the alleviation of suffering and pain and about control of hitherto uncontrollable realities like disease and decay. There is nothing wrong with this. Dooyeweerd's take on science and technology is not negative; on the contrary, he emphasizes the crucial role of technology in the development of Western culture.

However, technological advances often also unleash forces that amplify expectations. Advances hang in the air for some time, then suddenly—and often unpredictably—emerge. Such technological breakthroughs lead to a cascade of events. The history of medicine and psychiatry has seen several such serendipitous breakthroughs, including the discovery of antidepressants. These breakthroughs lead subsequently to an expansion of the field of applications (for instance, the use of antidepressants for anxiety disorders and bulimia nervosa). These expansions require more research. Pop-science in the meantime begins to glorify what is going on in the field, resulting in a renewed and sometimes impermissible heightening of expectations. This manipulation of expectations in turn may lead to the distorted and utopian atmosphere surrounding some new techniques and fields of science. This atmosphere is what was earlier referred to as the "dynamic" of a practice. This dynamic focuses the attention of scientists, clinicians, and policymakers on new technologies and innovations, thereby narrowing their focus and closing the circle of technology and (sometimes utopian) hopes. The expectations about psychopharmacology in the 1990s offer a good example of this cycle. New scientific findings led to increased hopes about the curability of mental disorder. This in turn brought about an immense increase in research efforts, with a very important market-driven component. All these developments together contributed to a narrowing of the clinical and research focus.

Scientism is therefore more than merely an interpretative frame; it is a power that has guided the field in a certain direction. It exerts a seductive appeal by narrowing the focus to what can be known by science and manipulated by technology. This appeal is exerted in many ways, today much less in the sphere of psychopharmacology and more by the suggestion of transparency in the way neuroscientific results are presented (in the form of images), by expectations about the role of big data and its promise of all-encompassing knowledge and control, and by the rise of genomics and its utopian promise to eradicate disease. Expectations feed longings, and these longings add to the credibility of scientistic assumptions—a credibility that is undeserved but no less practically effective.

It should be mentioned, however, that scientism indirectly made the profession also more aware of its moral basis. The counterforces against scientistic one-sidedness are many, as we saw in the previous chapters. And these counterforces have made many clinicians aware of the importance of a normative view on psychiatric practice. This is another way of saying that what qualifies normative practices like psychiatry is structurally given; it is a state of affairs that—ultimately—cannot be denied, in spite of suggestions to the contrary.

6.2.7 Conditioning norms and principles

Diagram 6.1 discerns three types of conditioning norm: social, economic, and legal. The term conditioning means "to function as a condition for; to fulfill a facilitating, enabling, and necessary role." Conditioning norms differ from qualifying norms in that they don't qualify the practice of (mental) healthcare as the practice it is. Psychiatrists and nurses should perform well in a social, economic, and/or legal sense, but their appropriate functioning in these spheres does not qualify them as psychiatrists or nurses. In other words, social, economic, and legal norms do not give the practice of psychiatry its typical moral meaning. Conditioning norms also differ from foundational norms in that professionals do not need to be experts in these spheres. The expert role is mandatory for what is foundational for medicine/psychiatry (i.e., medical knowledge and skills) but not for their functioning in social, economic, and legal contexts.

The recognition of conditioning norms and principles is initially based on common sense. Tensions in the practice of mental healthcare may help to uncover them, for instance when these tensions are caused by neglect or insufficient recognition of a principle, or by disproportional attention to one of them at the expense of others. If aspects are overlooked and not adequately dealt with, this will eventually lead to imbalances and stagnation in the development of a practice.

The norms and principles of the different aspects of psychiatric practice function simultaneously, whether they are qualifying, foundational, or conditioning. This idea is known as the principle of simultaneous norm realization. It was introduced by the Dutch economists T.P van der Kooy (1953) and, in his footsteps, B. Goudzwaard (1978, p. 65). The question is, of course, how to properly define the conditioning aspects.

Psychiatry as a discipline functions in *social* contexts, which include not only the micro-social context of the individual professional–patient relationship but also the meso- and macro-contexts of institutions and society at large, respectively. What is typical for the social sphere is interaction, relationship, belonging to, communality, respect, and etiquette. Social relationships build on the ability to communicate using language and signs. In Dooyeweerd's systematic philosophy, the lingual aspect therefore "precedes" the social aspect. There is also influence of "later" aspects on the social aspect, for instance influence of the legal and the moral aspect. Communal (social) experiences and interactions may acquire a legal component, for instance, when they should be safeguarded against improper exploitation and abuse. The sphere of social interaction ideally and ultimately finds its basis in trust and trustworthiness, which have a moral meaning. An example of a social relationship that is legally "deepened" and opened up is the relationships among residents in an apartment block who have signed a contract about the maintenance of the building. An example of a morally or even fiduciarily "deepened" relationship is that between friends.

Psychiatry also operates in *economic* frameworks. The economic point of view has become immensely important in current mental healthcare. It has its own lawfulness and inherent principles. In health economic accounts, efficiency is one of the defining key terms. The economic sphere is characterized by scarcity, i.e., the discrepancy between demand and supply and the need to make responsible choices given the limited amount of resources, time, and talents. Economic life is driven by the urge to achieve the maximum (or optimum) given the multiplicity of possibilities and the limited capacity to realize these possibilities (Hart 1984, p. 192). As this characterization suggests, the economic mode of functioning entails more than frugal and prudent management of financial resources. Functioning optimally in an economic sense involves responsibly dealing with virtually every form of scarcity. It is aiming to attain optimal value, not only financially but also in terms of other, softer values. In order to determine this optimal value, other normative principles must be taken into account. Goudzwaard (1978), a prominent Dutch economist who was influenced by Dooyeweerd's systematic philosophy, considers the notion of efficiency too shallow and asks for an opening up of the economic sphere via the regulative idea of stewardship. The focus of this approach is more on the fruit-bearing potential of economic activity for society as a whole than on maximization of financial profit for individual companies or entrepreneurs. This implies a different orientation for (mental) healthcare. Instead of one-sided emphasis on efficiency and economic survival of individual institutions, the economic aspect would include an invitation to maximize the total amount of a diverse series of values that are realized by the practice of mental healthcare.

Psychiatric practice also requires a *legal* framework, to regulate involuntary admission and treatment and to safeguard well-known rights such as informed consent, privacy, access to healthcare, and equal treatment. Characteristic of the legal aspect is the principle of justice. Justice is a complex concept. There is retributive justice, but also distributive and rectificatory justice. Dooyeweerd identifies retribution as the original meaning kernel of the juridical aspect of reality, but he immediately adds that the rigid and merciless nature of the primitive concept of retribution must be softened by the opening up of the judiciary sphere to other spheres. His account develops roughly along the lines that were sketched earlier in this chapter. Dooyeweerd suggests that in the process of opening up of the legal sphere, for instance, in its anticipation of the economic sphere, the rigid concept of retribution acquires the color of proportionality: one should give someone his or her fair share; maintaining a balance between individual interests and the interests of others. Later, in the anticipation of the juridical aspect of the moral sphere, justice acquires the connotation of support for those who cannot take care of themselves (NC II, pp. 129–140). The basis for this support lies in the intuition that, at the deepest possible level, humans are alike, whatever their social status and the evils they have done.

Most of the literature on justice in relation to healthcare is on the notion of distributive justice: the just allocation of scarce resources to those who need them most (for an overview, see Beauchamp & Childress 2013, Chapter 7, p. 249ff.). From the perspective outlined here, the concept of distributive justice refers to the economic underpinnings of acting according the principle of justice. It shows how morally informed legal notions guide the economic process of the fair distribution of resources. The topic of distributive justice is large and complex. The above may suffice to suggest that there is more to the legal aspect of healthcare than the processes and activities covered by the concept of distributive justice. In the opening up of the legal to the moral sphere other meanings of justice are going to resonate, such as society's duty to protect those who are weak and vulnerable and lack resources to defend themselves. These new meanings add an altruistic and asymmetric dimension to professional relationships in healthcare.

6.3 The normative practice approach and professionalism

It is time now for an example of how the NPA works in discussions about the current state of affairs in healthcare. I address two topics: the NPA in relation to professional codes (6.3.1) and the NPA in relation to the crisis in healthcare in general (6.3.2).

6.3.1 The NPA and professional codes: The Physician Charter

The NPA offers more than merely a professional code. Let me illustrate this with an example borrowed from the work of Pellegrino (2008, p. 157ff.), in which he discusses the statement on professionalism of the American Board of Internal Medicine (ABIM) Foundation, the American College of Physicians (ACP) Foundation, and the European Federation of Internal Medicine. This statement is titled *Medical Professionalism in the New Millennium: A Physician Charter* (2002). The Charter is a beautiful and succinct reaffirmation of the dedication of physicians to the principles of professionalism, with the explicit purpose of maintaining the "fidelity of medicine's social contract" in "turbulent times."

The statement begins with a preamble, which briefly addresses today's challenges: an explosion of technology, increasing influence of market forces, problems in healthcare delivery, bioterrorism, globalization, and wide variations in medical delivery and practice. It then refers to three fundamental principles: primacy of patient welfare, patient autonomy, and social justice (in fact, three of the four principles of Beauchamp and Childress). It then lists a set of professional responsibilities or commitments: a commitment to professional competence, to honesty, to confidentiality, to appropriate relationships with patients, to improvement of quality of care and access to care, to just distribution of finite resources, and a few others.

The general thrust of the Physician Charter is in line with our discussion earlier: The field of medicine needs a restoration of trust. Most of what the Charter says is about values intrinsic to healthcare. Every single one of these values, norms, and commitments is important enough to be highlighted and cherished. The Charter gives succinct suggestions and ideas.

However, the Charter is not a model; it does not offer a conceptual framework that puts the different norms and values into perspective. The reason for this is, first, that the intentions and normative criteria that are listed in the Charter lack inner coherence. They are presented as a set of desiderata for medical practice, not as a coherent perspective. What we are searching for in this book is a heuristic model of how the different norms and principles are related to one another. This model could then serve as a conceptual map that provides orientation in various discussions.

Another difference between codes such as the Charter and the NPA is that the Charter lacks deeper justification. One searches in vain for an underlying philosophy or worldview in the Charter. I admit that it would not be very realistic to expect this from such a declaration. My remark is not so much a critique of the Charter as it is a reminder that the profession needs more than a simple enumeration of norms, principles, and attitudes; it needs an overarching idea, some fundamental distinctions, and an analysis of how the different normative elements (or values) cohere. What is needed is a convincing story about how a normative practices type of analysis can provide medicine with the right ideas for its own moral and societal jurisdiction and justification.

The NPA addresses all these issues. It provides a coherent view of the different types of norm that play a role in (mental) healthcare, it gives a thorough and deep justification of the moral nature of medicine, it provides an answer to the crisis in trust in (mental) healthcare, and it specifies in detail how different types of norm interact among one another in the various contexts of (mental) healthcare.

6.3.2 The NPA and the crisis in mental healthcare

There appear be at least three sources of unease and tension about psychiatry:

1. The dynamic of increasing knowledge and technology, leading to a division of labor and a degree of specialization that makes patients feel lost in the system and that alienates professionals from their proper role.
2. The desire of the profession to keep control of its own dominion by emphasizing professional autonomy and the expert role and by redefining the professional domain, usually in more restricted biomedical terms.
3. The societal urge to keep the sector under control by requiring profitability, efficiency, and transparency.

Translated into the language of ground motives and the dynamic of practices, the above says that there is first the dynamic of modernization with its concomitant tendency to specialization and functionalism. This is expressed by point (1). There are, next, two counter-dynamics, one originating within the medical profession itself (2) and the other motivated by the desires and aims of other stakeholders (3).

Both reactions are mixed and have not been without inner contradiction. Medicine tried to remain faithful to its roots by restating its unselfish dedication to the patient, for instance in the Physician Charter. Psychiatrists did so, too. However, in their reactions to the unease among patients and in society, psychiatry has also shown signs of defensive selfishness. One example is the one-sided insistence on the expert role and on recognition of professional autonomy. This one-sidedness augments the decontextualization of the professional role and leads to a limitation of responsibilities to those that can be met on purely scientific and technical grounds. The relative neglect of non-epistemic and non-practical duties has proved to be insufficient to restore trust. Like other medical specialists, psychiatrists do not recognize that trust is based on more than fulfilment of one's expert role and a set of individual values. What is needed is a recognition of the full spectrum of norms and values, including those relevant to the social, economic, and legal aspects of the professional role.

My thesis is that the current crisis in mental healthcare can at least partially be explained by a relative neglect of the normative aspects of the professional role at the meso- and macro-levels. This neglect particularly pertains to conditioning norms and values. Psychiatrists have forgotten their role as health advocates and have paid too little attention to the broader societal implications of their functioning. I see this as one of the most important factors explaining why people still do not fully trust mental healthcare professionals.

The societal reactions have also been mixed and ambivalent. These reactions were meant to regain control and alleviate distrust, alienation, and disorientation in the complex system. However, the managerial countermeasures appeared to overlook their own side-effects in the form of a paradox of control. The measures aiming at control and re-establishment of trust often led to an increasingly defensive attitude among professionals and to a climate of suspicion among other stakeholders (i.e., patient groups, the government, supervisory bodies, and insurers).

There is, of course, no easy solution. What is needed is a change in the system of healthcare delivery. This change is not limited to what occurs in the consulting room, but should at least start there, too. Attuning to the patient not only means bringing into discussion what is known from a scientific perspective. It also means that other scenarios are discussed, patient scenarios especially, that the values that are represented by these scenarios are weighed, balanced, and made explicit. Shared decision making implies knowing, addressing, and challenging the fears, motivations, and ambivalences that steer the patient's predilections. In Chapters 7 and 9, I will discuss suggestions at the meso- and macro-level.

In summary, from the perspective of the NPA, the biomedical turn in the discussion about psychiatry's legitimacy has been more undermining than reinforcing because it one-sidedly sought the legitimacy of psychiatric practice in the foundational side of mental healthcare (science and technical skills). Overvaluation of this side easily led to underestimation of the importance of other aspects of the professional role, most notably empathic attunement to the interests and values that are at stake in everyday clinical decisions; and recognition of the societal role of the medical expert.

The societal response to the crisis of trust and the increasing volume of mental healthcare consisted of more control of the economic and social-institutional aspects of mental healthcare. We have seen how easily economic and institutional control led to managerialism and overemphasis on efficiency, at the expense of the qualifying moral aspect of mental healthcare. In terms of the NPA, managerialism consists of a role reversal between the conditioning and the qualifying norms: The efficiency norm takes the place of norms such as benevolence and beneficence. The balance is lost between the different normative aspects of mental healthcare, as became eminently clear in what I called the paradox of control. This paradox was a typical example of the suggestion made earlier: that imbalances, one-sidedness, and contradictions in the conception of a practice reveal what types of norm and value are relevant for that practice.

7

PSYCHIATRY IN CONTEXTS

7.1 Contexts, conceptions of professionalism, and the object of psychiatry

This chapter focuses on micro-, meso-, and macro-contexts of psychiatry and their relevance for discussions about the object and purpose of psychiatry. The NPA helps us keep an overview on the bewildering number of factors, developments, and ideals in current mental healthcare. The outcome of our analysis also bears relevance for the issue of the legitimacy of psychiatry.

I introduced this topic in the final part of Chapter 2. We saw there how the context of mental healthcare influences the profession's conception of the object of psychiatry, especially of the clinical approach to psychopathology. Later, I suggested that a stratification of contexts into three levels of interaction—individual, institutional, and societal—will help us make some further distinctions with respect to the object and purpose of psychiatry. I have suggested that each context produces its own conception of psychiatry's object and purpose.

In later chapters, another way of specifying contexts was introduced (i.e., in terms of types of conditioning norm and principle). In our exposition of the NPA, we saw how psychiatry should be viewed as a normative practice that is conditioned by social, economic, and legal norms, rules, and principles. These types of norm do not stand apart; they are, in fact, interlaced and function in conjunction with one another. What appeared to be needed was a careful analysis and assessment of their role in different healthcare practices. We discussed, for example, the legal aspect of the professional relationship and saw how this relationship is conditioned and made possible, but not qualified, by this aspect. Professional relationships undeniably have a juridical aspect. They are, for instance, based on a social contract that defines certain duties and grants certain jurisdictions. But this legal embedding does not stand on its own. It should, ideally, be opened up toward and deepened by the moral sphere, which is qualified by the aim of "doing good" and "taking care" of those who suffer and need help. This opening-up does not wipe out the typical legal/juridical aspect; it gives it a deeper meaning.

In this chapter, we further explore the interactions between contexts, conceptions of professionalism, and the object of psychiatry. Contexts co-constitute what professionals and professional groups are doing (i.e., what they see as the proper object of their care and how they define themselves in this caring role). This co-constituting can be split into the three levels of interaction just mentioned. On each of these levels of interaction, the NPA typology of norms and normative principles can be applied.

At the *individual* or *micro*-level, there is a wide variety of contextual factors with a potential impact on the how and what of psychiatry. The how refers to how psychiatrists and other stakeholders define their roles, and the what refers to the kinds of problem these professionals are dealing with. The object of psychiatry, what it considers to be its primary focus of attention, is, in fact, influenced via both the how and the what. Contextual factors have an immediate impact on the genesis and manifestation of disease and, thereby, on the object of mental healthcare (the what) (interaction A). But contexts also have an indirect and mediated impact. They codetermine how professions develop, how they define themselves, and how they are perceived by others (the how) (interaction B). These changing conceptions about the professional role influence the way patients communicate about their symptoms and signs (interaction C) (see Diagram 7.1).

At the *institutional* or *meso*-level, there is an interaction between psychopathology, professionalism, and the system of mental healthcare. With respect to the impact of institutional factors on conceptions of psychopathology (interaction A in Diagram 7.1), one may think of the role of labeling, the importance of medicalization and

Contexts, professional roles and the object of psychiatry

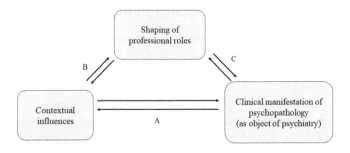

[A] Interactions between contextual factors and clinical manifestations of psychopathology
[B] Interactions between contextual factors and definitions of the professional role
[C] Interactions between professional roles and expression of psychopathology

DIAGRAM 7.1 Contexts, professional roles and the object of psychiatry

stigmatization, the induction of emotional and social dependence, the misattribution of common ailments as diseases, and recognition of the role of both the profession and mental healthcare institutions in addressing these issues (cf. Ikkos 2010). We can also focus, however, on institutional factors that bear relevance for conceptions of professionalism (interaction B in Diagram 7.1) and on the way clinical manifestations of psychopathology are influenced by changing conceptions about the professional role of psychiatrists (interaction C). I will propose a definition of the object (or purpose) of psychiatry from a meso-level or institutional perspective, which puts emphasis on meeting the *healthcare needs* of (future) patients and on the sustaining and improving of the *capabilities* of patients in a certain region (Daniels 1981).

Finally, at the *societal* or *macro*-level, there is an entire range of social and societal issues with an impact not only on how mental illness is expressed (interaction A) but also on how professions define themselves (interaction B) and on how changing conceptions of professionalism and of psychopathology interact (interaction C). Issues that are relevant in this context are loneliness and lack of social cohesion, social fragmentation, lack of social support, spiritual emptiness, and unresolved existential issues. These are issues with an impact not only on the expression and definition of mental illness (A), but also (indirectly) on the self-definition of professionalism (B) and what professions see as the object of their endeavors (C). It is in the interaction between society and mental healthcare as an institutional practice that the object of psychiatry appears in a new light. The emphasis now shifts from capacities and needs to distributive justice, i.e., to society's responsibility to provide access to care that meets standards that are sufficiently high—standards that evolve from a discussion between all relevant stakeholders (Daniels 1981; 2001). We will again see how normativity seems to be the forgotten dimension in the renewed negotiations about the social contract between medicine and society (Wynia et al. 1999). The chapter concludes by paying attention to service users, their experiences, and their role as patient experts. Whatever the outcome of the new healthcare arrangements, any future redefinition of professionalism should consider civic partnership as an inherent element of it.

7.2 The micro-level: The individual professional–patient relationship

There is a wide variety of potential contextual influences on the genesis and manifestation of symptoms of mental disorder and on the ability of the patient to cope with his or symptoms. Unemployment, lack of social support, trauma, bad socioeconomic circumstances, separation, stigma, discrimination, undernutrition, infectious disease early in life, and pre- and perinatal complications belong to the most important environmental factors with an impact on the genesis of mental disorder (Lewis et al. 2011).

The aim of this subsection is not so much to give a detailed overview of all these factors but to add to a conceptual understanding of the kind of influences we are dealing with. I first discuss the kinds of influence and then discuss the factors that determine those behaviors that count as specimens of disorder. In the final subsection, I focus more specifically on contextual factors, insofar as they are relevant for professional responsibility.

7.2.1 Contextual influences on the manifestation of psychopathology

Some distinctions may be helpful with respect to the first issue: kinds of influence. Let us briefly review the environmental factors just mentioned and categorize them in terms of modal kinds or types. Undernutrition, infectious disease, and pre- and perinatal complications are predominantly biological factors. Trauma, separation, and loss are psychological factors. Social support is socially qualified and unemployment economic qualified. Stigma and discrimination are a mixed bag; they consist of interactions with a social-psychological, legal, political, and/or moral meaning. All these factors have an impact on their own level: biological factors on the biotic mode of functioning, psychological factors on the psychic mode, and so on. However, as is well-known to clinicians, this point of entrance does not necessarily determine the mode of expression of the disorder. The initial biological disturbance may clinically come to expression in one's psychological functioning, for instance. Prenatal infections (biological) may come to expression in irritability and difficulties in concentration and learning (psychological). Adding to the complexity is the fact that contextual factors don't operate on their own but are mediated, balanced, and molded by other influences: coping mechanisms, personality strengths and weaknesses, social support, and core convictions. Some of these factors may have lasting effects on symptom formation; others have only temporary impacts. Contexts have also differential effects on how patients relate to their being ill (see Diagram 2.1). Contextual factors may have hardly any influence on the manifestation of illness (relation 1) but much influence on how patients deal with their illness (relation 2) or how they perceive their ability to cope with the illness (relation 5). These perceptions and expectations exert an indirect influence on the manifestation of psychopathology.

7.2.2 Contextual influences on what counts as psychopathology

With respect to the second issue—factors that determine which behavior counts as disordered—we must pay attention to the dynamic nature of interactions between the patient, the disorder, and the context. Instead of giving a general and abstract explanation, let me illustrate what is meant here with a vignette. It gives an impression of the kind and the complexity of interactions that are relevant for what counts as abnormal and/or specimen of a mental disorder.

> Anna is a married 35-year-old social worker with two small children. Until a year ago, when she gave birth to a healthy daughter, she worked in a daycare facility for elderly people. She suffers from ADHD (attention deficit type) and obsessive-compulsive disorder (OCD). The OCD is largely under control with appropriate medication and prolonged cognitive behavior therapy. The compulsions still take two hours a day, but are tolerable.

She was raised in a small village, where she also went to school. She was slow and easily distracted, but her ADHD was not really a problem. There were only ten to 15 children in the classroom, and she got lots of extra attention from the teacher, which was not a problem at all. With some delays, she succeeded in finishing her tertiary education as a social worker. The symptoms of ADHD became disturbing only after the birth of her second child, who cried a lot during the first three months. Gradually, Anna began to lose control of her daily activities at home. This lack of control influenced her OCD symptoms and gave rise to increased checking behavior and obsessive rumination.

Anna's mother, who was invited to (dis)confirm the diagnosis of ADHD, says that she knew from Anna's early childhood that there was something wrong with her daughter. She always suspected that her daughter had ADHD. "My daughter is like me. I have always known that my concentration is poor and that I have difficulty organizing things. I have learnt to cope with it and accept my limitations. I do things slower than others. I never allow others to urge me to do things faster." For Anna, her mother's way of coping worked for a while. However, since the birth of her second child, it did no longer. The children don't tolerate delays and her obsessive worries make it difficult to organize her day.

The story of Anna shows that context plays a decisive role in when and how symptoms become manifest and reach a level of intensity that is high enough to count as mental disorder. Anna's condition before the birth of her second child did not fulfill the criteria of ADHD (according to the DSM-IV and V). The small number of pupils in the primary school she attended, additional lessons from teachers, the tolerance of her parents, and her lack of ambition were among the many factors that prevented her tendency toward ADHD from developing into the full clinical manifestation of the disorder. Most of these contextual factors acted in a moderating and mediating way. Her mother and others interpreted Anna's behavior as different from others and weighed it as not disturbing enough to count as a disease. Her mother always said: "She has what I have and I can live with it, so there is no real psychiatric problem with her."

It is more difficult to decide whether there are also immediate contextual effects on the expression of Anna's symptoms. We have discussed this issue in general terms in Chapter 3. Classical biomedical accounts would locate Anna's problem entirely in her body and/or brain and consider contextual factors only as triggering causes (Dretske 1988). Interactional (relational) and system accounts are inclined to see Anna's problems as the expression of interactions. We have criticized the one-sidedness of purely biomedical approaches. However, it would be equally one-sided to see symptoms as only the expression of interactions between contexts and individuals. There exist, after all, tendencies within Anna herself that make her more vulnerable than others to develop ADHD. The answer to the question of whether there are immediate effects of the contexts on symptoms and their expression depends, in other words, on one's disease model and view on causality. According to the dispositional, flexible, and plural view that is defended in this book, it is easy to imagine situations in which contextual factors not only trigger, but also structure the manifestation of illnesses.

Considerations like these are also relevant for the assessment of depression, psychosis, personality disorder, and other mental illnesses. Contextual factors are relevant for the definition of thresholds for the severity and abnormality of symptoms. The DSM-IV says that symptoms of mental disorder should be severe enough to lead to "clinically significant distress," "dysfunction," and/or "impairment in social, occupational, or other important areas of functioning." The assessment of this distress, dysfunction and/or impairment depends on contextual factors; for instance, on what the context requires from the subject and on how early signs are interpreted by relatives and friends. People who need to focus their attention in their jobs will sooner fulfill the criterion of lack of concentration and will therefore earlier be recognized as depressed than people with less demanding jobs. Reassuring voices will be interpreted by some as innocent and informative and by others as sign of psychosis. Defining the threshold for abnormality may also be difficult because of looping effects. Symptoms of personality disorder, for instance, are notoriously difficult to weigh and assess. Think, for instance, of the criterion "having difficulty in making everyday decisions without an excessive amount of advice and reassurance from others" in dependent personality disorder. How excessive should the amount of advice and reassurance be to count as evidence of a dependent personality disorder? Assessment of this criterion must take local and cultural standards into account. But sooner or later this will lead to circularity and cultural bias. The social mechanisms that lead to the emergence of certain ideal types—for instance, the ideal of autonomy and independence—may turn out to be the same mechanisms that produce the cultural standards for the sanctioning or disapproval of certain behaviors, in this case, the rejection of dependence. There are many other instances in which definitions of what counts as mental disorder are caught in such circular formulations.

Does the NPA offer fresh insights into these issues? I think it does. It clarifies, for instance, why the presence of a mental disorder is not some bare and neutral fact. Fulfilling the criteria of mental disorder is not a value-free starting point for further diagnostic assessment and treatment planning. The NPA helps demonstrate that this fact, instead of being neutral, is in fact the product of a web of value-laden interactions. The NPA raises awareness of this value-ladenness and provides a better conceptual understanding of the kind of interactions and relations that are involved in this web. It offers a vocabulary to address the intrinsic normativity of these interactions and relations. It also gives a systematic and coherent picture of how the different types of relation and interaction cohere. By doing so, the NPA places psychopathology as well as the professional's role in a broader context. With the help of the NPA, professionals are better able to recognize and maintain the boundaries of the profession. They acknowledge that medical interventions are sometimes not the most appropriate response to the patient's problems.

7.2.3 Contextual influences on the professional role: An NPA approach

There are numerous contextual factors (legal, social, institutional, and administrative) that bear relevance for the definition and fulfillment of professional roles.

This has been widely recognized in the literature on the sociology of professions, medical education, and business administration and in position papers, reports, advices, and roadmaps issued by professional organizations, advisory boards, governmental agencies, and representatives of stakeholders. We saw how the ongoing division of labor has led to isolation of the professional, alienation from the patient, and fragmentation of the healthcare sector. Differentiation should keep pace with integration at all relevant levels. Professionals experience today how deeply their expert roles are embedded in complex, highly regulated, and often bureaucratic organizations (Mitchell & Ream 2015b). They begin to recognize that their roles need to become more varied, within and across the different social strata in which they perform their duties. Instead of a tendency to uniformity, current analyses foresee a tendency to plurality, with a proliferation of professional styles (Castellani & Hafferty 2006). Bloom et al. (2008) talk about new partnerships among representative bodies within the state, market players, and civil society organizations, including professional practices. What is negotiated is not only the content of care (i.e., the products) but also the terms under which these products are delivered. These terms define the rights, duties, and responsibilities of the relevant stakeholders. These negotiations occur not without tensions, ambiguities, and conflicts. Many healthcare professionals experience a split between the demand to care for their individual patients in an ethically responsible way and the demand to meet institutional and other standards of good care.

There is no blueprint for solving the puzzle of adjusting specific responsibilities to different types of negotiation and interaction. In an ideal situation, discussions about duties and jurisdictions are settled on the basis of a realistic assessment of what can be demanded from the various partners given their competence, their social (contextual) horizon, legal constraints, and their specific roles and responsibility in the delivery of care. In practice, this process is messy, ambiguous, and burdened by biases, preoccupations, and conflicts.

It is clear that the duties and jurisdictions of physicians at a micro-level differ from those who operate at other social levels. Differences in these duties and jurisdictions are based on differences in responsibility, which, in turn, are based on specific features of domains and social strata, types of interaction/negotiation, and goods that need to be realized.

Types of goods traditionally associated with individual patient–physician interactions are well-known. They include the following:

- meeting standards of excellence and/or good care, i.e., treatment that is safe, efficient, accessible, and in accordance with the best available scientific evidence
- informed consent, more precisely, the weighing of patient perspectives and professional judgments in negotiations about treatment options; the question is how the good of providing an evidence-based treatment should be weighed against preferences of the patient, given the risks and benefits of the different options

- provision of information to third parties in the context of assessments of disability or assessments of mental capacity
- balancing goods for the patient against goods for society (family, neighborhood, employer, insurance company, the state).

Today, these traditional goods must be embedded in broader frameworks of interlocking practices, which focus on a whole range of not strictly medical interests and topics, such as domestic violence, public safety, addiction, suicide, health education, advocacy, and access to care. In the literature, these practices are indicated with terms such as "collaborative communities" and "collaborative civic professionalism" (Adler et al. 2015). Current healthcare practices demand much more from professionals in terms of collaboration, leadership, and health advocacy than they used to. An important component of professionalism today is keeping the balance between one's civic and institutional responsibilities and one's responsibilities with respect to the expert role. This balancing is a second order competence and, in my view, part of the CanMEDS competence of professionalism.

This view is not undisputed, however. Some question, for instance, how far the imperative to stand up for one's patients and to defend their interests reaches. Professional responsibilities should not be confused with civic responsibilities, it is said. Professionals should not overstep their bounds in the civic sphere (Huddle 2013). But I believe this argument is one-sided. Today's healthcare arrangements do not ask doctors to give up their expert role and transform themselves into social workers or welfare promoters. What the new arrangements require is that professional expertise is adapted and creatively applied in other than strictly medical contexts, contexts in which medical problems interfere with labor, daily functioning, one's self-image, societal demands and expectations, and relationships with loved ones. Expertise should, in other words, be made relevant and applicable in these contexts. In the last chapter, we will return to this issue and discuss some innovations in mental healthcare.

7.3 The meso-level: The role of institutions

What role do institutions have in the construction of the object of psychiatry? And what role do they play in what we think doctors should do? Do they influence the expression of illness behavior, and, if so, how? What do institutions see as legitimate ground for the delivery of services in the form of mental healthcare? How do they influence definitions of the professional role? These are, again, very broad and difficult questions. I can only sketch a way of thinking about some of the broader conceptual issues.

7.3.1 Institutions from an NPA perspective

First, what are institutions? There are many definitions. One much quoted definition states that they are "systems of established and prevalent social rules that structure social interactions" (Hodgson 2006). This definition is broad: "Language, money, law, systems of weights and measures, table manners, and firms (and other organizations) are ... all institutions" (idem). Rules are in this context understood as "socially transmitted and customary normative injunctions or immanently normative dispositions, that in circumstances X do Y" (idem). Organizations are "special institutions that involve (a) criteria to establish their boundaries and to distinguish their members from nonmembers, (b) principles of sovereignty concerning who is in charge, and (c) chains of command delineating responsibilities within the organization" (idem).

What we can learn from these definitions is that the institutional embedding of psychiatry is broader, more multifaceted, and more pervasive than one would think. Institutions in the field of mental healthcare include not only hospitals, professional organizations, and patient groups but also municipalities, police departments, the legal system, insurance companies, medical language and literature, laboratories, research institutions, housing facilities, community centers, welfare organizations, churches, and relatives and friends. Each institution brings its own perspective on mental healthcare and has its own rules ("normative injunctions and dispositions").

One of the important functions of the NPA is to underscore that mental healthcare is a communal practice. It is not the practice of one group—of professionals, for instance—or of patients solely. It therefore does not embody and cherish the values of one group. The nucleus of the model is the concept of relationship; its focus consists of the inherent normativity of this relationship. We have worked from inside out, beginning with the individual professional–patient relationship and analyzing its different normative aspects (qualifying, conditioning, and foundational) (Chapter 5). In this chapter, we are drawing wider circles: first the circle of institutionally embedded relationships and then the circle of societally anchored relationships. Mental healthcare forms part of a web of relationships, which to a considerable extent are relationships among institutions. This web shapes mental healthcare as a practice and defines the object of psychiatry.

7.3.2 From individual well-being to service needs

There are many ways to approach this institutional embedding and its influence on the mental healthcare sector. Our focus here is on the object of psychiatric practice (A, Diagram 7.1) and definitions of professionalism (B, Diagram 7.1). My working hypothesis is that, at the institutional level, the object of psychiatry shifts from treatment of patients (micro-level) to responding to communal and regional service needs and to restoration and/or improvement of capabilities (meso- and partially also macro-level). This shift is not merely semantic; it is an expression of the different natures (or types) of relationship that constitute the practice of psychiatry at the institutional level. From an institutional perspective, relationships between physicians, nurses, and patients appear in a different light. They still aim at the well-being of the patient, but with more emphasis on fair allocation of resources, efficiency, and prevention of harm with respect to those people who are not able to take care of themselves (e.g., children, people with mental retardation, and those with chronic psychiatric conditions). Professional relationships are moreover embedded in a wider web of relationships with and among other stakeholders: the police, other local authorities, insurance companies, funding agencies, patient groups, hospitals and other medical facilities, housing corporations, transportation companies, and representatives of the general population. What characterizes meso-contexts is that stakeholders have diverging interests and that they collaborate in many ways.

Diagram 7.2 gives an indication of types of meso-context (economic, legal, social, administrative) and several examples of each type. Stakeholders must come to an agreement with respect to a variety of subjects. They not only negotiate about which treatments should be available for a population in a certain region but also about logistics, information and communication technology (ICT), housing, the availability of expensive technologies, access to other sources of support, and the conditions under which workers in healthcare must do their jobs. Many of these negotiations focus on responsibilities and/or jurisdictions: Who is responsible for what? Each stakeholder participates from a different perspective. Most of these perspectives belong to the conditioning sphere of healthcare (see again Diagram 7.2).

I will say a bit more about the interactions among these stakeholder perspectives insofar as they exert influence on the definition of the aims and the object of mental healthcare. I (initially) do this from the perspective of the concept of need.

I have said that healthcare facilities aim at the fulfilment of certain needs. Each institution has its own ideas about these needs, and these usually also overlap to a certain extent. What is interesting about the concept of need is that it helps us consider that needs at the level of the population are not the sum of the needs of all individual patients (Slade et al. 2011). At the level of populations, the definition of wishes and needs of other stakeholders than patients alone should be considered as well. In other words, in the translation of individual needs to collective needs and from these to service needs, more factors must be taken into account than are addressed at the individual level of provision of care.

What kind of healthcare facilities and healthcare system are needed to deliver the kind of care the various parties have agreed on? Which kinds of professionalism and of non-professional forms of support are needed for such care? How should needs be prioritized in a situation of economic prosperity or decline? What is the geographical and temporal horizon in the assessment of these needs? Are we defining them at a local, regional, or national scale? What is the time span: months, years, decades? These are the kind of questions that are relevant at this level.

The definition and assessment of needs also depend on the level of scientific knowledge and technology and on the availability of treatment facilities in a certain geographical area. Demands tend to follow supplies, despite all the efforts to reverse

Level of influence	Type of influence	Examples
Meso	Economic	Insurance companies (local arrangements)
		Local and regional funding agencies
		Local government (communities, provinces, regions)
		Collaborative networks on financial administration and logistics
	Legal	Regional regulations
		The police
		Collaborative networks on public safety
	Institutional/social	Hospitals/clinics
		Outpatient facilities
		Housing corporations
		Collaborative networks on triage, housing, and prioritization
	Administrative	Management of institutions
		Managerial rules and regulations
		Collaborative networks on administrative and logistic issues

DIAGRAM 7.2 Meso-level and types of influence

this sequence. Treatments that are available will be used, whatever they cost and however specialized they are. It is important to be aware of the influential role of science communication with respect to the perception of needs. New knowledge is communicated to the public, and new treatments are launched in popular media. Information and education of the public lead to what has been called proto-professionalization: the appropriation of professional knowledge by laypeople (de Swaan 1988). Proto-professionalization plays an increasingly important role in what people think they need (Dent 2006). Developing insights in the field of prevention and health education likewise influence what the profession is doing.

7.3.3 An NPA perspective on meso-contextual interactions and relationships

The NPA does not offer a blueprint for solving the many complex problems at this level of contextual aggregation. It offers, instead, a perspective, a way of thinking. I mention two points: The first concerns the relationship between the different contextual levels. The NPA embraces the idea that the individual professional relationship remains the nucleus of medicine and, therefore, of mental healthcare. Institutional arrangements are secondary; they exist to enable and support concrete, individual helping relationships. Medicine as an institution is no end-in-itself. It exists for the sake of patients. Self-evident as this may seem, it is far from superfluous to emphasize this in the context of current mental healthcare, given the increasing dominance and autonomy of large institutions in discussions about patient needs and distribution of services.

The second point follows from the first. It is about differences in language and in the definition of relationships. I emphasized the moral nature of professional relationships at the micro-level of analysis. I suggested that the transition toward the meso-level of analysis would require a shift in language and in the definition of relationships between stakeholders. This shift can be characterized as a move from a moral toward a predominantly economic and, to a lesser extent, legal interpretation of stakeholder relations. The NPA recognizes that relations at the meso-level differ from those at the micro-level. It acknowledges that important meso-level relationships are, indeed, primarily economically (or legally) qualified, though in a deepened sense. "Deepened" means in this context the same as what earlier was said about the legal aspect of professional relationships. The economic sphere should—just like the legal sphere—be "opened up" toward the moral destination of medical practice.

There is, in other words, nothing wrong with a predominantly economic definition of some of the relevant stakeholder relationships and with a legal definition of some of the other relationships. Think, for instance, of relationships between the CEO of a hospital, representatives of insurance companies, and officials of regional departments of health when they negotiate cost containment (economic), efficiency (economic), and access to care (legal). The point is that these meso-level interactions should enable and sustain the moral aims of medical practice, without colonizing and overgrowing the micro-world of individual physician–patient interactions. One of the messages of the NPA is a warning against a reversal of the order between contexts: meso-level interactions and relations exist to enable, sustain, and develop interactions in the micro-sphere; they are not ends-in-themselves. One other message of the NPA is that the norms and rules that guide meso-level interactions belong to the conditioning sphere. They do not qualify medical practice, neither do they belong to its core. Institutional arrangements and meso-level conditions should remain subservient to the micro-sphere, where individual practitioners try to fulfill the moral aims of medicine.

This has not always been recognized in recent years. Healthcare shows tendencies to succumb to the temptation to let meso-level relations and interactions dominate and overgrow individual relations between professionals and patients. We have discussed examples of this development earlier in this book. The NPA acknowledges the economic nature of many of the institutional arrangements, settlements, and relations between stakeholders. But it requires that these arrangements, settlements, and relations are respected and understood for what they are: conditions which constitute the conditioning aspects of medical practice. These arrangements, settlements, and relations ideally specify and actualize the conditioning (and not the qualifying) rules and norms for mental healthcare. They are necessary—without them modern healthcare would not exist—but they don't give healthcare its internal destination.

Let me illustrate the role of the NPA with a brief analysis of the role of the CEO in the board of a hospital. The CEO, obviously, has more and other duties and responsibilities than physicians within the hospital or in other practices. These differences can be traced back to differences in domain and in the types of goods associated with these domains. The domain of the CEO of the hospital is twofold and concerns, broadly speaking, the following:

a a the relation between the hospital and the practitioners to whom it provides employment
b the relation between the hospital as an institution and other players in the field, medical and non-medical, such as governmental agencies, the legal system, insurance companies, competing institutions, service users, and the public.

Much of what the CEO does aims at the improvement and strengthening of the conditions under which practitioners in the hospital deliver their services (ad a). The institution has the purpose of creating stable conditions for the delivery of these services. The duties and jurisdictions concern, therefore, the norms, rules, and principles that regulate the conditioning aspects of medical practices within the hospital. And these meso-level, institutionally anchored conditioning aspects are actualized and strived for in order to deliver services that do justice to the ultimately moral destination of healthcare (at the micro-level).

This means two things: First, it means that hospitals are not ends in themselves. They exist for a greater good: the care and treatment of people who suffer from illness and decline. Second, it means that what CEOs do is a good in its own right. Current medical practice is unthinkable without the guarantees the institutions like hospitals offer: housing, administrative support, technical equipment, contracts with insurers, platforms for teaching and education, and a living for its employees. In other words, the kind of good that is associated with the institutional domain and, more particularly, with the hospital as an institution, is that it provides safeguards with respect to the conditions under which healthcare can be delivered.

Both relationships (i.e., the relationship between the hospital and its employees [ad a] and the relationship between the hospital and external stakeholders [ad b]), have a relative autonomy. So, there are three spheres or practices that presuppose one another:

professional practice itself, intra-institutional practices and interactions, and practices and relationships between the hospital and other stakeholders. Each of the three spheres has its own relative autonomy and presupposes the others. Contexts can be specified in terms of domains or spheres of interaction. Each domain or sphere of interaction is associated with certain goods; these goods qualify the spheres of interaction. Stake-holders are responsible for the realization of these goods, depending on their role and responsibility. The spheres, as well as the conditioning norms they presuppose, are not self-contained, but related to, opened up, and determined by qualifying norms. In other words, the NPA suggests a certain order between the contexts. The promotion of the conditions that make healthcare possible, both intra- and extra-institutional, takes place with an eye on the destination of medical practice, which is to cure, to care, and to console. In the more technical language of the NPA: The norms and principles that guide intra- and extra-institutional relations of the hospital have a relative indepen-dence at their own meso-level, but are at the same time "opened up" in the direction of the qualifying aspect of the micro-sphere of professional interaction.

7.3.4 From needs to capabilities

One other way of analyzing the meso-sphere of interactions between professionals and other stakeholders consists of a conceptual analysis of key terms. One example of a key term is the notion of need itself. This notion is not undisputed, as we will see.

Needs are often defined in terms that depend on a utilitarian framework of understanding. In the philosophical literature on resource allocation in healthcare, this has been criticized, for instance by proponents of the capability approach, which was originally formulated by the political economist and Nobel prizewinner Amyarta Sen as a correction on one-sided utilitarian approaches to needs (Sen 1979; 1993).

Needs are often defined as desires for certain utilities or goods. Utility is an abstract term that refers to the relative value of a good or a service in terms of satisfaction (happiness; i.e., subjective utility) or benefit (income; i.e., objective utility). Goods are the object of needs; they are the things we desire. Needs aim at fulfilment of desires and attainment of goods. Goods can be measured and distributed under the guidance of utilitarian principles. Capabilities differ from both utility and goods. They differ from utilities because the utilitarian approach "uses a metric that focuses not on the person's capabilities but on his mental reaction" (e.g., the experience that one's desires are fulfilled). And they differ from goods because these are conceived as goods as such and "not from the perspective of what they do to people" (Sen 1979, p. 218). Utilities are, in other words, captured in terms of their potential to fulfill subjective desires and preferences instead of as realizations of values that constitute certain practices. And goods are conceived of as dissociated from the contexts in which they are actualized in the utilitarian approach.

Capabilities are abilities to do certain things. Examples are the ability to move, to meet one's nutritional requirements, to be clothed and sheltered, to have social contacts, and to be employed. They are, to use another phrase, combinations of functionings, things "a person manages to do or be in leading a life." The capability of a person reflects "the alternative combinations of functionings the person can achieve, and from which he or she can choose one collection" (Sen 1993). In this approach, quality of life can be assessed "in terms of the capability to achieve valuable functionings." The capabilities approach was initially developed to improve the study of economic development. Applications to the field of healthcare have begun to emerge (Law & Widdows 2008).

Two points should be noted: One is that the concept of capability is more flexible and context sensitive than other concepts, such as dysfunction or impairment. Capabilities are always "open to negotiation" and may "change from one context and individual to another" (idem). Sen thinks that this plurality and variety is an advantage that allows his approach to be applied in multiple contexts and within different value frameworks. The other point is related to the concept of need itself. The capabilities approach tries to surmount certain deficiencies of traditional utilitarian approaches, which emphasize fulfilment of subjective desires (happiness) and attainment of certain goods (income and welfare, in economic theory). The concept of capability puts more emphasis on value realization as a both an individual and a collective good. Value realization occurs in the form of achievement of functionings. This achievement of functionings is constituted by practices. Sen refers in this context to communitarian approaches, which see values as goods that are internal to practices (MacIntyre 1984).

Behind the capabilities approach, one finds a social philosophy and anthropology that considerably differs from the usual economic and utilitarian approaches. The capabilities approach criticizes the standard utilitarian approach because of its inherent tendency to disregard or minimize the enormous diversity between people—not only socioeconomic diversity, but also diversity in terms of their desires, their values, their traditions, and their temporal horizon. Instead of focusing on what they feel and realize in terms of income and welfare, like utilitarianists do, the capabilities approach puts more emphasis on what people do, are able to achieve, and deem important to do. This approach sees, in short, the achievement of functionings as embedded in social practices that embody certain values.

Applications of the capabilities approach to medicine are still relatively general and immature. It is too early to give a solid evaluation from the NPA perspective. Elements of the capability approach are adopted by the values-based healthcare (VBHC) approach, which will be discussed in more detail in the last chapter.

There are, at first sight, many points of convergence between the capabilities approach and the NPA. Both approaches emphasize the role of practices and the inherent good of functioning in these practices; both criticize one-sided emphasis on subjective preferences and definitions of goods in terms of such preferences. Both recognize that the struggle against disease is not an end-in-itself, but part of a larger practice. And both define the economic sphere as guided by value-sensitive intuitions and insights. My hesitations concern the broadness of the term capability and its lack of specificity with respect to the moral destination of medicine. Physicians and nurses are not welfare workers, neither do they aim at increasing well-being in general and in every imaginable respect. The goal of their efforts is more specific.

They serve the good of those who cannot sufficiently take care of themselves because of their illness or handicap. I can imagine solutions for this conceptual issue, but I am not aware of alternative definitions of capability that solve the problem of lack of specificity.

7.4 The macro-level: Interactions with society and culture

Needs and capabilities are not only defined by institutions; they are also shaped and interpreted by developments, interactions, discussions, and dynamics at a societal and cultural level. I can only give a brief excursion into this broad field and sketch the contours of a roadmap that might facilitate further exploration of this area. I focus on the interplay between societal (cultural, historical) factors and mental healthcare as a clinical, institutional, and social practice (relation B, Diagram 7.1) and, in particular, on the influence of this interplay on definitions of the object of psychiatry (relations A and C, Diagram 7.1). In what follows, I will again make use of the distinction between levels and types. Levels refer to the micro-, meso-, and macro-levels of analysis. Types refer to kinds of norm that are relevant for each of these levels (see Diagram 7.3).

7.4.1 Kinds of interaction between society, the profession, and the object of psychiatry

Before I proceed, I will outline the kind of interplay I am thinking about. I am referring to the following:

a   immediate effects of large historical, socioeconomic, sociocultural, and/or physical events (war, migration, physical disasters) on the incidence and prevalence of mental disorder; examples of relevant issues are loneliness, lack of social cohesion, social fragmentation, lack of social support, and all kinds of existential issue

b   interactions that define who needs care and thereby sanction certain behaviors and illness manifestations as deserving professional attention

c   interactions that shape the expression of symptoms

d   interactions that frame public awareness of psychiatric problems and help manage expectations about what mental healthcare can do

e   interactions that are meant to exert social control by means of medical labeling, registering, and/or reporting.

These are some of the influences and interactions between society and psychiatry. The list is not complete, and in many cases, there is more than one kind of interaction at the same time. Let me briefly review what is stated here.

Ad [a]. Large historical, socioeconomic, and/or physical events are a mixed bag, with war, migration (refugees), natural disasters, famine, and nuclear explosions as major contributors to mental health problems. Textbox 7.1 discusses an intriguing historical example: the fate of effort syndrome, which offers a clear picture of how wars not only

Level of influence	Type of influence	Examples	
Macro	Economic	National government	
		Insurance companies (nation-wide arrangements)	
		National funding agencies	
		Industry and other third parties	
	Legal	Laws and regulations with respect to	
		- financing of the healthcare system	
		- jurisdictions of professions	
		- mental capacity (a.o. the capacity to take one's own decisions)	
	Institutional	Government	
		Professional organizations	
		Service user groups	
	Administrative	Internal	Certification and accreditation
		Professional	Quality control
		Semi-governmental	Registration of demographic and public health related variables
			Different forms of quality control
		Governmental	Authorities for the enforcement of legislation
			Healthcare Inspectorate

DIAGRAM 7.3 Macro-level and types of influence

determine the incidence of mental disorder, but also the way symptoms are labeled and sanctioned. Without medical sanctioning, these soldiers could expect to be accused of malingering and, therefore, of desertion. The history of "shell shock" is an even more telling case, with around 300 death penalties for malingering and even some medically unexamined soldiers who were sentenced to death (Shephard 2000, p. 67ff).

Effort syndrome is a condition suffered by soldiers who departed the frontlines during the First World War, with physical symptoms such as fatigue, breathlessness, palpitations, and pain in the region of the heart (Glas 2003; Shephard 2000). Thomas Lewis, a British physician who took an interest in the condition, gives a figure of 70,000 such cases among British soldiers, 44,000 of whom subsequently received a war pension (Lewis 1940).

The story of effort syndrome began during the American Civil War, when Da Costa, a cardiologist, spoke about "irritable heart syndrome," thereby referring to soldiers who, sleep deprived and exhausted after long marches, developed unexplained palpitations, breathlessness, fatigue, and pain in the chest. During the First World War, soldiers with complaints like those in the American Civil War begin to return from the battlefields. Lewis became convinced that there was no real cardiac pathology in these cases, but nevertheless that the condition was physiological and should be taken medically seriously. The patients were simply unable to perform physically sufficiently, presumably—Lewis thought—as a result of some infection or other unnoticed organic process. Lewis developed a program of gradual exercise that enabled around half of victims to return to the front, a fact for which he was knighted by the British government in 1921.

Other terms that have come into use reflect similar uncertainties and ambiguities, with pseudo-organic terms such as "neurocirculatory neurasthenia" on the one end of the spectrum (Oppenheimer et al. 1918), seemingly neutral terms like "soldier's heart" and "Da Costa syndrome" (Wood 1941) in the middle, and psychological terms such as "war neurosis" (Mackenzie 1916; 1920) and "heart neurosis" at the other end of the spectrum. During the Second Word War, the discussion about effort syndrome re-emerged. Despite consensus about the incorrectness of the term "irritable heart," there was still no unanimity about what actually lies behind the syndrome. The story only ended after an elegant physiological experiment by Jones and Wood, in which lactate levels were measured after physical exertion (Jones 1948). The inability to deliver physical effort appeared to be related to psychic and not to physical factors. Patients with effort syndrome think that they are at the maximum of what their bodies can physically tolerate earlier than healthy controls do. Their blood shows lower lactate levels than that of controls at maximum performance. They seem, in other words, more vulnerable to the unpleasant side-effects of physical exertion. Jones' patients received a form of clinical group treatment with psychoeducation, exercises, and psychotherapy. This treatment was the first step in the development of the therapeutic community movement in the UK, initiated by the same Jones who performed the lactate experiments.

Ad [b]. By defining who needs psychiatric care and who does not, social and cultural factors help to establish the boundaries of mental healthcare as an institution.

Ad [c]. Socio-psychological and institutional factors codetermine the expression of mental disorder and the interpretation of its manifestations. Cultural factors influence how symptoms are shaped, profiled, and culturally coded. Cross-cultural psychiatry has taught important lessons about this shaping, profiling, and coding. Kleinman (1982), for instance, has shown that in many parts of Chinese society, the experience of depression is physical rather than psychological (see also Kleinman & Good 1985). Depressed Chinese people "do not report feeling sad, but rather express boredom, discomfort, feelings of inner pressure, and symptoms of pain, dizziness, and fatigue," classical manifestations of what was once called neurasthenia. Chinese immigrants in the United States find the diagnosis of depression morally unacceptable and experientially meaningless (Kleinman 2004).

Ad [d]. One major cultural influence is mental healthcare itself, which helps to frame the public's awareness of symptoms and risks. Mental healthcare shapes the expectations of the public about what it can do against these symptoms and risks. Shaping of expectations occurs by labelling, (mis)attribution of common ailments as diseases, and induction of emotional or social dependence (Ikkos 2011). Medicalization of common complaints is a large subject in the medical anthropological literature and in psychiatry. Horwitz and Wakefield have claimed that psychiatry has "transformed normal sorrow into depressive disorder" and "natural anxieties into mental disorders" (Horwitz & Wakefield 2007; 2012, respectively). Even, if their claims cannot fully be substantiated (Kendler 2008b), they are right in pointing at the framing of expectations and of the perception of risks and needs. Social theory has much to contribute to the understanding of illness perceptions and management of expectations (Kleinman 2010).

Ad [e]. A final, even more far reaching aspect of the interactions between psychiatry and society is indicated with the concept of biopower. This term was coined by philosopher Michel Foucault and later applied in social statistics and the social study of medicine. The idea is that statistics and other ways of registering biological and other medically relevant features may be used by the state and other agencies (insurance companies, for instance) for purposes of social control. We don't need to associate such control only with the brutal power that is exerted by totalitarian regimes (e.g., regimes of birth control or of eugenics programs). Subtler forms of such social control are now known under the heading of lifestyle politics and lifestyle programming: the influencing of health-related behavior by the government, insurance companies, the media and other agencies.

Interactions in which biopower in one form or another plays a role may also work in the other direction: citizens who claim certain social or economic privileges based on their biological or medical identity. Psychiatrists who report to the court or to agencies for pensions, payments, or certain facilities as compensation for disabilities are familiar with these cases at an individual level.

7.4.2 Medical identity: An analysis from the perspective of the NPA

An interesting example of an appeal to societally determined medical identity is described by Petryna (2002; 2004; see also Kleinman 2010), who studied the behavior of former victims of the Chernobyl disaster. Petryna introduces the term "biological citizenship" to understand what people do when they claim disability from the Chernobyl disaster. As a matter of fact, only a few hundred victims were certified as having really physically suffered from the exposure to radiation. However, a much larger group claimed compensation for symptoms they attributed to the disaster, although without clear physical evidence (see Havenaar 1996; see also Bromet & Havenaar 2007). These people suffered predominantly from the devastating social and economic effects—instead of the physical sequelae—of the disaster: uncoordinated transportation to other areas of Ukraine and Russia, disruption of family ties, lack of information, and later also job loss, lack of social recognition, failing healthcare and economic policies, corruption, and stigmatization by urban populations. Coding one's misery in medical terms seems an understandable reaction when legal, social, and economic safety nets are failing or absent (Petryna 2004).

I will pursue this subject a little further. In the literature on professionalism, one sometimes reads the suggestion that, historically, the medical profession has often been left untouched under dictatorial regimes. One of the reasons for this, it is argued, is that the medical profession is usually no threat to such regimes. According to some, another reason might be that the profession tends to be organized around a core set of values that make it relatively resistant to political manipulation. I am not so sure about the latter claim, given the long history of abuse of psychiatry under dictatorial regimes. But this is not the issue here. My point is conceptual and again related to the NPA. The NPA provides conceptual resources to withstand claims that psychiatry should be at the service of the state or whatever other political or economic power. It suggests a conception of mental healthcare that puts the individual patient–clinician relationship in the center and that positions institutions and society as wider circles around this core relationship. These circles shape the conditions that enable and support the individual professional relationship. The NPA emphasizes the moral nature of this core relationship and helps to identify the dynamics inside and outside the profession that enable, support, or threaten this core relationship. Health and healthcare are goods. These goods are not owned or possessed by one party (e.g., the state). They are communal. That is what the very notion of a normative practice means. The NPA is not a model for professionals alone; it is a model for a collaborative practice in which patients, doctors, nurses, and all other stakeholders participate. The NPA describes and defends the intrinsic normativity of mental healthcare as a practice and outlines a perspective on how the different levels of contextual embeddedness relate to one another and codetermine the object of psychiatry. It suggests that the wider circles just mentioned can be conceived as sub-practices. It suggests that these sub-practices may have a different (non-moral) qualification. This is no problem insofar as the focus of the sub-practices remains directed at—ultimately morally qualified—interactions at the individual level.

With respect to the Chernobyl disaster and its psychosocial aftermath, the NPA would point at the need for proper functioning of other safety nets. The model cannot *in abstracto* answer the question of whether doctors should be allowed to fool the system by giving fake diagnoses as legal basis for a form of compensation. But what the NPA can do is conceptually analyze the distortions in the functioning of society as a whole; help to identify deficiencies in legal, social, and economic forms of support; and show in which way these deficiencies put a burden on mental healthcare. One can imagine cases, for instance, the Chernobyl case, in which it is legitimate to expand the object of psychiatry, such that the profession gets involved in improper activities in order to repair deficiencies in other areas of society, solely for the good of people who otherwise would be much worse off. But the argument is slippery from a moral point of view and needs discussion on a case-by-case basis.

With respect to issues such as life style programming, biopower, and possibly defensible forms of medicalization, the NPA again does not give concrete answers. Instead, it outlines a direction in which the argument could go. For instance, with respect to lifestyle politics, the NPA might suggest that it pushes the profession across the edge of the ethical if it represents a policy of only one or two stakeholders (the state or a pharmaceutical company, for instance). This might be different if the policy is the result of a joined initiative in which all relevant stakeholders are heard and given justice; an objective that in real life will be very difficult (but not impossible) to reach.

Use of medical identity to claim certain social or economic privileges (biopower) sounds dangerous from an NPA point of view, since it alienates (mental) healthcare from its core. A possible defense could run along the same lines as the lifestyle programming discussion; that is, if all stakeholders would agree, and if it would not place too much burden on the practice of mental healthcare, limited forms of it could be permissible.

7.4.3 An NPA perspective on macro-contextual interactions and relations

This also holds for the macro-sphere (i.e., for the role of the state, the legal system, advisory and supervisory boards, policy groups, and service user groups). The domain to which these entities belong is diverse and concerns, for instance:

- the healthcare inspectorate
- laws and agreements that guarantee access to care, safety, informed consent, quality, jurisdictions of the profession, patient rights, and fair distributions of means
- agencies for health education (i.e., the framing of public awareness of mental health problems and of expectations about what mental healthcare can do)
- nationwide registration of illnesses for public health purposes
- prevention.

The list is not exhaustive, of course. From an NPA perspective, it is most important to see that relationships between the profession and the other authorities and representatives do not stand on their own and show an underlying logic. This logic can be explained in terms of a meshwork of types of norm (qualifying, conditioning, and foundational) and of modal distinctions between these norms. It can also be spelled out in the language of interlacements between different spheres of cooperation and communal action. The macro-sphere of cooperation and coordinated actions has its own relative independence and its own internal destination, like institutions in the meso-sphere. However, the relatively independent macro-scale relations and interactions reach their full meaning only by attuning to the ultimate destination of healthcare: the well-being of those who suffer from disease and illness.

Norms that determine the nature of these relatively independent spheres are therefore ideally opened up to the norms that qualify mental healthcare as practice. This opening up means that the practice that is described in terms of its normative structure keeps its own destination but enriched with elements from other spheres. Governmental agencies function in their legislating role in a juridical sense. But this juridical sphere is, ideally, opened up toward the ethical sphere. The practice of issuing laws will, in other words, remain qualified by legal principles. But legislators will ideally attempt to open up the juridical meaning of their laws and regulations to the sphere of ethics. By doing so, the lawgiver is not becoming a moral agent, and laws are not becoming moral commands. It is in his or her juridical functioning that the legislator will try to pave the way for a fully moral definition of the helping relationship, but this functioning remains juridical.

I think it is safe to conceive the principle of distributive justice as one of the most central and important principles for cooperation in the macro-sphere (Daniels 2001; 2013). Most of the (macro-) spheres of cooperation and coordinated action are meant to provide the conditions that make mental healthcare accessible, safe, efficient, and conforming to minimum standards of quality. The actualization of the different normative principles occurs first under the guidance of the principle of distributive justice. This principle in turn opens up toward the moral sphere, which aims at fulfilment of the ideal of beneficence (i.e., of doing good to the patient). The macro-sphere should, therefore, orient itself toward the meso- and micro-spheres of interaction. It is itself, basically, a conditioning sphere. So, what we add here is a new conceptual refinement. In Chapter 5, we described medicine and healthcare as practices with one destination and with a number of conditioning aspects. By broadening our perspective to the meso- and macro-levels of interaction, we are better able to acknowledge the relative independence of the different spheres of cooperation and interaction. Each sphere has its own responsibility and role. The overarching moral purpose of healthcare does not change. We are only better able to recognize that this purpose is realized by the interactions among a wide diversity of spheres of cooperation, each with its own internal destination. It is in this cooperation that all these different spheres (ideally) keep in touch with the overall aim of medicine and healthcare. Consider, for instance, a medical advisor at a ministry of health, who is convinced of the need and benefits of empowerment of patients. He or she will not personally undertake action as a campaigner. He or she will, instead, try to promote the conditions that make empowerment possible. This aim can be targeted by subsidies, legal reform, and additional regulations. These financial, legal, and administrative supports serve as enabling conditions for the good cause of patient empowerment.

7.4.4 Bureaucracy from an NPA perspective

Let me discuss one other example a bit more extensively: the increasing importance of administrative aspects in mental healthcare. Administration forms a considerable burden in many healthcare sectors today, as we have seen. Some of these forms of administration are new; others have existed for many decades. There are different forms of administrative accounting. I focus here on three forms of administrative accountability, corresponding with three goals: financial control, pursuit of safety, and warrants with respect to quality of care. These three goals refer to different stakeholders in the delivery of excellent and sustainable care.

Financial control refers—at the macro-level, among others—to the role of the government in maintaining the legal and economic framework of current healthcare. It also refers to the role of insurance companies, charity funds, and the industry in how healthcare is financed. Financial control is needed to put an end to the spiraling costs of (mental) healthcare.

Safety is an issue that is not restricted to the consulting room (micro-sphere); it is also and typically relevant to institutional (meso-level) and public health (macro-level) concerns. It refers to the role of internal rules within healthcare facilities (meso-level) and the role of supervisory bodies (macro-level). Today's obsession with safety is partially occasioned by carelessness in the healthcare sector itself (side-effects of medication and medical failures because of lack of communication between doctors and those who depend on their information). But it is also a societal phenomenon. Sociologist Ulrich Beck (1992) calls our society a "risk society." We increasingly try to avoid risk, despite the relative physical and economic safety of Western lives.

Quality of care, finally, is also an issue with aspects that go beyond the individual doctor–patient relationship. Accessibility of healthcare facilities is one of the important items in quality assessments. Efficiency and accountability are two other important issues. The supervision and control of these different elements predominantly takes place at meso- and macro-levels of interaction between stakeholders.

The bureaucratization of the public sector and of professionalism, together with the managerialism in public and private administration, offer interesting examples of the interaction between structure and dynamic, of the intersection of the different spheres (micro, meso, and macro), and of how these different spheres influence both the object of mental healthcare and the roles of the various stakeholders.

The weakening of trust in the medical profession has at least partially been attributable to individual scandals and improper behavior of the sector as a whole. The profession no longer succeeds in keeping up the image of impeccability and of an unconditional desire to put patients' interests above self-interest. At least equally important is a tendency to paternalism, which, in turn, is based on a wrong conception of the expert role. As a result of these developments, the prestige of the profession has diminished. To regain trust, the healthcare sector has had to accept additional forms of regulation beyond self-regulation. Examples of the new regulations are to be found in the sphere of patient safety (medication use, prevention of physical harm), transparency (electronic records, standardization in the form of treatment protocols, digital pre-scription of medication, registration of compulsory measures in mental healthcare), efficiency (registering of the activities of doctors and nurses and matching of these activities with treatment protocols), and efficacy (outcome monitoring and measuring of patient satisfaction). Healthcare providers are obliged to monitor and report about the various elements of the new agreements about all these different elements in the delivery of care.

At the same time, a combination of new treatment options and facilities, rapid technological innovation, and increasing expectations among the population have led to a steep increase in the costs of healthcare and mental healthcare. These costs put the system under pressure. Many countries allowed market incentives, with the purpose of stimulating efficiency and efficacy. Markets themselves, however, did not and still do not instill trust. They, in fact, tend to have an eroding effect on trust, especially in non-profitable segments of the market (Polder et al. 1996). Because of the market incentives, non-profitable segments appeared to need addi-tional safeguards against exploitation, misinformation, and insufficient care. These additional safeguards came in the form of rules aiming at the improvement of accountability, transparency, and quality of care. These rules came on top of the rules that were demanded to regain trust in the professionals themselves and which aimed at the reliability and transparency of the care process.

Despite the intention of governments and other stakeholders to deregulate the sector, the new agreements and rules laid the basis for the new bureaucracy. The profession's attempt to regain trust, on the one hand, and the need to put an end to the spiraling costs of healthcare, on the other hand, were the drivers behind an enormous increase in the administrative burden of healthcare providers. Nurses and doctors frequently need 30–40% of their time or more to fulfill their administrative duties today.

The modern professional should be quick and competent in shifting gears. This flexibility and competence to adapt are also required from other stakeholders. In the words of Mitchell and Ream (2015a, p. 332):

> Institutionalized professional work relationships are frequently subjected to coer-cive demands for specific task performance standards … To produce effective and efficient professional services within institutional settings, it is necessary to inte-grate employee duties to institutional managements, civic duties to stakeholders, legal duties to political regimes, and moral and fiduciary duties to clients.

Professionals, clients, and other stakeholders all have to learn to attune to the agenda of all others.

7.4.5 The role of service users

I suggested earlier that whatever care arrangements there will be in the future, successful arrangements will always require civic partnership of service users. This subject seems particularly important today. The position of service users has changed, and service user movements have become strong and important in most Western countries.

Earlier we saw that the profile of medical professionalism has changed and become more varied. This development is paralleled by increased variability and plurality in the profile of service users and service user movements. There are, broadly speaking, three definitions of the patient role: the classical role of the patient as a recipient of care; the new role of the patient as a service user, consumer, or client expert who is supposed to manage his or her own disease process; and the even newer role of the patient as user survivor, victim of stigma and of misuse of power (Speed 2006).

How service users defend their interests depends on their circumstances. The rise of service user movements was the result of increasing criticism of the paternalism of doctors in the 1960s. It brought about, after decades, legal reforms that improved the position of patients. Part of the criticism was driven by a strong anti-establishment ideology, which saw medicine as by definition an oppressive discipline with a "normalizing" function, even beyond the medical domain. In these ideological variants of criticism, medicine was considered to belong to the "establishment" and to possess alienating power: Once one had entrusted one's body (or mind) to representatives of the medical system, one longer owned one's body (or mind), and others—doctors and nurses—were in charge of the regulation and normalization of its functions, on the basis of a rationality that was thought to be far beyond the patient's comprehension. The ensuing expropriation, ideologically driven critics said, deprived service users of their most fundamental rights, including freedom and integrity of the body. One other important side-effect of the same ideology was that the healthcare system created its own reality in the form of medicalization (Charland 2013).

It is well-known that this ideology became especially influential in psychiatry. However, the antipsychiatry movement did not develop uniformly in Europe (Bracken & Thomas 2005). In most countries, it succeeded in its goal (i.e., legal reform and a firmer establishment of patient's rights). As a result, in some countries (including the Netherlands and Scandinavia), the criticism toned down, and service user groups developed into collaborating parties with a well-established position in debates about healthcare policy. In other countries (the UK, Canada, and the US, for instance) the situation was more mixed, with elements of both normalization and radicalization. Some service user groups were ready to collaborate with professionals, the government, and other stakeholders; others were renamed and called themselves user survivor groups while clinging to a firm anti-establishment agenda (Bracken & Thomas 2013). In Italy, the situation became even more confusing. Legal reform led here to a split in mental healthcare, with a very small proportion of it delivered along the lines of the traditional medical model and a larger proportion along the lines of an anti-authoritarian, democratized community model. There were also, finally, countries in which patient movements never became very strong, and still other countries (Germany, for instance) in which patients' rights were already quite securely established.

7.5 Conclusion

So, here we are. Contemporary healthcare is more than a meeting between professionals and those who need professional help. There is a wide variety of contexts and roles outside their consulting rooms in which professionals need to make sense of their knowledge and skills. Professionals can only be relieved from the burdensome task of accounting for what they do when they regain the trust of patients and other stakeholders. This will not occur when professionals withdraw from the broader contexts just mentioned and keep basing their jurisdictions solely on their expert role. Restoration of trust will only occur when professionals really open up to what other stakeholders say and aim at and when they adopt responsibility in these broader contexts. In the last chapter, I give some suggestions and advice about how this can be done.

8

PHILOSOPHICAL BACKGROUNDS

8.1 Introduction

This chapter provides the philosophical background of the normative practice approach (NPA) and locates this approach within the broader field of value-sensitive approaches to psychiatry.

In the first part, I delve somewhat deeper into the systematic philosophy of Dutch philosopher Herman Dooyeweerd. His work is less known in the philosophical world and needs a more extensive introduction, since it has been important for the initial formulations of the NPA. I draw on Dooyeweerd's idea that norms are intrinsic, i.e., structurally given, and make use of some of his distinctions between types of norm and principle. I place Dooyeweerd's work in the context of other, more recent appropriations of his work (Chaplin 2011; Mouw & Griffioen 1993; Verkerk 2004; Verkerk et al. 2015). This discussion provides additional background for the previous chapter, in which the stratification of contexts and the typification of types of norm and principle relevant for these contexts was dealt with.

I then focus on other philosophical approaches to the issue of normativity of professional practices, especially Alasdair MacIntyre's defense of virtue ethics and virtue-ethical approaches to professionalism; Charles Taylor's idea that goods are not arbitrary options, but formative for who we are in the different practices that constitute our lives; and Ricoeur's suggestion that moral authenticity and trustworthiness require attunement between a particular practice and who we are as persons (MacIntyre 1984: Ricoeur 1990; Taylor 1989). Emphasis on this last element leads to a self-relational approach to moral responsibility, which influenced our analysis of the relationships within and between professionals and patients (Chapter 3). The NPA builds on MacIntyre's idea that goods (or norms) are "internal to practices." It adopts Taylor's idea that goods are not products of arbitrary choices. It also acknowledges the implicit reflexivity of normative practices, as outlined in the work of Ricoeur.

8.2 Herman Dooyeweerd

Who was Dooyeweerd, and what were his most important ideas? Herman Dooyeweerd (1894–1977) was one of the founders of what has become known as reformational (or "neo-Calvinist") philosophy. He developed his philosophy in the interbellum, in an intellectual climate characterized by uncertainty, deep divides between philosophical traditions, and the presentiment of decline of Western culture. The chair of the Royal Dutch Academy of Arts and Sciences once called him "the most original philosopher the Netherlands has ever produced, Spinoza himself not excepted" (Langemeijer 1964, cited in Kalsbeek 1970, p. 10). Dooyeweerd studied law and philosophy. He had a brief career in public administration before he became secretary of the Abraham Kuyper Foundation, a precursor of the scientific institute of one of the Christian political parties in the Netherlands before the Second World War. From 1926 until his retirement in 1965, he was professor of philosophy and history of law at the Vrije Universiteit in Amsterdam.

He wrote extensively and had an almost encyclopedic knowledge not only of philosophy and the history of philosophy (especially neo-Kantianism and ancient philosophy) but also of the sciences of his time, especially mathematics, physics, biology, law, and the social and political sciences. Most of his ideas in systematic philosophy were developed and refined via interaction with the sciences (Dooyeweerd 1953–1958).

To understand Dooyeweerd's philosophy, it is useful to keep in mind that it is built up around two main themes: (1) the distinction between different modal aspects (or ways of functioning) and (2) the idea that all human activity is rooted in what he calls the "heart," which denotes a concentration point within our existence, out of which our ultimate concerns originate. In the following sections, we discuss first the theory of modal aspects, then the theory of entities or "individuality structures," subsequently the concepts of law and cosmic order, next the idea of heart and, finally, what Dooyeweerd saw as the fundamental flaw of Western philosophy and science: its absolutization of the theoretical attitude of thought.

8.2.1 Modal aspects

Dooyeweerd tells in an interview that his idea of modal diversity came to him in a flash during a walk in the dunes somewhere around 1921 when he was overwhelmed by the astonishing diversity and the incredible coherence in the way things exist and function (van Dunné et al. 1977, p. 37). Everything exists in different ways, which are both distinguishable and interconnected in our ordinary experience of the world. A flower, for instance, exists in a spatial, in a physical, and in a biotic way: It occupies a certain space, it has physical properties (such as mass), and it functions as a biotic entity because it grows, blossoms, and reproduces. Flowers may also exist in other spheres or aspects, for instance in the economic or the aesthetic aspect. They then function as economic or aesthetic object, respectively. They are bought (economic) or valued because of their beauty (aesthetic).

All these different ways of functioning are weaved together in a seemingly self-evident and natural way in our everyday experience. We don't even notice the differences. However, we can become aware of them in certain contexts in which a particular feature stands out or when we step back and reflect on the differences. A flower seller, for instance, is more aware of certain physical properties of plants and flowers (e.g., their strength and weight) because he or she has to handle them. Consumers, by the same token, may be more interested in how flowers function in the aesthetic and the economic aspect. It is similar for wounds: Patients will be inclined to focus on the pain they cause and how ugly they look, whereas a physician will primarily be interested in specific features of a wound, including its size, color, and heat. Dooyeweerd calls the most general ways (or kinds) of existing or functioning aspect, or modal aspect, functions, modal functions, or (more technically) law spheres. The term modal does not refer to logic (modal logic) but to the Latin term *modus*, which means way of existing or functioning. Everything functions in several spheres, not one sphere at a time, diachronically, but in all spheres synchronically, in an orderly way and in close conjunction. A sphere is not a layer, an ontic cross-section so to say, within an entity. It is a way of functioning or existing of the thing itself as a whole, it is not a part or component of the thing.

Things function in these spheres in basically two ways: as subject or as object. Flowers exist (function) within a numerical, a geometrical, a physical, and a biotic sphere, as we have seen. This means that, in their existing, flowers manifest discreteness (numerical), spatial continuity (geometrical), physical qualities (mass, energy), and biotic qualities like generation and a tendency to self-preservation. In these four spheres (numerical, spatial, physical, biotic), flowers function as subject, i.e., they manifest these qualities themselves, actively. Flowers also function in other spheres, that is, as objects, for instance as object of scientific analysis (logical), as products that can be bought or sold (economic), or as objects with aesthetic qualities (aesthetic). In all these other spheres, flowers function passively in their interaction with human beings.

Modal aspects refer to kinds of property instead of properties per se. The term property is usually understood as referring to an instantiation of a more general category. When I say "This car is black," "black" is a property of that car. It is an instantiation of the general category of blackness, namely, the instantiation of the general category of blackness in this car. Modes or modal aspects refer to these general categories, i.e., to kinds of property, not to concrete and individual instantiations. The distinctness of these kinds has something to do with the distinctness (or "sovereignty") of laws and/or lawful principles, according to Dooyeweerd. More precisely, the distinctness of kinds of property should be considered as a reflection of the irreducible distinctness of laws in the ways they determine what exists and occurs.

The idea of distinctness is an extension of thoughts that were originally formulated by the thinker who inspired Dooyeweerd probably most: Abraham Kuyper, a theologian, philosopher, statesman, and journalist. Kuyper developed the idea of sphere sovereignty to understand how different social spheres can overlap and at the same time retain a relative independence. The activities of the church and of the state overlap, but state and church are at the same time sovereign in their own spheres. This is because both obey their own normative principles. These normative principles are ultimately not manmade, but intrinsic to our social existence and "given," although, of course, influenced by culture and local circumstances. Dooyeweerd applied this sociological principle of sphere sovereignty to all kinds of law. The cosmos we inhabit manifests an order with a manifold of laws. Each of these laws belongs to a particular type, and these types represent modal spheres.

Dooyeweerd devoted an entire volume of his opus magnum to the analysis of and distinction between these modal aspects (Dooyeweerd 1953–1958, Vol. II). He distinguished not two or three but as many as 14 (later 15) modal aspects, each with its own typical character or meaning. It is important to notice that the aspects are not layers or components or whatever other form of substantial existence in an entity. They are modes of existence or functioning; they concern the "how" and not the "what." In the next section, we will see what Dooyeweerd has to say about the what (i.e., about entities and their structure).

In Dooyeweerd's systematic philosophy, the modal analysis precedes and is more fundamental than the analysis of entities. Dooyeweerd is, of course, aware of the fact that most scientists are primarily occupied with entities (i.e., with part–whole relationships and with the interactions and relations between particular types of thing). He nevertheless maintains that science starts by selecting a particular modal point of view. It is only after having gone through "the gate of modal analysis" that the scientist studies the relationships between and within things. This modal point of view can be any modal aspect; it does not have to be similar to the modal aspect that qualifies the thing in question. Physics became a science, not by adopting a physical point of view, but by applying mathematical principles to physical phenomena.

8.2.2 The difference between modes and entities

Not recognizing the relevance of the distinction between modes and entities is the cause of much trouble in the sciences, according to Dooyeweerd. Mental phenomena, for instance, are often conceived of as expressions of a mental part, layer, or component within the organism. In other cases, they are seen as products that are causally brought about by some mechanism in the brain. This mechanism is usually considered to be non-mental. Both ways of conceptualizing mental phenomena are problematic in the Dooyeweerdian view.

The implicit assumption of the first position (mental phenomena as expressions of the existence of a mental "layer" or "part") is that if there are mental properties and functions, they can only exist if there is also some mental "stuff" that serves as bearer of these properties and functions. This view leads inevitably to a form of mind–body dualism, which is very unattractive for most scientists and philosophers today (and for Dooyeweerd, too). From a Dooyeweerdian point of view, the argument is based on a non-sequitur, namely, a confusion between the modal and the entitary point of view. Mental properties and functions are not just mental; the phenomena they are referring to are always also synchronously biological, social, and moral, to mention only a few of the most obvious other candidate spheres. The term mental is already a bit confusing because it refers to so many kinds of psychological activity and experience. But all these psychological kinds of functioning presuppose entities (processes) that realize them, and these entities also have other qualifications: they involve the working of certain brain circuits (biotic), they presuppose molecular and metabolic processes in these circuits (physical), and they have a developmental history with psychic, social, cultural, and moral characteristics. In short, mental phenomena are activities, processes, and actions that function in all modal spheres. To see them as immaterial expressions of an immaterial "part" within the organism is mixing the modal point of view (their modal qualification) with the entitary point of view: the psychological aspect of the thing (thought, feeling) is held to be a proof of the existence of a psychic thing (entity) in us. Dooyeweerd strongly opposes this position and would also be very hesitant to speak of levels or layers as ontic realities. Such layers don't exist in reality and are, in fact, the product of the ontologizing (or reification) of a modal point of view. We can distinguish biological, psychological, social, and moral aspects in our functioning as human beings. But that doesn't allow us to conclude that we are composites that are built up of biological, psychological, social, and moral components (layers, levels, or parts).

The implicit assumption of the second, more popular, position (mental phenomena as products of an underlying mechanism or brain process) is also based on confusion between the modal and the entitary point of view, but differently. The point is here that mental phenomena are, first, isolated and, second, conceptualized as products of the preceding operation of another entity or component in the organism, usually the brain, which is conceived as a biotic entity. The problem becomes then how to conceive of the transition from the biotic to the mental. How can non-material mental phenomena be the output of material biotic processes in the brain? The difficulty is, again, the result of a conceptual confusion between modes and entities. Psychological qualities of someone's behavior are first reified to manifestations of a mental reality (a "mind stuff") and subsequently conceived of as the (causal) product of another reality, the brain, which, in turn, is conceived of as a material (physical or biological) substance or organ. The conflation of the modal and entitary point of view leads, in other words, to reification of both mental and bodily (brain) processes and to the artificial separation between production process and product.

The picture of the brain as an organ that produces mental phenomena is as old as the sciences of psychology and psychiatry. It is problematic because it construes causal relationships between processes that, in fact, logically and factually imply one another. Psychological phenomena are always mediated by brain processes and cannot be separated from these processes. Mental processes are embodied; their existence can never be seen apart from this context of embodiment. Brain functioning is also by definition embedded in the functioning of the nervous system as a whole, both the central and the peripheral system. This nervous system functions in its interlacements with the body. The body, in turn, functions in its interlacements with all other aspects of who we are: persons who are interacting with their physical and social environment. This relatedness and these interactions are not secondary to but constitutive for what it is to be a brain, to function as a brain, and to function as a person with a brain and a whole lot of psychological capacities. The production metaphor is therefore wrong. It suggests that mental processes and brain processes are separated in time and that they belong to a different order, logically and factually. Mental (psychological) properties indeed fundamentally differ from physical or biotic properties, but these differences are no proof of entitary distinctness.

8.2.3 Dooyeweerd on laws, order, and transcendental ideas

Let us return to the relationship between modal aspects and laws. The distinctness of kinds of property, we have said, reflects the irreducible distinctness in the way laws determine what exists and occurs. What is meant by this statement?

Dooyeweerd is a (kind of) realist with respect to laws and, consequently, to order. He holds, more precisely, a transcendental view of laws. In the transcendental view, laws exist as conditions, without which the things for which they hold would not exist. The term transcendental refers to fundamental concepts and/or conditions that need to be presupposed in order to conceive of certain states of affairs in the world as real and existing. This necessity is not only logical—as in the Kantian, idealistic version of transcendental philosophy—but also ontological, or cosmological, as Dooyeweerd prefers to say. The absence of these transcendental conditions would render impossible not only logical thinking but also our everyday experience and even existence itself. The existence of flowers, for instance, requires (i.e., necessarily presupposes) laws or lawful regularities in the spatial, physical, and biotic sphere. We have a pretheoretical understanding of plants as living things. This intuition of what it is "to live" or "to be living" is translated into biological (i.e., theoretical) terms. But this theoretical approach to what it is for a plant to live falls short. We have numerous theoretical concepts (physiological, biochemical, molecular) referring to what it is to live or to be living, but none of them fully grasps the meaning of living. In order to do justice to the pretheoretical intuition that the biotic aspect is fundamentally distinct from the physical and spatial aspects of the flower, we need a notion of modal distinctness that neither reduces biotic distinctness to cultural and/or subjective habits (as in constructivist epistemologies) nor identifies it with things in the world that can be objectified and conceptually grasped (as in rationalistic or scientistic ontologies). The proper meaning of being biotic cannot theoretically be deduced or scientifically be defined. The meaning of what it is to live transcends, so to say, the logical conception of living.

An analogy with beauty may be helpful in this respect: Beauty as a real-life phenomenon entails more than what is meant by the theoretical concept of beauty. What it is for a piece of music or poem to be beautiful cannot be defined in a scientific way. I am not referring to a distinction between subjective and objective understanding, but to the distinction pretheoretical ("holistic") and theoretical ("reduced") ways of understanding. Scientific concepts only highlight the logically graspable aspects of things. Concepts are logical artefacts. However, beauty is more than its concept. The logical concept of beauty is a derivative of beauty in its full sense. What beauty is can hardly been expressed, even in ordinary language. Beauty must be experienced; it emanates as an enigmatic quality of our experience. It is there, undeniable, and we can approach it in different ways: by undergoing the experience, by scientific study of all sorts, by practicing the relevant form of art, or by learning from what others say about their experiences. But, in all these instances, we never grasp a fixed conceptual structure behind or within the phenomenon itself. We intuit that there is something special and distinct in the phenomenon of beauty, but we cannot define it.

Let us now, for the sake of the argument, presume that beauty is the essential feature of the aesthetical aspect. Then, Dooyeweerd would say something like this: Just as the essential feature (or "meaning kernel") of the aesthetic aspect cannot be grasped conceptually, theoretically, or scientifically, so too the essential feature of the biotic aspect cannot be conceptually, theoretically, or scientifically defined. This also would hold for all the other aspects: They have essential features that transcend their scientific/theoretical conceptualization. These features should rather be conceived of as presupposed (i.e., as being always already there) than as products of theoretical/philosophical reflection. This is what Dooyeweerd has in mind when he speaks about the irreducible nature of the modal aspects.

In the above, we have connected Dooyeweerd's conception of law with his ideas about modal aspects, especially their logical and cosmological irreducibility. We can now see why this connection can be made. The lawful order is not a logical, but a transcendental order; it is an order that we should presuppose as being necessarily there in how things behave and are, according to Dooyeweerd. Laws hold, which means that they determine how things exist.

Transcendental conditions are special in the sense that they refer to realities of which we have a pretheoretical intuition but to which we have no immediate epistemic access. Our pretheoretical intuitions can be deepened and explicated into theoretical, philosophical intuitions. But these intuitions remain fallible. They do not form a firm conceptual, logical foundation for any possible science. They function more as invitations to thinking and interpretation. Behind these considerations looms the old (Kantian) distinction between concept and idea. Concepts can be grasped by pure (i.e., theoretical or scientific) reason; they can accurately be defined. Transcendental ideas cannot accurately be defined; they are intuitions or invitations. They offer a clue about what transcends theoretical understanding and what nevertheless should be supposed as true and existing within theoretical understanding, for example, the irrevocable distinctness between the different modes of functioning.

It will be clear that Dooyeweerd's conception of law differs from what scientists use to call law (or principle) or lawful regularity/pattern. Scientific laws are interpretations, or approximations, of a lawful order. They are not the order itself. Dooyeweerd's notion of law and of a lawful order are (transcendental) boundary concepts for theoretical thinking. Dooyeweerd suggests that scientists and philosophers need to presuppose the existence of a lawful order to make sense of the regularities and causally relevant relations they discover in their sciences. It is based on the (transcendental) presupposition that there is such order, that scientists are able and entitled to discern the more mundane laws of their respective branches of science, he says. The laws that the sciences discover are interpretations, fallible attempts to grasp the order of reality.

Let us now take one final step with respect to this notion of transcendental order. We have strong pretheoretical intuitions, Dooyeweerd says, about the fundamental diversity of reality, a diversity that finds its origins in a cosmic order that transcends our logical mode of knowing and of which we also have no empirical proof. In a similar fashion, Dooyeweerd also speaks of other important (transcendental) features of our knowledge, experience, and existence, especially of the coherence, unity, and origin of the cosmic order we inhabit. The fundamental diversity in our experience of reality reflects the fundamental distinctness of laws and how they hold. There is, however, also and at the same time a fundamental connectedness between the things in the world and between us and the world. This experience of connectedness reflects what is theoretically expressed by the term coherence, as a transcendental idea. Coherence and diversity belong together; they are two sides of the same coin and indicate the first transcendental idea. The experience of meaning—the fact that things refer to one another, together with the suggestion that their connectedness reflects a deeper wholeness and unity—is the pretheoretical precursor of the transcendental idea of unity, which is the second transcendental idea. This sense of unity and wholeness requires in turn a notion of origin of meaning, according to Dooyeweerd. This is expressed in the third transcendental idea, that of an origin of meaning. Diversity (in conjunction with coherence), unity, and origin are the three most fundamental ideas or transcendental presuppositions of our experience of reality and of reality itself.

8.2.4 Do we still need this philosophy?

I am aware that many readers will have difficulty swallowing these statements. The question arises whether we really need this difficult and unpopular transcendental conception of law and of an underlying lawful order. What are Dooyeweerd's arguments? Isn't it sufficient to maintain a much more pragmatic notion of law, such as the notion of laws as models for the lawful regularities we notice in the object under study or laws in the sense of the regularities (equations, statistical probabilities), constants, and definitions scientists work with in their everyday practices?

Let me give two responses to these doubts, one more pragmatic, the other more fundamental. The pragmatic response runs as follows: Maybe we don't need Dooyeweerd's strict notion of law in the everyday practice of laboratory research, or while digesting large amounts of data, as in genetic or epidemiological research. But some of Dooyeweerd's core concerns are always on the table, especially his concerns about diversity, coherence, and wholeness (unity). Ultimately, scientists must face the question of how their findings should be interpreted and fit into a larger picture of the world. Old, well-known questions will then recur. What does this hypothesis or theory mean with respect the object under study? What does it say in a larger context? Are the reductions valid and to what extent? Coherence and wholeness are always on the agenda, not only in science itself but also in its applications. References to these broader notions inevitably emerge when scientists tell their stories to colleagues or the broader public. Pointing out what we know about the brain, the origin of the universe, or our genes inevitably brings the scientist to a point where his or her implicit assumptions can no longer be kept private. Ultimate questions about coherence, wholeness, and meaning can never completely be evaded, particularly not outside the laboratory or other research settings.

There is also a more fundamental, philosophical reason for Dooyeweerd's difficult, transcendental route. The argument for cosmic order and for the (modal) distinctness of laws is indirect and, in fact, a philosophical conjecture, he would say, and it is a conjecture that is defensible given the unattractiveness of some of the alternatives. Trying to account for what we know without presupposing the ideas of order and law sooner or later leads to inconsistency, he suggests. More precisely, without the presupposition of a (transcendental) cosmic order, our philosophical position would easily slip either toward a nominalistic or toward a rationalistic position. Nominalists traditionally say that laws only exist in our minds. Rationalists think that the order of reality is intelligible and that laws can be accessed and known by (theoretical) reason.

Both positions are unattractive for Dooyeweerd. He rejects nominalism because it removes the point of contact between the sciences and everyday experience. For Dooyeweerd, pretheoretical intuitions are important, not because they are always true, but because they shed light on the different forms of distinctness (and coherence) in the cosmic order. This distinctness (and sense of coherence) is lost as soon as the scientific attitude is adopted. From a more practical perspective, nominalism is also unattractive because it is so much in contrast with the common-sense realism of most scientists. Their hypotheses are conjectures about what they think really exists. Nominalism with respect to laws would, in other words, introduce a contradiction into the heart of the empirical sciences.

Dooyeweerd's resistance against rationalism is mainly based on and, in fact, coincides with his objections against classical realism (as espoused by Aristotle and the scholastics). Classical realism supposes that we can grasp the order of reality with our intellectual faculties. The capabilities of our intellect, in other words, comply with the intelligibility of reality. Dooyeweerd rejects this position because it ultimately absolutizes theoretical reason, or, more precisely, the theoretical attitude of thought. For Dooyeweerd, theoretical reasoning is always a derivative of our everyday understanding of the world. What is lost in the theoretical attitude is the "indissoluble interrelation" among the modal aspects, which present themselves as completely interwoven within our everyday experience (NC I, p. 3). This everyday understanding is, of course, less precise and more subject to error than scientific knowing, but it is characterized by a holism, as well as a sense of diversity, that is very characteristic for our understanding of the world and that fades away as soon as the scientific attitude is adopted. The experience of coherence and diversity is so fundamental that we cannot go behind it, neither by reasoning nor by experience; and not even by a scientific reconstruction of the phenomenological properties of our experience.

Dooyeweerd's position may still raise many questions. For instance, it seems to thrive on what some would call a certain mysterianism (i.e., on pretheoretical intuitions that only partially can be made explicit in the form transcendental ideas). Let me concede that for readers with a primarily empirical scientific interest, philosophical details about the status of transcendental conceptions are less relevant. However, what remains is that something is lost when scientists adopt their scientific attitude and that it is crucially important to acknowledge this. What is lost is, basically, the pretheoretical awareness of diversity, coherence, and wholeness that is typical for our everyday mode of knowing.

Today our scientific image of the world has in many respects merged with our pretheoretical understandings. It is very much in line with Dooyeweerd's philosophy to see this as a challenge, as the inevitable counterpart of the differentiation of our culture and not as something which is inherently wrong or deplorable. Today, it is important to recognize such mergers and to investigate what they imply and mean.

8.2.5 Dooyeweerd on the "heart"

Let us finally turn to Dooyeweerd's other core idea, which concerns our functioning as humans, individually and collectively. It is Dooyeweerd's deep conviction that all human functioning is ultimately rooted in what he calls the "heart." The heart is the concentration point of our existence. The term refers to the idea that we humans are driven by fundamental concerns, motivations, commitments, and convictions. These commitments and convictions are not only individual psychological realities; they have an existential and moral/spiritual core and typically aim at what is beyond the horizon of our knowledge and experience (something "greater than us"). The heart itself is not something that can be studied with empirical means; it is presupposed, and it expresses itself in all human functioning, most clearly and explicitly in the worldview of a person.

Dooyeweerd's Christian, neo-Calvinist inspiration is definitely important in this idea of rootedness in the "heart" and of striving beyond the horizon of our knowledge and experience. However, Dooyeweerd goes to great lengths to defend the universality of the idea of the heart as origin of an existential/religious dynamic. This idea is not a philosophical translation of insights taken from a local religious tradition but refers to a reality that is structurally given. All human beings are inclined to transcendence, so to speak, independent of their ethnicity or religion. This inclination is ingrained and structurally given. Philosophy cannot answer the question of what (or who) it is that this existential dynamic is aimed at. It can only argue that the deepest and most central human commitments focus on an ultimate meaning of which the source cannot be grasped, explained, or experienced. Dooyeweerd calls this source "origin" or "origin of meaning." This source of meaning lies beyond the horizon of experience and reflection.

The difficulty with conceptualizing the notion of the heart is that it cannot be equated with functioning in one or another modal aspect or be identified with a part of our biopsychosocial existence. It is not the same as aesthetic feeling, or moral sensitivity, or religious openness, although these may represent what is "in" our hearts. We could call the functioning of the heart a "dynamic," which itself is not bound to one modal aspect and which resonates with a person's character, morality, ethos, and worldview. If the modal aspects are plotted on the Y-axis, then the activity of the heart could be plotted on the X-axis. Followers of Dooyeweerd have described this as a relation between structure and direction. Structure refers then to modal functioning (Y-axis) and direction to the existential, moral, and/or religious dynamic within a person, group, or culture (X-axis).

8.2.6 Dooyeweerd on absolutization

From the above, it requires no great leap to understand where things go wrong for Dooyeweerd in philosophy and in the sciences. This occurs when philosophers or scientists ignore the transcendence of the notion of order and the transcendental nature of the ideas of diversity/coherence, unity, and origin. This ignorance inevitably leads to identification of some aspect of reality with what these transcendental notions stand for and represent. This identification means that something within reality (say, elementary particles and the laws they are subjected to) is held to be the ultimate foundation (origin), the most unifying element (unity), and/or the ultimate binding principle (coherence) of reality. Dooyeweerd calls this absolutization. Absolutization occurs when an aspect or part of reality is set apart and dealt with as if it is self-sustaining (as substance), has a meaning by itself, and is the ultimate source (origin) of unity and coherence in the world. This absolutizing is the same as what earlier was called "reification."

Absolutizations are characteristic for what Dooyeweerd calls "immanence" philosophies, which consider one element or aspect of the world as the basic material and/or most fundamental explanatory principle for all that exists. The -isms in the sciences refer to such absolutizations (physicalism, biologism, psychologism, and so on). Other examples are less bound to one modal aspect and related to major themes in cosmology, epistemology, or anthropology: the absolutization of individual freedom, for instance; or the exclusive reliance on reason and scientific thinking; or utopian ideas about the malleability of the social and cultural world.

It is one of the main thrusts of Dooyeweerd's philosophy to unmask these absolutizations. It is his philosophical bet that the absolutization of an aspect (or part) of reality always leads to inner contradictions in one's overall conception of reality. This is because absolutization by itself is already a form of reality distortion. Distortions resulting from absolutization inevitably lead to tensions in one's overall picture of reality and, therefore, to what Dooyeweerd calls inner antinomies. One-sided emphasis on scientific and/or technological control for instance causes problems in one's concept of freedom. One-sided emphasis on human freedom is incompatible with the idea that we are in many ways determined by our biology and culture. This also holds for the analysis Western culture. Long before Adorno and Horkheimer published their landmark study *Dialektik der Aufklärung* (*Dialectic of the Enlightenment*) (Adorno and Horkheimer 1947), Dooyeweerd had already pointed out that there is a fundamental tension between technocratic control and individual freedom, or between "the ideal of science" and the "ideal of personhood" (being a free person). This tension or polarity is irresolvable without a fundamental critique of the presumed autonomy of scientific reason. Dooyeweerd speaks in this context of an irresolvable dialectic in the ground motive of our culture. The root of this dialectic is a dogmatic adherence to the idea of the autonomy of (scientific) reason. A real critical philosophy will adopt a reflective attitude toward its own biases, including the bias of a one-sided scientistic look at reality.

Dooyeweerd entertained an extensive dialogue with scientists and philosophers during his time—neo-Kantians, positivists, and phenomenologists alike—to show the inter-antinomies in their thinking. His most important target was the absolutization of theoretical thought itself. It is the presumed autonomy of theoretical reasoning that lies at the heart of the crisis in philosophy and the culture of his days, he says. Scientism can be seen as a variant of this absolutization. Scientism is the view that it is science and science alone that gives us access to true knowledge of what exists. Philosophers and scientists who accept and proclaim this idea tend to think that their work is critical, independent, and objective. Dooyeweerd's thesis would instead be that their work is not critical enough. The presumption of the supremacy of the theoretical view on the world is biased; it forgets that all human activity, theoretical thinking included, is always rooted in attitudes that embody a broader conception of reality. Adherents of scientism insufficiently recognize that the scientifically abstracted aspects of reality they are studying (elementary particles, molecules, cells, and the relationships between them) are not identical to reality itself, and knowledge about other aspects of reality always remains insufficient and inadequate (albeit probably more precise, in certain respects) if caught in terms of these particles, molecules, cells, and their relations. The reductive physicalism that feeds current variants of scientism has transformed legitimate reduction into illegitimate reductionism. This transformation is what Dooyeweerd means by absolutization.

8.3 A virtue-ethical approach to practices

The virtue-ethical concept of practice is attractive because it is substantive and concrete. Moreover, it offers an alternative to some of the weaknesses of two other main traditions within moral theory: duty ethics (or deontology) and utilitarianism (or consequentialism). I briefly indicate general points of disagreement and then translate these general points to the debate on normative practices and professionalism. Many of these issues have already been addressed in previous chapters, albeit from a different angle. I go into slightly more detail with respect to the virtue-ethical approach because it is well-known and shares a considerable amount of common ground with the theory of normative practices as developed in this book.

8.3.1 The virtue-ethical critique on duty ethics and principlism: Alasdair MacIntyre

Virtue-ethical approaches criticize duty ethical, or deontological, approaches to ethics as too formal. The rules and principles duty ethicists discern are so abstract, general, and thin that their interpretation can be manipulated in virtually any direction (MacIntyre 1967, p. 198). This manipulability worry already existed in the 19th century in the form of a critique on the most well-known version of deontology (i.e., Immanuel Kant's), which put the categorical imperative at the center of moral deliberation. On the basis of the categorical imperative, people could defend opposite behaviors by subtly changing of the conditions under which a general rule could be applied. Today, this critique is still heard in the form of a warning against the "potential for avoision" of deontological principles (Alexander & Moore 2016).

A second criticism against duty ethical approaches is that they have a tendency to interpret principles and norms in a legalistic way, as if they merely function as external constraints. One vigorous criticism of duty-oriented (or principlist) approaches to moral issues in medicine can be found in the work of Pellegrino (2008, p. 157), who laments the lack of reflection on the moral foundations of professionalism. Reflection on medicine should start with a philosophical analysis of what it is to be sick, he says, and then proceed by making explicit why the relationship of a doctor with a sick person is intrinsically moral. Without this broader foundation in medical philosophy, medical ethics ends up with lists of virtues and duties that lack inner necessity and coherence. For Pellegrino, a natural law approach along Aristotelian and neo-Thomist lines offers the most promising route to such a fundamental reflection.

There is a striking similarity between these criticisms and the worries about the concept of professionalism discussed in Chapter 5. There, we heard Margolis' (2015) plea for a medical professionalism based on fiduciary duty. The adjective fiduciary refers to the need for duties to be supported by inner conviction (or character, as virtue ethicists would say) and by a commitment that reaches deeper than merely respect for laws. The suggestion is as subtle as it is important. Duties alone are not enough; they are too thin and external to serve as the basis for a restoration of trust.

Similar concerns have also been expressed about the principlist approach of Beauchamp's and Childress (2013) (Holm 1995; Rauprich 2008). Their influential *Principles of Biomedical Ethics* describes how moral problems in medicine can be made manageable by relating them to the four medical ethical principles: autonomy, beneficence, doing no harm, and justice. These principles are, so to say, mid-level constructs, somewhere in-between views at the level of moral philosophy and the common morale (Rauprich 2008). Lee (2010) calls the four principles "thick in status" but "thin in content." The thinness of the principles indicates that they lack content and that their application allows much interpretative variation in concrete cases; thick in status means that the principles nevertheless play a strong prescriptive role.

Concerns about the thinness of duties may be legitimate, but this does not mean that laws, or even administrative regulations, are unimportant. They are undeniably of crucial importance. Laws and regulations are conditional, however. Without them, medical practice in its current form could never have gotten off the ground. But, as recent discussions have shown, medical practice needs more than this; not only legal entitlement but also trust. The latter requires trustworthiness, faithfulness, commitment, and dedication. This is what Margolis means when he says that duties need a fiduciary complement. Doctors are only believed when they themselves believe in what they are doing (for a similar analysis in industrial contexts, see Verkerk 2004). In summary, the objection against deontological accounts is that they leave us with a thin and legalistic notion of morality; this objection is echoed in recent discussions about professionalism, for instance in the argument for an enriched ("fiduciary") notion of duty.

8.3.2 The virtue-ethical critique on utilitarianism: Charles Taylor

Consequentialism (or utilitarianism) has other weaknesses. It sees norms and rules as self-chosen ideals or goals (i.e., as the product of subjective desires) and therefore as external to practices. One of the perennial issues in utilitarian approaches concerns the question of what it is that brings people to the point that they give up their natural inclination to egoism and create space for cooperation with others. This was already an issue in Hobbes' initial formulations of contract theory, and it is still a widely debated issue in evolutionary accounts on altruism and morality. The very notion of a (social) contract presupposes a minimal amount of trust. The question has always been whether this minimal amount of trust can be accounted for in terms of utilitarianism itself.

The issue of trust is in turn related to the utilitarian view of the good. Utilitarianism is the theory that conceives moral behavior as the pursuit of the greatest amount of happiness for the greatest number of people. This pursuit is usually framed in the form of rational-purposive action, i.e., in a rational account of the relation between means and ends. Means and ends are not intrinsically coupled in this approach, for instance by tradition or by the inner logic of practices. They are coupled based on rational deliberation about the most effective balance between the two. For the field of labor this implies, as we have seen, an instrumentalistic and functionalistic approach to work and to professionalism.

Proponents of virtue ethics have criticized this instrumentalism. They put the discussion about it in the broader context of the position of the moral subject. What is typical for the utilitarian subject is, as Charles Taylor has called it, the "nakedness" of the self, i.e., its lack of intrinsic connectedness with the goods it attempts to realize, its individualism, and its lack of embeddedness in traditions and communities. Goods have become optional, says Taylor; they are the arbitrary object of our subjective choices. It is the arbitrariness of our choices that lies at the basis of the experiences of meaninglessness and emptiness that are so typical for our era (Taylor 1989, Chapter 1).

Or, paraphrasing the words of another important virtue ethicist, Alasdair MacIntyre, goods are the things we say "hurrah" to. This is what emotivists say. Emotivism is the doctrine that all evaluative and moral judgments are nothing but expressions of preference, attitude, or feelings. MacIntyre sees emotivism as dominating the style of today's moral debate. "Good" means the same as "I approve of this, do so as well" (MacIntyre 1984, p. 12). Characteristic for these and related doctrines is the instrumentalist conception of the relation between the subject and its goods.

Functionalism, instrumentalism, and dissociation between persons, means, and ends are the key terms that capture some important features of today's moral landscape. We have seen that these terms precisely refer to the issues that were the targets of the assault on professionalism. Increasing specialization in terms of knowledge and skills; ongoing division of labor; the growing role of technology; and the expansion of the logistic, financial, and managerial infrastructure for all sorts of professional activity have all contributed to the alienation of the professional from his or her proper role. The relation between doctors and their role has become technical, instrumental, and increasingly driven by market mechanisms. Health is becoming a commodity and healing the instrumental activity that aims at the provision of this commodity. Accountability is more and more guaranteed by the actions of third parties, instead of by the ethos of professionals themselves. Physician competence is defined in terms of outcome criteria and of levels of performance, dissociated from the "telos" of a practice. Even the concept of excellence has become externalized (I refer to what has been said earlier about competences and transferrable skills).

With respect to the solutions that have been proposed, there are similarities between what virtue-ethicists like Charles Taylor propose and the analyses and suggestions that were made with respect to professionalism as a normative practice. The virtue-ethical variant of social ethics and political philosophy is known as communitarianism. Communitarianists like Charles Taylor plead for new forms of social engagement. Taylor thinks that the modern subject is not completely dissociated from his or her spiritual sources. These sources traditionally provided the motivation and inspiration to counteract tendencies to egoism, indifference, and exploitation. New forms of social engagement have a chance if society finds a way to re-establish and invigorate the connections with these sources. This inevitably occurs in a pluralistic way today.

We have heard similar responses to the assault on professionalism. This assault should be counteracted by policies that aim at restoration of trustworthiness, and this was thought to be possible based on new forms of collaboration between varying combinations of stakeholders. Current (mental) healthcare is characterized by a plethora of new forms of collaboration among patients, clinicians, insurers, and representatives of healthcare organizations and the public administration.

Collaborative care is even the name of one of these initiatives. Trust and civic partnership belong to the most cherished keywords in the negotiations about these new forms of collaboration.

In summary, the main objection of virtue ethicists to utilitarian accounts of morality is that they leave us with a moral subject that is dissociated from its intrinsic connection with certain goods. This critique returns in today's assessments of medical professionalism, which shows strong tendencies to functionalism and instrumentalism; the doctor as person has become dissociated from his or her role. The solutions that are proposed in both contexts—the general-societal and the professional context—look similar. Goods are conceived of as embodied in certain practices. Communitarianists stimulate new forms of civic partnership and reconnection with the spiritual sources of one's civilization. Professionals are invited to participate in renegotiations of parts of the social contract between mental healthcare and society.

8.3.3 Virtue-ethical accounts of practices and the NPA: Paul Ricoeur

The normative practice approach (NPA) shares some common ground with the virtue-ethical approach to mental healthcare. Let me enumerate some points of convergence. Both approaches:

- emphasize the intrinsic nature of norms
- are substantive as well as practical
- find their resources in what real people in real-life situations tell about their hopes, concerns, and fears
- are sensitive for the inherent ambiguities of life
- are motivated by an ideal, an overarching goal, i.e., restoration of a certain ethos for the professions and a shared sense of pursuing a common good.

Instrumentalist accounts of professionalism have difficulty accounting for the fact that professions embody values that go beyond those of bureaucratic control and market-driven self-interest. Of course, individual professionals can have their personal values, but however high spirited these may be, they will fail to have an enduring impact on professional practices so long as they are not really embedded in these practices. The NPA emphasizes that values and normative principles constitute the practice of medicine. Norms and values are, in other words, not a subjective addition to a practice that is value neutral in itself. They are not the icing on the cake but the very cornerstones of these practices. Delineating the inherent and shared values and normative principles of a practice is precisely what both virtue ethicists and adherents of the NPA aim to do.

Despite these important commonalities, there are also some differences that need to be addressed. The NPA puts less emphasis on tradition than virtue ethics and has a more positive appreciation of the process of modernization, i.e., the cultural-historical process of social differentiation and integration with its division of labor and its impressive developments in the sphere of technology, science, and economy. The NPA welcomes this process of differentiation and integration and sees it as valuable and important by itself. This positive appreciation does not imply, of course, that the negative sides of the modernization process (alienation, fragmentation, and functionalism) are disregarded.

Unlike virtue ethicists, adherents of the NPA approach are less inclined to locate normativity in traditions and to bind it to communities and character. They also tend to see normativity as an intrinsic quality of relations between subjects and their practices and between subjects within these practices. The normative practice approach is, in other words, more interested in "structure" than in tradition and character. This focus on structure leads, as we have seen, to a refined meshwork of types of norm and normative principle. Each type appeared to have its own function; not statically, but as part of a process of opening up (or closing down) of the practice under study. With respect to (mental) healthcare, we made use of a distinction between foundational, conditioning and qualifying norms/principles.

One other element is the tendency of the NPA to see the normativity of practices not as carved in stone but as a response to what is needed and appropriate in the relevant context. This responding is both self-relational and a reflection of a fundamental openness to what is needed, even (and especially) if this feels unfamiliar, different, and difficult. In philosophical terms, I am drawing a connection between Ricoeur's self-relational approach to personhood and Dooyeweerd's notion of the heart as the sphere of existence out of which our deepest responses, attitudes, and aspirations emerge (see also Glas 2010). This connection is needed because it deepens our understanding and enriches our vocabulary. So far, the dynamic of practices has mostly been conceived of as an unfolding of the inner normative structure of practices (Dooyeweerd). However, the phenomenology of this dynamic needs other, richer, and more plural descriptions. Our deepest motivations are reflected in our attempts to respond to what is needed; in how we attune to other people in their varying conditions; and in our ability to tolerate, recognize, and value the "otherness" of others (Ricoeur). This tolerating, recognizing, and valuing is not easy; it may deprive me of my egocentrism, my certainties, and what I consider to be self-evident.

Let us step back for a while and take up again the thread from Chapters 1 (section 1.4) and 4 (section4.4), in which Ricoeur's self-relational and self-referential account of personal identity was reviewed. We introduced the distinction between *idem* identity and *ipse* identity. Classical accounts of personal identity almost exclusively focus on *idem* identity (i.e., on sameness). Sameness comes in two variants: numerical and qualitative. Numerical identity, or singularity, refers to the bare fact that there is only one who is me (with my unique fingerprints as a bodily expression of that fact). Qualitative identity refers to a general quality or feature that is considered to define a fundamental aspect or property of what it is to be a person. Examples of such features are having a memory of oneself, having a personality, and self-consciousness. Both numerical and qualitative identity, however, are one-sided in that they only refer to sameness. Sameness is about *what* we are, not *who* we are, people with stories, memories, disappointments, and hopes. Who we are is determined by how we relate to ourselves. This is what is meant by the ipseity. Ipseity means selfhood or being oneself. We need ipseity to express who we are. We are not merely things in the world or bundles of properties or functions, but human persons. We are not re-acting, but acting, i.e., persons who speak, interact, interpret and, by doing so, give testimony of who we are, as self-designating beings.

In everyday life, answers to the question "who am I?" usually intersect with answers to the question "what am I?" Answers with respect to "the who" influence "the what," i.e., the way people shape and define specific features of their personhood. The intersection between *ipse* and *idem* manifests itself both in the singularity and the sameness of people. It is expressed in the singularity of persons because it is only me who can be held responsible for acts done by me. It is expressed in the form of sameness when people remain faithful to themselves. The ipseity of the person brings us, in other words, via a transformed and deepened meaning of *idem* into the sphere of personal responsibility, authenticity, and faithfulness to oneself. I interpret this as an echo of Dooyeweerd's idea of interdependence between structural unfolding and the existential dynamic. The idem refers to structural features of one's personhood in different circumstances, the *ipse* to the dynamic of the unfolding I–self relationship, when the self opens up to what is the needed in these circumstances.

With this, Ricoeur highlights a dimension of self-relatedness that goes beyond character and virtue and therefore beyond virtue-ethical approaches to the moral subject. Ricoeur invents a new term to address this dimension: attestation. Attestation is the ultimate expression of self-referential and other-directed responsibility. It is a difficult and somewhat ambiguous concept, in the sense that it refers to both witnessing (being a witness; bearing witness to) and to an elementary sense of being-called-on. Both meanings of attestation refer to otherness. The self, in its very self-relational structure, cannot do without the otherness to which it is attuned. The openness towards otherness is expressed by listening to others, to their narratives, and to what resonates between the lines; by assuming an attitude of responsibility; by allowing others to disturb my life, to pull me out my comfort zone and to deprive me of self-evident and self-sufficient certainties. The self is oneself as another; that is, a self that strives for an openness that is both based on and the expression of the otherness of those whose fate I bear witness to and for whose lives I adopt responsibility by allowing them to urge me to take care of them and to struggle for their well-being.

9

CONCLUSION: FUTURE PROSPECTS

9.1 Where are we?

In Part I of this book, we saw that a scientistic defense of the legitimacy of psychiatry falls short and that we need a richer model of psychopathology. We have also seen that this model is intrinsically relational and that normative aspects form an intrinsic part of these relations. In Part II, we argued for a normative practices approach, which distinguishes between types of norm and between types of (interlocking) context and practice, each context/practice with its own constellation of values and normative principles. We analyzed the normative structure of psychiatry at three contextual levels (micro, meso, and macro), and we investigated the impact of interactions at each of these contextual levels on the object and internal destination of psychiatry. Doing well to the individual patient (*beneficence*) appeared to be the aim of psychiatry at the micro-level. At the meso-level, we identified the concept of *service need*; care arrangements at this level typically aim at meeting the needs for healthcare services of a population in a certain region. At the macro-level, the emphasis shifted to an enriched ("opened-up") notion of *distributive justice*: Governments should guarantee a minimum level of care for every citizen, and, by doing so, express a fundamental solidarity between people. This level of care can be specified in terms of quality, access, safety, rights, and sustainability. Healthcare is a good that should be distributed fairly to those who need it most.

We have, furthermore, argued that there is a certain order between the contexts. The term context refers here, again, to the activities and interactions that constitute the various practices at each contextual level. These practices have their own internal dynamic. Each should optimally be attuned to other practices. All practices together ultimately aim at healthcare as a moral good. This means that healthcare-related activities at meso- and macro-levels should never be conceived as ends-in-themselves, but rather as enabling and sustaining the ultimate internal destination of medicine, which is: doing well to individuals who suffer from disease, impairment, and/or handicap.

To clarify the complexity of the professional role in different contexts, we paid considerable attention to the relationships among contexts, the object of psychiatry, and definitions of the professional role. The self- and context-related approach of psychopathology requires a flexible, broad, and dynamic view of the professional role. Recognition and appreciation of the responsibilities of all the legitimate stakeholders leads to adaptation and fine-tuning of professional roles and to careful definition of how parties relate to one another.

The analysis in Chapters 5 and 6 made it clear that psychiatrists can no longer base the legitimacy of their role solely on their expertise and should seek a broader foundation for their duties. It was suggested that the legitimacy of the activities of professionals and professional groups increasingly depends on the way they interact with and attune their responsibilities to other stakeholders, patients included. So, it is in the quality of their interactions with other stakeholders that psychiatrists and other mental healthcare workers find the grounds for justified trust, i.e., the trust of citizens, funding agencies, representative bodies, and the state. This is not a new situation. Professions have always been based on trust. This trust was and is partially based on the expertness of professionals and partially on the value transactions on which the social contract between medicine and society is based. These value transactions are guaranteed by and depend on the quality of the relations between the profession and other parties. The current contract differs from its earlier versions in that the role of other parties has become much more prominent. Today's value transactions are much more influenced by the voices of patients and patient groups, by public images of mental healthcare, by insurance companies and other funding agencies, and by the legal system.

In summary, the contextually expanded normative practice approach to psychiatry leads not only to a highly dynamic and flexible conception of the professional role but also to a plea to adopt public responsibility for the quality of one's interactions with patients, their representatives, and other stakeholders.

In this chapter, I broaden the focus and locate the normative practice approach in the context of other value-sensitive accounts of psychiatry. I first investigate how other value-sensitive perspectives on psychiatric practice contribute to the understanding of psychiatry as a normative practice. I investigate how these other accounts add to the precision and validity of the NPA and, conversely, how the other concepts and accounts may gain focus and coherence in light of the NPA.

I then briefly go into the prospects of the self- and context-oriented approach to psychopathology as developed in this book in light of new concepts, such as precision medicine, personalized medicine, P-4 medicine, person-centered psychiatry, and the like.

In the third part of the chapter, I discuss the implications of the contextualized version of the NPA and of the self- and other-oriented approach to psychopathology for residency training in psychiatry (see also Glas 2018). Recognition of normative aspects of psychiatric practice requires certain competences and attitudes. I discuss these competencies and make some suggestions about the future of psychiatric education.

In the last part, I focus on the existential dimension of professionalism (see also Glas 2017b). Openness of the professional about his or her own role fulfilment—one's ideals, but also one's ambivalences and insufficiencies—may prove to be a decisive factor for the patient to open up him- or herself. In other words, awareness of and the ability to communicate about the self-referentiality of professional role fulfilment may help the patient to feel accepted and understood. Tensions and ambivalences with respect to this openness and sensitivity in the current system of mental healthcare are discussed.

This chapter, like previous ones, focuses on psychiatry as a clinical practice, not as a science. About the science of psychiatry, a different but related normative analysis could be performed, including an analysis of the way psychiatry as a science understands itself and its context. This is not the topic for this book, however. Relevant developments in the science of psychiatry will be discussed when this is needed for a better understanding of what is going on in the clinical practice of mental healthcare.

9.2 Other value-sensitive approaches to the delivery of healthcare

In this section, I broaden the focus and locate the normative practice approach, as well as the self- and context-oriented approach to psychopathology in the context of other value-sensitive accounts of psychiatry, most notably value-based psychiatry (VBP; Fulford 2008; 2011; Woodbridge & Fulford 2004), values-based healthcare (VBHC; Porter 2009; 2010; Porter & Teisberg 2006), and recovery oriented approaches (Slade 2009). I pay attention to popular notions, such as self-management and shared-decision making; emerging new paradigms, including positive psychology, personalized medicine, and precision medicine; and a couple of new approaches to the organization of mental healthcare, such as flexible assertive community treatment (FACT) and resource group assertive community treatment (RACT), Open Dialogue, integrated care, and positive psychology. Instead of discussing all these accounts, concepts, and approaches at length, I focus on how the different perspectives contribute to an understanding of psychiatry as a normative practice.

9.2.1 Values-based practice (VBP)

Values-based practice was initially developed as an approach to clinical decision making. Medical decisions are increasingly made against the background of complex and conflicting values, says Fulford (2008, p. 11). This complexity is characteristic not only for the clinical encounter but also for other areas. Think, for instance, of negotiations and interactions that focus on quality, effectiveness, efficiency, prevention, public health, and quality of life measurement. Empirical evidence is not immediately applicable in all these areas and needs translation. Values are the missing link between evidence and practice. They determine the relevance of scientific insights and of the protocols and guidelines that are based on them. Fulford speaks of a two-tiered approach to healthcare. Evidence-based medicine and values-based practice are complementary and support one another.

Fulford has developed his view over the years, from his *Moral Theory and Medical Practice* (1989) via the workbook *Whose Values?* (Woodbridge & Fulford 2004) and many papers and chapters (for instance, Colombo et al. 2003; Fulford 2004; 2008; 2011; Fulford & Benington 2004) to a whole range of initiatives in the field of policymaking, education, research, collaboration, and publication, not only in psychiatry, but also in other areas of medicine. It is no exaggeration to say that VBP has become one of the most, if not the most, influential philosophical approach to mental healthcare. Among its successes is the establishment of the *NIMHE* (National Institute for Mental Health in England) *Values Framework*, which defines a number of key principles of VBP. This framework has become the basis for several policy and service development initiatives in the United Kingdom.

Fulford describes VBP as a primarily skills-oriented approach. It is based on insights from various sources: analytic philosophy, linguistic analysis, bioethics, phenomenology, hermeneutics, and quantitative and qualitative empirical research. It also offers a process for working more effectively with complex and conflicting values in medicine (Fulford 2008). Fulford builds on R.M. Hare by describing values as action-oriented prescriptions. These prescriptions are:

> [W]ider than ethics and include all the many ways in which we express positive and negative evaluations, including preferences, needs, wishes, etc., as well as ethical values. (Fulford 2011)

VBP has always been strong in its emphasis on diversity and on inclusion of the service user perspective. It is practically oriented and responsive to empirical evidence. It embraces a democratic style of discussing and of searching for common ground.

There are ten key elements that characterize VBP: four practice skills (awareness, reasoning, knowledge, and communication), two models of service delivery (user centered and multidisciplinary), three ideas about the relationship between VBP and evidence-based practice (EBP) (see below), and partnership, i.e., the idea that decisions should be taken by service users and providers of care together. The three ideas about the relationship between VBP and EBP are the two-feet (or two-tier) principle, indicating that decisions are based on facts and values together; the "squeaky wheel principle," suggesting that values are especially noticed when there is a problem; and the interdependence between science and values, which, for example, is shown when scientific insight creates choices in healthcare that call into play different values.

The heterogeneity of these different elements illustrates that VBP is much more than merely a philosophical framework. Its innovative potential lies in a radical choice for practice, for diversity, and for the contextualization of insights from many different corners in philosophy and the humanities. VBP does not offer a model, but a toolbox of insights, concepts, and methods that helps clinicians, policymakers, and managers explore their respective fields of expertise and interact with one another. VBP does not guide one toward an ideal-typical conception of healthcare, but it also does not preach that "anything goes." With its emphasis on diversity and principles of democracy, VBP prohibits racial exclusivism and expresses an inclination toward support for the vulnerable and the weak. VBP also shows high esteem for shared canons; it locates itself, for instance, explicitly within boundaries that are drawn by national and international ethical guidelines. It also advocates for conceptual rigor and fine-grained analysis of the logical structure of arguments and ideas. All this prevents VBP from becoming relativistic.

How does VBP relate to the view on professionalism developed in this book? I see the two approaches mostly as complementary and overlapping, but with differences in emphasis. It is interesting and important that VBP and NPA both characterize themselves as offering more than just another approach to medical ethics. Earlier in this book (6.1.1), we explained why the notion of normativity, as we use it in this book, entails more than moral norms and principles only. A similar broad concept of value is expressed by VBP when it defines values as action prescriptions that are relevant for the whole range of interests, preferences, evaluations, needs, and wishes people may have. There are also points of divergence between the two approaches. One is that the NPA is more explicit about the nature of normativity and, especially, about the different types of normativity. It distinguishes between differences in the roles of norms and normative principles. They may, for instance, function in a foundational, a qualifying, or a conditioning sense. There also appeared to be more than one type of norms within each of the three broader categories. VBP, contrariwise, has a more explicit focus on policy and policymaking in a wide variety of contexts. It offers a fascinating perspective on how philosophy can be put into practice.

The most important point of divergence is that the NPA has the explicit aim of overcoming the duality between facts and values and between evidence-based and values-based practice, whereas VBP seems to take these dualities for granted. One sometimes gets the impression that the implicit acceptance of these dualities by adherents of VBP has a primarily strategic goal, i.e., that of convincing adherents of the EBM paradigm, whether in science or in the quarters of policymakers and business administrators. From an NPA perspective, there is no such large divide between science and professional practice; science can, in fact, itself be interpreted as a professional practice, albeit with different aims and a different normative structure than clinical practice. Contexts are everywhere. There is no value-free, context-free, universally applicable knowledge in science or elsewhere. What VBP says about the task of values for clinical practice, i.e., that they help to bridge the gap between knowledge and practice, can be extended to other contexts as well and, especially, to science. What concepts, hypotheses, theories, and empirical findings mean for relevant groups in their contexts is a matter of interpretation, of weighing of evidence in light of the values that are relevant in the various contexts.

9.2.2 Values-based healthcare (VHBC)

Despite the similarity between their names, values-based healthcare (VBHC) offers a totally different, much more economical and policy-oriented view on how values can be conceptualized (and operationalized) in the context of healthcare than VBP.

The concept of VBHC was born out of unease with the unexplained and unpredictable variation in costs and outcomes in healthcare (Porter & Teisberg 2006; 2007). Skyrocketing costs in healthcare led to a preoccupation with cost shifting and cost reduction. Porter and Teisberg (2007, p. 1104) describe the usual reflex among policymakers, executive officers, and business administrators, which is to reduce costs by increasing productivity and efficiency. Another reflex is the merging of institutions to gain more bargaining clout on rates and to sign up more physician groups to guarantee referrals. Both authors are very critical about these reflexes and the kind of competition that results from them. It leads to healthcare practices in which "each player in the system gains not by increasing value for the patient but by taking value away from someone else." Healthcare organizations tend to measure costs and outcomes around departments, physician specialties, discrete service areas, and line items such as drugs and supplies (Porter 2010). Such outcome measures are not a reflection of quality for the patient. Instead, they reflect benefit to the organization and the financing of care.

Porter and Teisberg (2006) warn against competition based on the wrong outcomes. Costs and outcomes should be measured around the patient. They urge creation of value-based competition on results. The current system is disastrous because it strives for zero-sum competition. This is the type of competition in which one player's win is another's loss. They propose, instead, positive-sum competition, which is about creating and improving value, defined as "more customer benefit per dollar spent." Values need to be defined in terms of outcomes over the entire care cycle of a disease or health problem and over various dimensions (see later). Patient value is defined as outcome divided by the costs.

Physicians must lead the system change that is needed. After all, they are the ones who can increase the value of care. Changes in the system of healthcare delivery should be "market driven but physician led" (Porter & Teisberg 2007).

There are three principles on which the change toward a value-based system is grounded:

1. the goal of the change is to increase value for patients
2. care delivery should be organized around medical conditions and care cycles
3. results are measured.

Measuring outcomes is a big issue in current mental healthcare. In his *New England Journal of Medicine* landmark paper, Porter (2010) proposes a three-tiered hierarchy in measuring outcomes. Each tier has two dimensions or levels. These dimensions or levels are measured with the use of one or more specific metrics. On top (tier 1 outcomes) are survival (first dimension) and the health status that is achieved or retained (second dimension). Survival can be measured over various periods appropriate to a given medical condition. In cancer care, one- and five-year survival periods are common metrics. For other conditions, it is not always the duration of survival per se that matters. In older patients, for instance, other outcomes may weigh more heavily. The other dimension, the health status that is achieved or retained, includes relevant aspects of one's functional status and freedom from disease (or symptoms).

Second tier outcomes are related to the recovery process. The first dimension concerns the time to recovery and to return to normal or best attainable activities. If needed, this time dimension can be split into various phases. The other, process-related dimension of tier 2 consists of the disutility of care or treatment process in terms of discomfort, complications, efficiency, and diagnostic and other errors and their consequences.

Tier 3 outcomes focus on the sustainability of health. The first dimension captures recurrences of the disease or long-term complications. The second dimension refers to new health problems that occur because of treatment. These health problems are not side-effects of treatment (these are measured in tier 2) but new problems. Examples include increased incidence of secondary cancer after treatment for breast cancer or risk of complex fracture after knee replacement. New health problems may also come in the form of the long-term consequences of a given treatment. Examples of such consequences are premature osteoporosis in breast cancer and loss of mobility due to inadequate rehabilitation in knee replacement.

Since 2006, Porter and Teisberg's concept of values-based healthcare (VBHC) has developed into a worldwide movement, with local groups, initiatives, and advisory boards developing strategies to implement changes in clinical governance, outcome measurement, and financing of care. The key issue of VBHC is how to find a coherent, fair, and adequate notion of patient value. It is the aim of VBHC to bring together and do justice to the entire range of quality parameters. But how should this be done? How should VBHC develop a coherent set of quality parameters, when these parameters find their roots in such heterogeneous contexts (micro, meso, and macro), are operationalized and used by so many parties with so different duties and responsibilities (providers, insurers, professional groups, patients, and patient movements), and refer to such a wide variety of aspects of the care cycle (outcome, process, and structure)? And can the intrinsic quality of the caring practice itself also be part of the calculation. Can this intrinsic (moral) quality be measured?

It is encouraging that patient values and patient experiences are central in the VHBC movement. They "open up" the managerial, financial, and social constitutive elements of healthcare to patient value as a moral good. My worries are about the role of the overarching framework; that is, does it merely serve as a (conceptual, philosophical) guiding idea? Or does it function as the early version of a new managerial blueprint? From an NPA perspective, these two should be distinguished. The NPA would welcome the first interpretation (guiding idea) and would hesitate with respect to the second (blueprint). This is because blueprints usually lead to new one-sidedness. They are unavoidable but always risky. They are unavoidable, because, ultimately, professional groups, policymakers, insurance companies, and other representative bodies must coordinate their activities and come up with healthcare plans, public health policies, long-term assessments, and so on. But these plans, policies and measurements are always translations of a general, undoubtfully valuable idea into the practical and one-sided language of products, processes and their technical, logistic, and social infrastructure. VHBC operationalizes outcomes in terms rooted in macro- and regional economics, business administration, and logistics. The risk is not the translation itself, which is unavoidable, but lack of recognition of what is lost in the translation. There exists a gap between the rich notion of outcome ("patient value") that served as a guiding idea and the primarily managerial version of VBHC after the translation and operationalization of guiding ideas. I do not reject VHBC as an overarching perspective on outcome- or quality-driven healthcare. I only warn that VHBC in its operationalizations may easily slip back into one or another well-known variant of managerialism. At the end of the day, parties should agree about how to run healthcare from an encompassing perspective. At that moment parties will be inclined, like in the old days, to focus on measurable performance, efficiency, and sustainability, i.e., they will focus on results and on enabling factors at the conditioning side of healthcare. There is nothing wrong with this focus as such. However, it should always be made subservient to the ultimate internal destination of healthcare, which is to heal the sick and to serve the weak. Values related to the conditions for healthcare must be balanced with the moral aims of helping relationships themselves.

In summary, the NPA offers three insights that help to sharpen the focus of the VHBC:

- It locates the VHBC at the meso- and macro-levels of organization of healthcare, and it suggests that this approach interprets its role as serving the internal, moral destination of healthcare at the micro-level of organization.
- It highlights that the VHBC approach will mainly impact the conditioning aspects of the practice of healthcare and that these aspects should, ultimately, be opened up toward and be subservient to the moral aims of medicine.
- It emphasizes the intrinsic normativity of relations that constitute healthcare practices, a normativity that is, in turn, characterized by the attuning of responsibilities of parties.

I am aware that this attuning of responsibilities usually does not consist of a peaceful exchange of preferences and opinions. It is, in fact, often determined by struggles between competing interests, differences in the valuing of these interests, manipulations of this valuing, and messy powerplay. But this unfortunate reality should not detract us from endorsing a normative practice approach.

From a conceptual point of view, it is important to underscore that values are not things, or characteristics of things. They are not out there; they become real in interactions, by filling in the space between oneself and others and between oneself, one's interests, and those of others.

We touch here the deepest dimension of the discussion about values and their relation to the intrinsic normativity of professional and other relations: values—that is, what we experience and interpret as valuable—are both intuited as intrinsic normative dimensions of practices and creatively developed and embodied in the interactions that constitute these practices. I use this double terminology—of intuiting and developing—to illuminate and retain the idea that the gaps between oneself and one's ultimate concerns and between oneself and others and their ultimate concerns will never be closed. This incongruence is not merely an imperfection; it is a "place" that invites professional creativity to give shape to and to reshape "the valuable." It is in this shaping and reshaping that participants respond to the intrinsic normative dimensions of their relationships.

Parties always have their own perspectives on values, even the same values. To mention one obvious example, successful treatment is operationalized differently by clinicians and by consumers. Reconciling these differences remains a challenge. Clinicians are inclined to think in terms of symptom reduction, consumers in terms of reduction of discomfort, pain, and fear. The practice of consultation, diagnosis, and treatment is based on the attuning of the roles of both the clinician and the patient. This is why we introduced the NPA not as a blueprint or a set of guidelines but as a heuristic framework that may help orient discussions and shed light on possible guiding ideas and normative dimensions of the clinical encounter. The NPA offers no quick fix for negotiations about seemingly irreconcilable issues. It guides participants to ideas and intuitions about the aims and the meaning of their interactions and negotiations. It calls them to search for connectedness and develop responsible behavior with respect to intuitions that guide participants toward these aims and meanings. This guidance leaves room for new interpretations and creative reappraisal of what matters in each situation.

To identify outcome with patient value is, therefore, both worthwhile and begging the question. Values are the expression and embodiment of interactions. It is in the interaction, i.e., in the actualization of the in-between between people with different roles, concerns, and responsibilities, that values are actualized and made explicit. There is not one stakeholder who owns the discussion or defines the values, even not from an overarching perspective. How values are articulated depends on who speaks, on who is speaking on behalf of whom, in which context, at which moment, and under what kind of jurisdiction or responsibility. There is, I repeat, no real overarching perspective, no comprehensive plan, no blueprint, no model, not even a normative practice model, except as a guiding idea. The NPA offers no more than a heuristic framework or a set of such guiding ideas. This explains why, in the further elaboration of the NPA, we put the notions of responsibility and of attuning of responsibilities so centrally. The concept of responsibility acknowledges both the irreducibility of what one is up to, one's relationship with a certain good, and the distance between this calling and its factual and proper realization. Following the NPA means that, by definition, the work is always in progress. Conceived in this way, patient values and outcomes are not measurable things, once and for all, but the temporary result of negotiations between responsible parties.

I am not here arguing against the measurement of outcomes. On the contrary, new technologies and forms of data management offer dazzling possibilities to inform responsible agents about what is going on in terms of outcome, process, and structure. The issue is that this information is not merely information; it is not neutral and meaningless input for intricate decision processes. Information provided by data-management systems and routine outcome monitoring devices acquires meaning in the negotiations and interactions between relevant parties. The same can be said about other outcomes.

To close this section, it should be mentioned that the normative practice approach itself may profit from VBHC as a comprehensive approach. VBHC offers suggestions for further refinement of the NPA, for instance in the idea that patient value is bound to a temporal horizon (tier 2, first element). VBHC is also exemplary in its attempt to do justice to the full complexity of the current healthcare system. I am not sure that most adherents of the approach stick to my more philosophical interpretation of patient value. Attempts to develop integral quality measures are important and worthwhile, provided that they themselves are properly valued (i.e., as comprehensive measures of what is happening on the conditioning side of medicine).

9.2.3 Recovery-oriented approaches

The recovery-oriented approach has become a preeminent crystallization point for discussions about the interdependence among contexts, professional roles, and the purposes of mental healthcare. The approach began as a consumer movement in the late 1980s. It was affected by the impact of long-term outcome studies, which suggested a course for chronic psychiatric conditions such as schizophrenia that was more positive than had previously been thought possible (Harding et al. 1987; Jablensky et al.1992). The widespread idea that schizophrenia is associated with an almost uniform, unfavorable outcome with gradual intellectual and socioemotional decline was proved to be wrong. Warner (2004) mentions percentages of complete recovery in 20–25% and of "social" recovery in still another 40–45% of patients. Complete recovery is defined as "loss of psychotic symptoms and return to pre-illness level of functioning" and "social recovery" as a regaining of "economic and residential independence and low social disruption." This distinction was complemented with the analogous distinction between clinical and personal recovery. The recovery movement is interested in the latter. Anthony (1993) describes recovery as follows:

> [A] deeply personal, unique process of changing one's attitudes, values, feelings, goals, skills, and/or roles. It is a way of living a satisfying, hopeful, and contributing life even within the limitations caused by illness. Recovery involves the development of new meaning and purpose in one's life as one grows beyond the catastrophic effects of mental illness.

This focus on personal recovery means for the professional at least a fundamental change in attitude. In the words of Slade (2010):

> [R]ecovery is not about "getting rid" of problems. It is about seeing people beyond their problems—their abilities, possibilities, interests and dreams—and recovering the social roles and relationships that give life value and meaning.

From here, it is no great leap to see connections with related concepts and notions such as empowerment, self-management, shared decision making, peer support, and the patient as expert (Roberts & Wolfson 2004). The recovery movement puts much emphasis on patient narratives, on the sharing of tacit knowledge among patients, and on positive psychology. Its different approach to psychopathology requires a different role for the psychiatrist (Slade 2009). The professional becomes a participant in the life of the patient, and he or she acts more like a personal coach than an expert. The professional is, in fact, all three: expert, coach, and friend.

The question is, of course, how clinicians should strike the balance between these different roles. A position statement by consultant psychiatrists of the South London and Maudsley NHS Foundation Trust and the South West London and St George's Mental Health NHS Trust (2010) says that psychiatrists must offer their professional skills and knowledge; however, they are at the same time invited to learn from and value the patient in their role as experts by experience. When they do so, the position statement says, psychiatrists are no longer the distant and authoritative experts they used to be. They are now supposed to:

> [P]rovide the service user with resources (information, skills, networks, and support) to manage their own condition "as far as possible" and to help him to "get access to resources" he or she needs to live his or her life. (idem, p. 20; cf. Roberts & Wolfson 2004, p. 41)

These formulations represent an intermediate position between the extremes of a classical expert role with limited attention for the person, the context, and the "deskilled" professional some representatives of the user survivor movement envision, i.e., the professional who has given up the expert role and behaves as a coach, participant, and/ or friend. Proponents of the latter approach justify their devaluation of the expert role by suggesting that this role is inextricably linked with misuse of power, alienation, and oppression. It is, in other words, not possible to separate the expert role with its emphasis on proper scientific foundations from the oppressive ideologies behind it.

I think this is one-sided. Factual abuse of power never justifies neglect of important conceptual distinctions. I remind the reader of the epistemic distinctness of philosophical knowledge (paradigms, worldviews, and ideologies), scientific knowledge, and clinical expertise (the expert role) discussed in Chapter 1. Based on the fundamental epistemic difference between philosophical, scientific, and clinical practical knowledge, it is possible to argue against the conflation between the expert role and any kind of ideology. The medical profession may have historically misused its power on ideological grounds, and there may still be areas in (mental) healthcare in which ideologies, scientific rationalizations, and clinical applications are inextricably entangled and form an alienating and oppressive power. But there is no necessary or conceptual relationship between this ideology and the expert role. Factual situations should not be interpreted as disconfirmation of plausible and self-evident epistemic distinctions. On the contrary, these distinctions should serve as a safeguard against improper use of authority and power.

The recovery movement shows some striking similarities with the approach developed in this book. It is based on a contextual view of psychopathology that takes into account not only the patient's micro-world but also the patient's meso- and macro-worlds. It defends a pluralistic view of professional roles and relates these roles to the different aims of psychiatric practice. It emphasizes that patients do not coincide with their illnesses and that professionals do not coincide with their professional roles. It views illness as a personal journey with an aim (i.e., reconnecting clients with their sources of value and meaning). The recovery approach delineates in a natural way how individual service user–professional interactions can relate to developments in the larger (meso- and macro-) world. It puts social inclusion high on the agenda. This is relevant and informative for the normative practice approach, especially its conceptualization of the relation between contexts and the objects and aims of mental healthcare. The NPA could profit from case-based descriptions of how the relation between the micro- and the meso-/macro-world of the patient is established in recovery-oriented forms of mental healthcare. The NPA, by way of contrast, has an elaborate and precise view of how the different normative dimensions of mental healthcare should be interpreted and positioned with respect to one another.

The conceptual framework the NPA offers could be helpful for a thorough rethinking of the recovery approach, especially the question of how the different professional roles relate to one another. The recovery approach is right when it suggests that the broadening of the clinical perspective—by focusing on recovery of social relationships and the societal roles of clients—also leads to changes in the definition of the professional role. But, as far I can see, the recovery theorists have difficulty answering the question of whether, how, and to what extent expert knowledge is relevant in the pursuit of the social aims of mental healthcare. Can the promotion of social inclusion not better be accounted for by social workers or other workers in mental healthcare? What does their psychiatric expertise mean with respect to the social and advocacy roles psychiatrists are supposed to have in the recovery model?

9.2.4 Other points of view

Professional roles in psychiatry have become and are still becoming more varied, within and across the different social strata. Castellani and Hafferty (2006) predict, as we have seen, a proliferation of professional styles. This is also what stands out in other, more recent approaches to professionalism in psychiatry (see Bhugra & Malik 2011; and especially Schmutzler & Holsinger 2011).

Differences in duties and jurisdictions are based on differences in responsibility, and these, in turn, on differences in domain (or object) and the type of good that must be realized in that domain. Ideally, the discussion about duties and jurisdictions is settled on the basis of a realistic assessment of what can be demanded from the various partners given their competence, social horizon, legal constraints, and their specific role in the delivery of care. In practice, this process is messy and full of ambiguities, tensions, and conflicts.

It seems obvious that the duties and jurisdictions of physicians at a micro-level differ from those of doctors at other social levels. However, this does not mean that single professionals may forget their social responsibility and concern for public health. On the contrary, many of the recent policy statements and professional standards put social responsibility and altruism high on the agenda. This responsibility is split into two broad dimensions: patient advocacy and provision of health information.

To sum up, future psychiatrists understand that significant parts of their work should be devoted to the following:

- Patient advocacy: Even professionals working in private practices have a role to fulfil in the public domain.
- Informing patients, their families, and the public: The provision of relevant and trustworthy information about health and illness becomes increasingly important in times in which treatment options increase and most patients have (online) access to other, not always trustworthy, sources of information.
- Self-care: Physicians learn to take care of themselves better by maintaining balance between professional duties and their private lives; they should also search for sources of (additional) emotional, social, and spiritual support. This is important in the light of the increasing number of overburdened professionals.

Schmutzler and Holsinger (2011) build on work by Priester (1992), who distinguished a number of essential and instrumental values in professionalism. Priester described a transition from a conception of professionalism that centers around the notion of professional autonomy to an understanding of professionalism that considers fair access the most important value, alongside other essential values like quality, efficiency, respect, and patient advocacy. The key denominator in the new value-oriented framework for professionalism that Schmutzler and Holsinger (2011) envision is still the healthcare practitioner who shows commitment and responsibility, not only toward the patient, but increasingly also toward the healthcare system itself and toward society. Healthcare professionals should fundamentally see themselves as an integral part of the healthcare system. Their professional lives will more than ever be intertwined with their personal lives (Schmutzler & Holsinger 2011, p. 124). Their caring attitude will be expressed not only by correct diagnosis and treatment but also altruism and patient advocacy.

Underlying these changes is a transition from an essentially legal approach of the patient–physician relationship to a more personal, social approach. Instead of viewing the patient–physician relationship as based on a contract regulating the interactions between providers and consumers of some good, this relationship is now fundamentally captured in terms of partnership. The transition coincides with the transition from self-management (previously) to shared decision making (currently). Self-management obviously highlights patient autonomy, whereas shared decision making focuses on the element of partnership. The general idea with the notion of shared decision making is not only that decisions are made together, but, more precisely, that physicians help patients to recognize their needs and assist them in making responsible choices. To accomplish this, professionals should adopt the perspective of their patients and imagine what the various treatment options and proposals might mean for them. Partnership conceived in this way comes close to the notion of a covenant. Covenantal relationships have a moral meaning that transcends mutual agreement between parties. This meaning comes to expression in commitment, personal engagement and trust.

To conclude this section, I want to mention and briefly discuss some new approaches to the process of delivery of mental healthcare. Most of these approaches have considerable consequences for the professional role. Some of them focus on particular aspects of the care cycle, others on particular patient groups, and still others on both. There are, for instance, models that emphasize the importance of continuity of care, such as the model of integrated care (MIC; Theodoridou et al. 2015). Other models, especially the collaborative care model (CCM), focus on collaboration between primary, somatic, and specialized care (APA&APM 2016; Katon et al. 1995). In this approach, multidisciplinary groups of professionals provide care in a coordinated fashion and take responsibility for a defined subset of the population of patients. There are also approaches aimed at certain patient groups. Assertive community treatment (ACT; Stein & Santos 1998), for instance, and its Dutch variant, flexible assertive community treatment (FACT; van Veldhuizen 2007), focus on patients with severe and long-lasting mental disorder, including addiction, mild mental retardation, and/or social needs such as homelessness and social isolation (Killaspy & Rosen 2011; Nordén et al. 2012). The aim of the (F)ACT methodology is to prevent further deterioration and to build a network of services around the patient, with the aim of enabling patients to fulfill certain social roles. In the newer resource group, assertive community treatment (R-ACT) patients, their relatives, acquaintances, neighbors, colleagues, and other people of special importance are themselves members of the team and form a so-called "resource group" (Falloon et al. 2004). Variants of this approach are known as optimal treatment, integrated care, integrated psychiatry, and integrated mental healthcare. In some variants, there is a larger and a smaller resource group. In these cases, the large group meets no more than five times a year, whereas the small group may meet up to once a week (Nordén et al. 2011; 2012). The formation of these resource groups is a logical consequence of the idea that patients (and their relatives) should participate in their own treatment. Patients and those who support them need help not only to define the goals of treatment but also the means by which these goals are achieved.

Even more radical approaches choose from the start a different definition of the helping relationship. One example is the Open Dialogue approach to psychosis (Seikkula & Olson 2003; see also Thomas 2011). Open Dialogue finds its origin in the Finnish mental healthcare system and takes place in communal practices organized in social networks. It draws on Bakhtin's dialogical principles (Bakhtin 1984) and is rooted in the tradition of Bateson, specifically in the Milan school of family therapy (Selvini-Palazzoli et al. 1960). Two concepts, originally described by the Finnish community psychiatrist Pakman (2000), are central in the Open Dialogue approach, i.e. poetics and micropolitics. Poetics refers to the process of care, which is guided by the principles of tolerance of uncertainty, dialogism, and polyphony of social networks. These principles are an echo of concepts that are central to the Milan approach: circularity, hypothesizing, and neutrality. The term micropolitics refers to the larger institutional practices that support this way of working. These larger practices are seen as part of the system and not merely as entities that provide conditions for healthcare.

9.3 Prospects of the self- and context-oriented approach to psychopathology

The move toward new forms of professionalism is supported by and founded on new views on the concepts of health and illness. We discussed several newer approaches to the concept of disease in Chapter 3, especially neo-mechanistic and network approaches, RDoC, and enactivistic models. We concluded that perso-nalized network analysis comes closest to the ideal of a truly person-centered approach to psychopathology. It promises, in fact, a blended form of science and clinical practice: science *within* practice.

These were the broad outlines. In the subsequent chapters, we mainly focused on the clinical approach to psychopathology. We argued that it is inherently self- and context dependent. The question in this section is how this clinical approach should be positioned and evaluated in light of paradigms that have recently emerged in medicine: precision medicine, stratified medicine, personalized care, individualized care, and P-4 medicine.

Let me first explain the terms. Precision medicine aims at treatments targeted to the needs of individual patients based on genetic, biomarker, phenotypic, or psy-chosocial characteristics that distinguish a given patient from other patients with similar clinical presentations (Jameson & Longo 2015). Initial formulations of the concept emphasize the predictive potential of genetics (Collins & Varmus 2015). Later variants included the other "omics," such as epigenomics, transcriptomics, proteomics, metabolomics, and other factors, such as biomarkers and clinical and contextual features (Fernandes et al. 2017).

Individualized care and personalized care are usually taken to mean the same as precision medicine. Stratified medicine is primarily associated with the identification of subgroups of patients with a specific disease who respond to a particular drug or, alternatively, are at risk of side-effects in response to a certain treatment (Schumann et al. 2014).

The general idea of all these concepts is to move away from symptom-based taxo-nomies towards the characterization of individuals in terms of multilayered systems (ESF 2012). These layers encompass the entire range of constitutive elements, from molecules to behavior. Precision medicine uses the principles of systems biology, a branch of systems theory that focuses on biology (molecules, cells, and, tissues) and consists of the computational and mathematical modeling of complex biological systems. These systems are represented as dynamic states of networks (Palsson 2011).

P-4 medicine goes one step further and is based on the view that, because the distinction between knowledge producers and knowledge recipients is becoming less rigid, patients and citizens now function both as producers and end users of data (ESF 2012). Medicine will become P-4 medicine: predictive, preventive, personalized, and participatory. A core goal of personalization is the following:

> [T]o acknowledge the position of patients and citizens at the centre of the endeavour, not merely as receivers of care but as active contributors of data and as participants in the process of decision-making. (ESF 2012, p. 14; cf. Hood & Friend 2011; Weston & Hood 2004)

From the perspective of the self- and context-related approach to psychopathology defended in this book, these are refreshing conceptual improvements. From a philosophical point of view, the caveats that were discussed in Chapter 3 (section 3.1.8) can be repeated. How do researchers make sense of data that are generated at system levels that are supposed to be overlapping? How should they adequately and responsibly interpret all the information? How, in other words, do they know that different types of network analyis (gene-protein networks and symptom networks in Alzheimer's disease, for instance) are about the same explanans?

The overarching idea in P-4 medicine (i.e., the blending of science and practice as a result of patient empowerment and the establishment of new, interdisciplinary networks of researchers, patients, and other stakeholders) is appealing. But how realistic is it? There has been some research on the effectiveness of public involvement in the establishment of research agendas in health technology assessment, and this research suggests that some caution is warranted. Citizens' panels have proved capable of generating sets of ethical and social values (Bombard et al. 2011). However, their role has appeared to be more difficult to define when they had to balance scientific standards and the perspective of healthcare policymakers (Gauvin et al. 2010).

The term "person-centered care" sounds as if it were a form of personalized care, but it is something completely different. It aims at no less than a reformulation of the central mission of medicine, by recognizing the person as its fundamental focus and not simply a carrier of disease. It is holistic and informed by the wisdom from great ancient civilizations and recent developments in clinical medicine and public health. Mezzich (2011) proposes to define person-centered medicine (PCM) as:

> [M]edicine *of* the person (of the totality of the person's health, including its ill and positive aspects), *for* the person (promoting the fulfilment of the person's life project), *by* the person (with clinicians extending themselves as full human beings, well-grounded on science and with high ethical aspirations) and *with* the person (working respectfully, in collaboration and in an empowering manner through a partnership of patient, family and clinicians). The person here is conceptualized in a fully contextualized manner, consistent with the

words of philosopher Ortega y Gasset, I am I and my circumstances. (see also Mezzich 2007; Mezzich et al. 2016; Miles & Mezzich 2011)

Andrew Miles, editor in chief of *Journal of Evaluation in Clinical Practice*, and philosopher Michael Loughlin recognize the "resonant voice" of Paul Tournier in the rise of person-centered medicine (Miles & McLoughlin 2011). Tournier (1898–1986), who is the founder of the so-called "medicine of the person," propagated an integrative approach in medicine by situating clinical interventions in the context of psychological understanding and pastoral counselling (Tournier 1940; see also Cox et al. 2007). Mezzich also mentions the person-centered approach to psychotherapy of Carl Rogers as source of inspiration.

Miles and Loughlin view person-centered medicine as the successor of evidence-based medicine (EBM). They state that EBM "has ... been ... incapable of incorporating patients' values and preferences into clinical decision making when these are in conflict with EBM's evidence" (idem, p. 532). They add:

> [I]t seems incontrovertibly clear from raised voices worldwide, that patients are no longer prepared to be "dealt with" or "processed" by technicians in applied bioscience, but wish rather to be attended by scientifically trained advocates who recognize their problems not only at an organic, but also at an emotional and spiritual level and who, in addition, then proceed through shared decision making to tailor treatment for the patient through a medicine of, for, by and with the patient. (idem, p. 534)

This sharp criticism is consonant with the views developed in this book with respect to clinical consultation and the individual patient–physician relationship. It is less clear, however, what kind of research would best fit with PCM, what kind of evidence person-centered psychiatry needs, and how, from a holistic perspective, old and new scientific evidence is used in shared decision making. This book suggested the unravelling of causal trajectories in analyses of personalized networks as a promising way to connect scientific evidence, contexts, and person-centered care.

Person-centered medicine resembles approaches that emphasize the positive aspects of health. A recent example of this latter approach is offered by the Dutch researcher Machteld Huber (Huber et al. 2011), who argues that we need a positive and dynamic concept of health, a concept that is "based on the resilience or capacity to cope and maintain and restore one's integrity, equilibrium, and sense of well-being." Because definitions draw us to boundaries and to a precision that might be unhelpful, she proposes the formulation of a general framework instead of a definition, i.e., a framework that gives a characterization of an agreed direction in which to look. Health is, then, "the ability to adapt and to self-manage, in the face of social, physical, and emotional challenges." This initial formulation serves as starting point for a fresh conceptualization, in which a set of dynamic features is distinguished. These features are operationalized in measurable bodily, mental, and social dimensions (Huber 2014; Huber et al. 2016). Six dimensions are discerned:

bodily functions, mental functions, a spiritual/existential dimension, quality of life, social and societal participation, and daily functioning. Huber's approach has been adopted by the (Dutch) Federatie van Medisch Specialisten (Federation of Medical Specialists; 2016) in its vision document on the future of medical specialists and by the (Dutch) Committee Innovation Healthcare Professions & Education (2016).

Huber's predilection for a positive approach to health is part of a broader and rapidly expanding movement, which has become known as positive psychology. Positive psychologists emphasize the forgotten but crucial role of positive factors, not only in cure and care but also for healthy psychological development and functioning. Positive psychology calls for "massive" research on human strengths and virtues, such as happiness, hope, wisdom, creativity, future mindedness, courage, spirituality, responsibility, autonomy, perseverance, and self-regulation (Seligman & Csikszentmihalyi 2000).

Positive psychology's approach to health and illness is congruent with the main thrust of this book, with the proviso that it does not lead to ignorance of the extreme vulnerability of service users who are most dependent on professional care. The emphasis of positive psychology on the patient's potential for self-care, resilience, and creativity are a welcome correction on the image of the helpless and dependent patient that may have colored (some of the) old-school views on psychiatry. But it should not lead to new one-sidedness and disregard of the fragility and fundamental lack of balance and inner strength in many patients with severe chronic mental illness.

9.4 Psychiatric education

In this section, I briefly discuss some implications of the contextualized version of the NPA, as well as the self- and context-oriented approach to psychopathology for residency training in psychiatry.

Let me begin by stating that we already live in a different world than two or three decades ago. Until then, virtually nothing had been published on medical specialists' education. Medical specialists were supposed to learn from their role models, to practice under supervision, to do exams on the scientific and technical basis of their disciplines, and, by doing so, gradually gain competence and responsibility. Since then, residency training has considerably changed. Most countries in the Western world have adopted a competence-based training curriculum as a reaction against overemphasis on the medical expert role. This implied a shift in focus, with more focus on communicative, organizational, collaborative, and reflexive skills (Frank 2005; Royal College of Physicians and Surgeons of Canada 2015).

What also changed was the role of ICT. Digital exchange of information has rapidly entered the scene and dominates medicine and medical education. Medicine is developing into network medicine. This will also hold for mental healthcare and medical education. The care cycle will be organized closer to where people live, in networks consisting of diverging disciplines. Technology will play an increasingly important role in these networks. Wearables, smartphones, and other forms of registration will lead to unprecedented levels of health surveillance. Similar developments are currently occurring in medical education: new forms of instruction, the setting up of new learning environments (digital learning environments, skills labs, and e-communities), together with an awareness of differences in learning styles and new definitions of educational outcome. In the words of Wilkes (2015):

> The educational outcomes that we have traditionally held as sacrosanct (memorization and good test taking) have changed. There is no need to memorize long lists of items anymore. Everything can be easily found on a smartphone. Every dose, every nerve connection, every anatomic bone, every metabolic pathway is on a smartphone or tablet. What students need to learn is how to think critically, how to reason, how to be ethical, and how to communicate and connect with people.

Reports on future professionalism also point at changes in the relationship between medical professionals and service users. For instance, the *Shape of Training Review: Securing the Future of Excellent Patient Care* by the British Medical Council (BMC 2013) states that patients will increasingly be seen as citizens who are expected to develop health-related skills from an early age. Professionals have a role in teaching these skills. Professionals themselves will live a life of permanent learning, in teams, organizations, and networks. These networks will connect health education with research and daily practice with policy.

Changes in the definition of professional role impact medical education. New terms emerge in this context: "new professionalism" (Belar 2013), "T-shaped professionals" (cf. Hansen & van Oetinger 2001), and interprofessional professionalism collaborative (IPC) (Stern 2006; see also Hammer et al. 2012; Holtman et al. 2011; Stern & Papadakis 2006). Hargreaves describes new professionalism as a synthesis of professional and institutional development. In an early article on primary and secondary school education, he defines it as following "a movement away from the teacher's traditional professional authority and autonomy towards new forms of relationship with colleagues, with students, and with parents." He foresees that these relations will become more intense and collaborative, involving "more explicit negotiation of roles and responsibilities" (Hargreaves 1994). This is a shift in social tradition, involving a movement from individualism to collaboration, from hierarchies to teams, from supervision to mentoring, from liaison to partnership between training institutions and professional organizations, from authority to contract, and from survivalism to empowerment.

Hansen and van Oetinger (2001) develop a similar concept for professionalism in business administration. The new manager is "T-shaped." The vertical line indicates the expert role, with its narrow focus but in-depth insight. The horizontal part represents the entire range of communicative, collaborative, and organizational skills that enable the manager to interact with relevant stakeholders. Dutch medical specialists adopted the idea of T-shaped professionalism in one of their vision documents about the medical specialist role in 2025 (Federatie 2016). They argue that future caregivers should have skills to collaborate in networks with other physicians, nurses, psychologists, social workers, patients, and their representatives. Interprofessional collaboration is also a priority in the education of psychologists. In the words of former American Psychological Association Executive Director of Education Cynthia Belar (2013): "[I]f we are to maintain the public trust, our health-care system needs a 'new professionalism' that emphasizes interprofessional collaboration, shared values and shared accountability."

Interprofessional professionalism is defined as follows:

> Consistent demonstration of core values evidenced by professionals working together, aspiring to and wisely applying principles of, altruism and caring, excellence, ethics, respect, communication, accountability to achieve optimal health and wellness in individuals and communities. (Stern 2006, p. 19)

These developments and new concepts underscore one of the main messages of this book: We need a richer, more nuanced approach to professionalism than traditional technocratic, scientistic, or administrative and/or managerial views suggest. Two features are especially important for new professionalism and its future. The first is value sensitivity, which includes awareness of meaning. The second is training of attitudes and skills that enable professionals to give shape to their social responsibility (collaboration, communication, advocacy, and health education). Both characteristics are based on recognition of the value-laden aspects of psychiatric practice and are, evidently, not meant to detract from the lasting importance of the medical expert role.

With respect to value sensitivity and awareness of meaning, I would like to point to the importance of the competence of clinical judgment. The NPA cherishes clinical judgment, conceived as the ability to consider all relevant (self- and context-related) relations and interactions in the patient and in oneself as a professional (see Diagram 2.1). It consists of the ability to weigh and balance the (value-laden) implications for cure and care of all these relations and interactions. Clinical judgment is an embodiment of the sensitivity and wisdom required to do justice to the complexity of the patient's problems and to the normative aspects of psychiatric practice. New forms of data generation offer new challenges. Advances in smartphones and wearable biosensors enable gathering of real-time psychological, behavioral, and physiological data in increasingly precise and unobtrusive ways. Data-mining techniques offer unprecedented numbers of associations. In and of themselves, these data and associations are meaningless. There is an increasing need for adequate interpretation and ascription of meaning. Clinical judgment entails the capacity to interpret what is measured. It is, ideally, rooted in an attitude of wonder, respect, and discernment. This attitude presupposes empathy, compassion, and openness, the prerequisites for value sensitivity. This value sensitivity functions as sounding board for the needs of patients.

The second characteristic, the ability to exhibit social responsibility, requires open mindedness with respect to one's role in broader contexts (Birden et al. 2014). Future psychiatrists should be flexible with respect to organizational change, but at the same time firm with respect to their basic convictions. They must regard patients as civic partners. They are able to give a normative account of the legitimacy of the profession, for instance in discussions with meso- and macro-level stakeholders. But they should also defend patients and their rights against threats from their emotional, economic, and social environments. They should be able to represent the voice of the patient in the public arena, when needed and appropriate. They, alone or in professional groups, should be ready to establish new partnerships between representative bodies within the state, market players and civil society organizations. They will be engaged in negotiations that no longer solely concern the content of care, but also and increasingly the terms under which these products are delivered (Bloom et al. 2008). These terms define the rights, duties, and responsibilities of the relevant stakeholders. Because there is no blueprint for these duties and responsibilities, lots of persistence and creative imagination are required to fulfill this difficult job.

This account sounds high spirited. Is it not also naïve? Do we still have a civil society that is willing and effective in endowing professional groups with the kind of professionalism that is outlined here—a professionalism that reminds us of the professionalism of the early days, with its strong moral claims? Are professionals themselves not divided in this respect? Do they agree on the content of their commitments and views and on whether and how to express these commitments and views? Is there one dominant form in which the concept of responsibility can be revived in our ages of experts and large organizations (Brint 2015)?

I agree with Brint (2015) that the answer to these questions is not self-evident:

> In my view, it will not be possible to revive social trustee professionalism—or any derivation from it—in an effective and honest way without emphasizing the centrality of professional skill and the moral potential inherent in the social relationships affected by skill. It will also not be possible without appreciating the fundamental significance of organizations for absorbing society's claims on professionals and for shaping the contours of professional responsibilities. Finally, it will not be possible to do so without acknowledging the contested terrain of social responsibility and the role of non-professional actors in definitions and redefinitions of this terrain.

These are wise words. A persistent focus on the humanness of the relationship between the professional and the patient is not enough. Whatever reformulation there will be of social professionalism, it should at least retain a strong link with the expert role. In other words, restoration of trust depends on solid proof of professional skills and valorization of these skills in a variety of contexts in which these skills may manifest their inherent moral potential. This is only possible in (institutional) contexts, which are varied and large enough to absorb all relevant societal claims and expectancies. The shaping of these contexts, their priorities and targets, should be seen as the outcome of negotiations in which "non-professional actors" also participate. Therefore, the outcome of the discussion about values is not settled beforehand. It will depend on who participates, on the content of these negotiations, and on how professionals participate.

9.5 The existential dimension of professionalism

In a book on person-centered psychiatry, one may expect to focus not only on the personhood of the patient but also on the professional as a person. In sections 5.2.2 and 5.2.3, I have already discussed relation [E] (of Diagram 5.1), which referred to the impact of who one is as person on how one relates to one's professional role. In this section, I especially focus on the existential aspects of this self-relating, in conjunction with a discussion about the interpersonal relation between the patient as person and the professional as person.

Let me first explain what I mean by existential. Existential are those aspects of one's self-relating that refer to the whole of one's existence (at a certain point in time) and to one's fundamental intentions, motives, commitments, and concerns at that moment. Existential are therefore those features of one's self-relating that reveal who one is, really and authentically. Existential aspects of self-relating cannot always be made conscious or produced by an act of volition. The purpose of this section is not to urge professionals to be more open to their patients or to colleagues and to disclose the existential motivations of their functioning. Instead, I mean to say that the existential dimension is given, that it exists by definition, in a structural sense, *a priori* if one wishes. Terms like commitment, dedication, passion, soul, inspiration, meaningfulness, hope, ethos, and connectedness to one's ideals indicate how the existential aspect of self-relatedness may become manifest. These terms refer to drives of the person as a whole and to ultimate concerns at the horizon of one's life as professional (Glas 2017b). I add that these are the positive terms. Existential aspects of self-relatedness can also be negatively colored, e.g., when one's attitude is dominated by cynicism, indifference, untrustworthiness, or inauthenticity.

Professionals do not need to be aware of the existential dimension of their self-relatedness. This is pointed out by the philosopher Sören Kierkegaard, in his discussion of the importance of "indirect communication" and in his plea for correspondence between the "how" and the "what" of one's communications (Kierkegaard 1846, pp. 72–80). If it is true that the manner of communicating is fundamental to what is communicated, then this is also of crucial importance for the physician–patient relationship. It means that not only the message should be true but also the messaging. The "truth" of messaging is called trustworthiness; it refers to the messenger (the professional, in this case). Can I as a person take responsibility for what is said? Is it consistent with my view on my professional role? Is it an expression of sincerity and commitment to the patient's good? These are the kind of questions physicians—ideally—try to answer when they reflect about their functioning.

In other words, the thesis of indirect communication implies that in professional activity, there is always something co-communicated about how the professional relates to his or her own role. This "co-communicating" often occurs implicitly, by the tone of one's voice, by gestures, facial expressions, muscle tone, and one's attitude. Over the years, professionals learn to recognize and use this co-communicating better. Not all forms of co-communication are existential, of course. Countertransference reactions are a typical example, i.e., implicit or explicit feelings, likes and dislikes, attitudes and concerns that reveal more about the personality of the therapist than about the problem of the patient.

Patients often say that the turning point in their therapy came when the professional him- or herself was temporarily unable to persist in the professional role, such as moments of shared silence, in which the therapist implicitly communicates that he she is unable to say anything for whatever reason (inner confusion, powerlessness, or strong feelings). This also includes moments of sadness and grief in which the therapist cannot hide his or her own grief, or spontaneous "unprofessional" and/or surprisingly "honest" reactions to what the patient says. These examples illustrate a more general point, i.e., that perhaps the most essential aspects in the encounter between patient and professional can hardly be spoken about and are nevertheless undeniably present. The professional is, as a rule, no expert in existential issues.

There are, of course, psychiatrists who deny that dealing with these issues should be part of the expert role. However, we have seen that the existential dimension is structurally given and that it reveals important information about the professional's stance toward his or her own role. Psychiatrists and psychotherapists cannot close their eyes to the obvious, i.e., that dealing with illness is a personal struggle for the patient and that handling the professional role is ultimately an equally personal endeavor. Professionals must deal with these undeniable states of affairs in one way or another, just like patients have to deal with their illness. Denying or ignoring one's implicit stance toward one's professional role is no solution. This learned ignorance will also be co-communicated between the lines (e.g., as "difficult territory" or as a subject to be avoided).

A related ambiguity exists with respect to the relationship between patient and professional as persons, in Diagram 5.1 the unaddressed arrow between the patient as a person and the professional as a person (left side of the diagram). This relationship is for many patients the most important one in the therapeutic encounter. At the same time, it is often the least supported by the expert role. We are discussing a reality that hardly can be addressed because there is so little legitimacy for the professional to do so.

I don't believe there is any completely satisfactory solution to this ambiguity. It is the inevitable byproduct of modernization, with its division of labor and its refined distribution of increasingly limited responsibilities. No wonder many patients—and sometimes also professionals—long for a premodern, romantic inclusiveness and wholeness with its own perils.

That said, I would like to add that it is possible to remain within the boundaries of the professional role and yet address the existential dimension of the patient's problem and also—in a slightly more restrained manner—discuss some of the existential aspects of one's own role as a professional. The professional may create room for a conversation about what the illness means in the context of the person's life. He or she may address existential themes such as hope, longing, connectedness, meaning, gratefulness, consolation, doubt, suffering, anxiety, and powerlessness. This may be done straightforwardly, but also in a subtler way, by listening and by making explicit what is said between the lines.

Professionals may learn to deal with questions about their own roles. They may show how they reflect on their own roles. They may change their stance toward those roles and communicate about this change with their clients. They may display a certain freedom with respect to this stance. They may learn to play with this by explicitly changing hats. When patients don't want to comply with an evidence-based intervention because of some personal ("idiosyncratic" as doctors call it) reason, the professional may say:

> Well, this is what I have to say when I put on my professional hat. I can understand that you have difficulty with this, when I look from your perspective. But I think that, even within your perspective, it makes sense to consider what I proposed a moment ago.

In other words, by explicitly relating to their own role and by communicating about it (i.e., their own different stances toward their role), professionals show openness and freedom with respect to their roles. This freedom will be (co-)communicated to the patient and often affect the patient's stance toward his or her own condition. This also holds for the existential dimension in the professional interaction: The better professionals are able to recognize and address existential themes within their own roles, the better they will be able to address the existential dimension in the illnesses of their patients.

Of course, there are boundaries to these attempts. It is often not necessary or advisable for doctors to share their own views on life and/or political convictions, at least not where these views and convictions have no obvious relationship with how doctors perform their expert role. Most patients are not primarily interested in these views and convictions. What they expect is sensitive and critical wisdom of doctors. I see this wisdom as a second-order competence that is part of the broader competence of professionalism.

Openness of the professional about his or her own role fulfilment, ideals, ambivalences, and recognition of insufficiencies may, however, in some case prove to be a decisive factor for the patient to open up him- or herself. Ambiguities and ambivalences with respect to this openness are in a certain way inevitable, given the pressures of modern healthcare, especially on medical specialists. It will usually be impossible to avoid any kind of communication about these pressures and how they affect one's commitments and views.

Allow me to close by saying that this book was written out of a passion for patients and for the discipline of psychiatry. Psychiatry's secret is contact and connection with the patient, with oneself, and with the communities that fuel our understanding of and sensitivity to values. As a resident, I learned to open up to the patient while remaining in touch with myself, as a person and as a professional. When my professional experience increased, I learned how institutional and societal issues resonate in my contact with the patient. Nevertheless, openness is what counts: openness to the patient, openness to myself, despite the turbulences within the system, resistant against wishful thinking of policymakers and firm with respect to temptations to withdraw and give up medicine as an ultimately moral endeavor. What counts is searching for what really matters, with the patient and for the patient. Changes in décor—societal, financial, qua governance—are inevitable and resonate in how I relate to myself as a professional. But they are not all decisive. I try to relativize their importance; I withstand them where needed, and they will leave my openness and enthusiasm untouched, whatever occurs.

REFERENCES

Abbott, A.D. (1988). *The System of Professions: An Essay on the Division of Expert Labor*. Chicago: University of Chicago Press.

ABIM Foundation, ACP–ASIM Foundation, and European Federation of Internal Medicine (2002). Medical professionalism in the new millennium: A physician charter. *Annals of Internal Medicine*, 136: 243–246.

Adler, P.S., Heckscher, C., McCarthy, J.E., and Rubinstein, S.A. (2015). The mutations of professional responsibility: Toward collaborative community. In: D.E. Mitchell, R.K. Ream (Eds.), *Professional Responsibility: The Fundamental Issue in Education and Healthcare Reform*, pp. 309–326. Advances in Medical Education 4. New York: Springer.

Adorno, T.W., Horkheimer, M. (1947). *Dialektik der Aufklärung*. Amsterdam: Querido.

Alexander, L., Moore, M. (2016). Deontological ethics. *Stanford Encyclopedia of Philosophy* (Winter 2016 Edition), Edward N. Zalta (Ed.). https://plato.stanford.edu/ archives/ win2016/entries/ethics-deontological/ [retrieved 04-09-2017].

Allen, B.P., Potkay, C.R. (1981). On the arbitrary distinction between states and traits. *Journal of Personality and Social Psychology*, 41: 916–928.

Amador, X., David, A. (2004). *Insight and Psychosis: Awareness of Illness in Schizophrenia and Related Disorders*, 2nd ed. Oxford: Oxford University Press.

American Psychiatric Association (APA). (1980). *Diagnostic and Statistical Manual for Mental Disorders*, 3rd ed. Washington, DC: American Psychiatric Association.

American Psychiatric Association. (1994). *Diagnostic and Statistical Manual for Mental Disorders*, 4th ed. Washington, DC: American Psychiatric Association.

American Psychiatric Association (2013). *Diagnostic and Statistical Manual for Mental Disorders*, 5th ed. Washington, DC: American Psychiatric Association.

American Psychiatric Association & Academy of *Psychosom Med*. (APA&APM) (2016). *Dissemination of Integrated Care within Adult Primary Care Settings: The Collaborative Care Model*. Washington, DC: American Psychiatric Association.

Anthony, W.A. (1993). Recovery from mental illness: The guiding vision of the mental health service system in the 1990s. *Psychosocial Rehabilitation Journal*, 16: 11–23.

Anthony, W.A. (2000). A recovery-oriented service system: Setting some system level standards. *Psychiatric Rehabilitation Journal*, 24: 159–169.

Aristotle. Nicomachean ethics. In: *The Complete Works of Aristotle. The Revised Oxford Translation* (Ed. by J. Barnes). Book II. Princeton, NJ: Princeton University Press, pp. 1829–1967.

Arnold, M.B. (1960). *Emotion and Personality*. New York: Columbia University Press.

Ashcroft, R.E. (2003). Current epistemological problems in evidence-based medicine. *Journal of Medical Ethics*, 30: 131–135.

Austin, C.P. (2018). Translating translation. *Nature Reviews | Drug Discovery*. Advance online publication, 20 April.

Baier, A. (2004). Feelings that matter. In R.C. Solomon (Ed.). *Thinking about Feeling: Contemporary Philosophers on Emotions*, pp. 200–213. Oxford: Oxford University Press.

Bakhtin, M. (1984). *Problems of Dostojevskij's Poetics: Theory and History of Literature*, Vol. 8. Manchester: Manchester University Press.

Beauchamp, T.L., Childress, J.F. (2013). *Principles of Biomedical Ethics*, 7th ed. New York: Oxford University Press.

Bechtel, W. (2008). *Mental Mechanisms: Philosophical Perspectives on Cognitive Neuroscience*. New York: Psychology Press.

Beck, J., Young, M.F.D. (2005). The assault on the professions and the restructuring of academic and professional identities: A Bernsteinian analysis. *British Journal of Sociology of Education*, 26(2): 183–197.

Beck, U. (1992). *Risk Society: Towards a New Modernity*. London: Sage Publications.

Belar, C. (2013). A new professionalism. *Monitor on Psychology*, 44(7): 48.

Belsky, J., Pluess, M. (2009). Differential susceptibility to environmental influences. *Psychological Bulletin*, 135(6): 885–908.

Bennett, M.R., Hacker, P.M.S. (2003). *Philosophical Foundations of Neuroscience*. Malden/Oxford: Blackwell.

Bermudez, J.L., Marcel, A., and Eilan, N. (Eds.) (1995). *The Body and the Self*. Cambridge: MIT Press.

Bhugra, D., Malik, A. (Eds.) (2011). *Professionalism in Mental Healthcare*. Cambridge: Cambridge University Press.

Bircher, J. (2005). Towards a dynamic definition of health and disease. *Medicine, Healthcare and Philosophy*, 8: 335–341.

Bird, A., Tobin, E. (2015). Natural kinds. *Stanford Encyclopedia of Philosophy*. http://plato.stanford.edu/archives/spr2015/entries/natural-kinds/ [retrieved 30-04-2015].

Birden, H., Glass, N., Wilson, I., Harrison, M., Sherwood, T., and Nass, D. (2014). Defining professionalism in medical education: A systematic review. *Medical Teacher*, 36: 47–61.

Blashfield, R.K. (1986). Structural approaches to classification. In: T. Millon, G.L. Klerman (Eds.). *Contemporary Directions in Psychopathology. Toward the DSM-IV*, pp. 363–380. New York/London: Guilford Press.

Bloom, D.E., Cafiero, E.T., Jané-Llopis, E., Abrahams-Gessel, S., Bloom, and Weinstein, C. (2011). *The Global Economic Burden of Noncommunicable Diseases*. Geneva: World Economic Forum.

Bloom, G., Standing, H., and Lloyd, R. (2008). Markets, information asymmetry and healthcare: Towards new social contracts. *Social Science & Medicine*, 66: 2076–2087.

Bolton, D., Hill, J. (1996). *Mind, Meaning, and Mental Disorder: The Nature of Causal Explanation in Psychology and Psychiatry*, rev. ed. 2006. Oxford: Oxford University Press.

Bombard, Y., Abelson, J., Simeonov, D., and Gauvin, J.P. (2011). Eliciting ethical and social values in health technology assessment: A participatory approach. *Social Science & Medicine*, 73: 135–144.

Boorse, C. (1975). On the distinction between disease and illness. *Philosophy and Public Affairs*, 5: 49–68.

Boorse, C. (1976). What a theory of mental health should be. *Journal for the Theory of Social Behaviour*, 6(1): 61–84.

Boorse, C. (1977). Health as a theoretical concept. *Philosophy of Science*, 44: 542–573.

Borsboom D. (2008). Psychometric perspectives on diagnostic systems. *Journal of Clinical Psychology*, 64: 1089–1108.

Borsboom D., Cramer, A.O.J. (2013). Network analysis: An integrative approach to the structure of psychopathology. *Annual Review of Clinical Psychology*, 9: 91–121.

Borsboom, D., Cramer, A., and Kalis, A. (2018). *Brain* disorders? Not really ... Why network structures block reductionism in psychopathology research. *Behavioral and Brain Sciences*, 24: 1–54.

Borsboom, D., Cramer, A.O.J., Schmittmann, V.D., Epskamp, S., and Waldorp, L.J. (2011). The small world of psychopathology. *PLoS ONE*, 6: e27407.

Bracken, P., Thomas, P. (2005). *Postpsychiatry: Mental Health in a Postmodern World*. Oxford: Oxford University Press.

Bracken, P., Thomas, P. (2013). Challenges to the modernist identity of psychiatry: User empowerment and recovery In: K.W.M. Fulford, M. Davies, R. Gipps, G. Graham, J. Sadler, ... and T. Thornton (Eds.). *Oxford Handbook of Philosophy and Psychiatry*, pp. 123–138. Oxford: Oxford University Press.

Brint, S. (2015). Professional responsibility in an age of experts and large organizations. In: D.E. Mitchell, R.K. Ream (Eds.). *Professional Responsibility: The Fundamental Issue in Education and Healthcare Reform*. Advances in Medical Education, Vol. 4, pp. 89–107). New York: Springer.

British Medical Council (BMC). (2013). *Shape of Training Review: Securing the Future of Excellent Patient Care. Final Report of the Independent Review* (led by Professor D. Greenaway). London: British Medical Council.

Broadbent, J., Dietrich, M., and Roberts, J. (Eds.) (1997). *The End of the Professions? The Restructuring of Professional Work*. London/New York: Routledge.

Bromet, E.J., Havenaar, J.M. (2007). Psychological and perceived health effects of the Chernobyl Disaster: A 20-year review. *Health Physics*, 93(5): 516–521.

Bunge, M. (2003). *Emergence and Convergence: Qualitative Novelty and the Unity of Knowledge*. Toronto: University of Toronto Press.

Cartwright, N. (1999). *The Dappled World: A Study of the Boundaries of Science*. Cambridge: Cambridge University Press.

Cartwright, N. (2011). The art of medicine: A philosopher's view of the long road from RCTs to effectiveness. *Lancet*, 377: 1400–1401.

Castellani, B., Hafferty, F.W. (2006). The complexities of medical professionalism: A preliminary investigation. In: D. Wear, J.M. Aultman (Eds.). *Professionalism in Medicine: Critical Perspectives*, pp. 3–24. New York: Springer.

Cesuroglu, T., van Ommen, B., Malats, N., Sudbrak, R., Lehrach, H., Brand, A. (2012). Public health perspective: From personalized medicine to personal health. *Personalized Medicine*, 9(2): 115–119.

Chaplin, J. (2011). *Herman Dooyeweerd: Christian Philosopher of State and Civil Society*. Notre Dame, IN: Notre Dame University Press.

Chaplin, W.F., John, O.P., and Goldberg, L.R. (1988). Conceptions of states and traits: Dimensional attributes with ideals as prototypes. *Journal of Personality and Social Psychology*, 54(4): 541–557.

Charland, L.C. (2013). Why psychiatry should fear medicalization. In: K.W.M. Fulford, M. Davies, R. Gipps, G. Graham, J. Sadler, ... and T. Thornton (Eds.). *Oxford Handbook of Philosophy and Psychiatry*, pp. 150–175. Oxford: Oxford University Press.

Christoff, K., Cosmelli, D., Legrand, D., and Thompson, E. (2011). Specifying the self for cognitive neuroscience. *Trends in Cognitive Sciences*, March 15(3): 103–112.

Clark, D.A., Beck, A.T. (2010). *Cognitive Therapy of Anxiety Disorders: Science and Practice*. New York: Guilford Press.

Cloninger, C.R. (2004). *Feeling Good: The Science of Well-being*. New York: Oxford University Press.

Collins, F.S., Varmus, H. (2015). A new initiative on precision medicine. *New England Journal of Medicine*, 372(9): 793–795.

Colombetti, G. (2014). *The Feeling Body: Affective Science Meets the Enactive Mind*. Cambridge/London: MIT Press.

Colombo, A., Bendelow, G., Fulford, K.W.M., and Williams, S. (2003). Evaluating the influence of implicit models of mental disorder on processes of shared decision making within community-based multi-disciplinary teams. *Social Science & Medicine*, 56: 1557–1570.

Committee Innovation Healthcare Professions & Education, National Healthcare Institute. (2016). *Summary: A Paradigm Shift in Perception, Learning and Action. Boundary-crossing Learning and Educating in Healthcare and Welfare in the Digital Age*. Dieman: Zorginstituut Nederland.

Cooper, M.W. (1992). Should physicians be Bayesian agents? *Theoretical Medicine*, 13(4): 349–361.

Cox, J., Campbell, A.V., and Fulford, K.W.M. (2007). *Medicine of the Person: Faith, Science and Values in Healthcare Provision*. London: Jessica Kingsley.

Craver, C.F. (2007). *Explaining the Brain: Mechanisms and the Mosaic Unity of Neuroscience*. Oxford: Oxford University Press.

Craver, C.F., Darden, L. (2013). *In Search of Mechanisms: Discoveries across the Life Sciences*. Chicago: University of Chicago Press.

Cruess, R.L., Cruess, S.R. (1997). Teaching medicine as a profession in the service of healing. *Academic Medicine*, 72(11): 941–952.

Cusveller, B. (2004). *Met zorg verbonden. Een filosofische studie naar de zindimensie van verpleegkundige zorgverlening*. Amsterdam: Buijten & Schipperheijn.

Cutler, P. (Ed.) (1998). *Problem Solving in Clinical Medicine: From Data to Diagnosis*, 3rd ed. Baltimore, MA: Lippincott Williams & Wilkins.

Damasio, A.R. (1999). *The Feeling of What Happens: Body and Emotion in the Making of Consciousness*. Orland, FL: Harcourt Inc.

Damasio, A.R. (2010). *Self Comes to Mind: Constructing the Conscious Brain*. New York: Pantheon Books.

Daniels, N. (1981). Health-care needs and distributive justice. *Philosophy and Public Affairs*, 10: 146–179.

Daniels, N. (2001). Justice, health, and healthcare. *American Journal of Bioethics*, 1(2): 2–16.

Daniels, N. (2013). Justice and access to healthcare. *Stanford Encyclopedia of Philosophy* (Spring2013 Edition). Edward N. Zalta (Ed.). http://plato.stanford.edu/ archives/spr2013/entries/justice-healthcareaccess/ [retrieved 04-05-2015].

de Haan, S. (2015). *An Enactive Approach to Psychiatry*. Doctoral dissertation: University of Heidelberg.

De Swaan, A. (1988). *In Care of the State*. Cambridge: Polity.

Deegan, G. (2003). Discovering recovery. *Psychiatric Rehabilitation Journal*, 26: 368–376.

Dennett, D.C. (1995). *Darwin's Dangerous Idea: Evolution and the Meanings of Life*. New York/London: Penguin Books.

Dennett, D.C. (1998). The Leibnizian paradigm. In: D.L. Hull, M. Ruse (Eds.). *The Philosophy of Biology*, pp. 38–51. Oxford/New York: Oxford University Press.

Dent, M. (2006). Patient choice and medicine in healthcare: Responsibilization, governance and proto-professionalization. *Public Management Review*, 8(3): 449–462.

Dent, M., Whitehead, S. (Eds.) (2002). *Managing Professional Identities: Knowledge, Performativity and the "New" Professional*. London: Routledge.

Dooyeweerd, H. (1953–1958). *A New Critique of Theoretical Thought*, Vols. I–IV. Amsterdam/Paris/Philadelphia, PA: Presbyterian and Reformed Publishing Company.

Dretske, F. (1988). *Explaining Behavior: Reasons in a World of Causes*. Cambridge, MA: MIT Press.

Eddy, D.M. (1996). *Clinical Decision Making: From Theory to Practice*. Sudbury, MA: Jones & Bartlett Publishers.

Engel, G.L. (1977). The need for a new medical model: A challenge for biomedicine. *Science*, 196: 129–136.

Engel, G.L. (1980). The clinical application of the biopsychosocial model. *American Journal of Psychiatry*, 137: 535–544.

Eraut, M. (1994). *Developing Professional Knowledge and Competence*. London: Falmer Press.

Erde, E.L. (2008). Professionalism's facets: Ambiguity, ambivalence, and nostalgia. *Journal of Medicine and Philosophy*, 33: 6–26.

European Science Foundation (ESF). (2012). *Personalised Medicine for the European Citizen: Towards More Precise Medicine for the Diagnosis, Treatment and Prevention of Disease (iPM)*. http://archives.esf.org/ fileadmin/Public_documents/ Publications/Personalised_Medicine.pdf [retrieved 06-09-2017].

Evans, C.S. (2006). Who is the other in *The Sickness unto Death*? God and human relations in the constitution of the self. In: *Kierkegaard on Faith and the Self*. Waco, TX: Baylor University Press.

Evetts, J. (2003). The sociological analysis of professionalism: Occupational change in the modern world. *International Sociology*, 18(2): 395–415.

Falloon, I., Montero, I., Sungur, M., Mastroeni, A., Malm, U., ... and Geyde, R. (2004). Implementation of evidence-based treatment for schizophrenic disorders: Two-year outcome of an international field trial of optimal treatment. *World Psychiatry*, 3: 104–109.

Farah, M.J. (2012). Neuroethics: The ethical, legal, and societal impact of neuroscience. *Annual Review of Psychology*, 63: 571–591.

Federatie van Medisch Specialisten. (2016). *Visiedocument Medisch Specialist 2025. Ambitie, vertrouwen, samenwerken*. Federatie van Medisch Specialisten: Utrecht.

Fernandes, B.S., Williams, L.M., Steiner, J., Leboyer, M., Carvalho, A.F., and Berk, M. (2017). The new field of "precision psychiatry." *BMC Medicine*, 15: 80–85.

First, M.B., Pincus, H.A., Levine, J.B., Williams, J.B.W., Ustun, B., and Peele, P. (2004). Clinical utility as a criterion for revising psychiatric diagnoses. *American Journal of Psychiatry*, 161: 946–954.

Fonagy, P., Gergely, G., Jurist, E.L., and Target, M. (Eds.) (2002). *Affect Regulation, Mentalization, and the Development of the Self*. New York: Other Press.

Francken, J.C., Slors, M. (2017). *Neuroscience* and everyday life: Facing the translation problem. *Brain and Cognition*. http://dx.doi.org/10.1016/j.bandc.2017.09.004.

Frank, J.R. (Ed.) (2005). *The CanMEDS 2005 Physician Competency Framework: Better Standards. Better Physicians. Better Care*. Ottawa: Royal College of Physicians and Surgeons of Canada.

Frank, J.R., Jabbour, M., Tugwell, P., et al. (1996). Skills for the New Millennium: Report of the Societal Needs Working Group CanMEDS 2000 Project. *Annals Royal College of Physicians and Surgeons of Canada*, 29: 206–216.

Frankfurt, H. (1998). *The Importance of What We Care about: Philosophical Essays*. Cambridge: Cambridge University Press.

Freidson, E. (2001). *Professionalism: The Third Logic*. Chicago: University of Chicago Press.

Friedman, M. (1962). *Capitalism and Freedom*. Chicago: University of Chicago Press.

Frijda, N. (1986). *The Emotions*. Cambridge: Cambridge University Press.

Fuchs, T. (2000). *Leib, Raum, Person. Entwurf einer phänomenologische Anthropologie*. Stuttgart: Klett-Cotta.

Fulford, K.W.M. (1989). *Moral Theory and Medical Practice*. Cambridge: Cambridge University Press.

Fulford, K.W.M. (1999). Nine variations and a coda on the theme of an evolutionary definition of dysfunction. *Journal of Abnormal Psychology*, 108: 412–420.

Fulford, K.W.M. (2000). Teleology without tears: Naturalism, neo-naturalism, and evaluationism in the analysis of function statements in biology (and a bet on the twenty-first century). *Philosophy, Psychiatry, Psychology*, 7: 77–94.

Fulford, K.W.M. (2004) Ten principles of values-based medicine. In: J. Radden (Ed.). *The Philosophy of Psychiatry: A Companion*, pp. 205–234. New York: Oxford University Press.

Fulford, K.W.M. (2008). Values-based practice: A new partner to evidence-based practice and a first for psychiatry? In: A.R. Singh, S.A. Singh (Eds.). *Medicine, Mental Health, Science, Religion, and Well-being. Mens Sana Monographs*, 6(1): 10–21.

Fulford, K.W.M. (2011). The value of evidence and evidence of values: Bringing together values-based and evidence-based practice in policy and service development in mental health. *Journal of Evaluation in Clinical Practice*, 17(5): 976–987.

Fulford, K.W.M., Benington, J. (2004). VBM: A collaborative values-based model of healthcare decision-making combining medical and management perspectives. In: R. Williams, M. Kerfoot, (Eds.). *Child and Adolescent Mental Health Services: Strategy, Planning, Delivery, and Evaluation*. Oxford: Oxford University Press.

Gabbard, G.O. (2010). *Long-term Psychodynamic Psychotherapy*. Washington, DC: American Psychiatric Publishing, Inc.

Gabbard, G.O., Roberts, L.W., Crisp-Han, H., Ball, V., Hobday, G., and Rachal, F. (2012). *Professionalism in Psychiatry*. Washington, DC: American Psychiatric Publishing, Inc.

Gadamer, H.G. (1960). *Wahrheit und Methode. Grundzüge einer philosophischen Hermeneutik* [1975]. Tübingen: J.C.B. Mohr (Paul Siebeck).

Gallagher, S. (2000). Philosophical conceptions of the self: Implications for cognitive science. *Trends in Cognitive Sciences*, 4(1): 14–21.

Gallagher, S. (2005). *How the Body Shapes the Mind*. Oxford: Oxford University Press.

Gallagher, S. (Ed.) (2013). *The Oxford Handbook of the Self*. Oxford: Oxford University Press.

Gallagher, S., Shear, J. (Eds.) (1999). *Models of the Self*. Exeter: Imprint Academic.

Gascoigne, N., Thornton, T. (2014). *Tacit Knowledge*. London/New York: Routledge.

Gauvin, F.P., Abelson, J., Giacomini, M., Eyles, J., and Lavis, J.N. (2010). "It all depends": Conceptualizing public involvement in the context of health technology assessment agencies. *Social Science and Medicine*, 70: 1518–1526.

Geddes, J.R., Harrison, P.J. (1997). Closing the gap between research and practice. *British Journal of Psychiatry*, 171: 220–225.

Geertsema, H.G. (2004). Analytical and reformational philosophy: Critical reflections regarding R. van Woudenberg's meditation on "aspects" and "functions." *Philosophia Reformata*, 69: 53–76.

Gendlin, E.T. (1996). *Focusing-Oriented Psychotherapy: A Manual of the Experiential Method*. New York: Guilford Press.

Gill, C.J., Sabin, L., and Schmid, C.H. (2005). Why clinicians are natural Bayesians. *British Medical Journal*, 330: 1080–1083.

Glas, G. (1989), Descartes over emoties. Het spontane en het instrumentele lichaam in de cartesiaanse antropologie. *Philosophia Reformata*, 54: 4–28.

Glas, G. (1991). *Concepten van angst en angststoornissen. Vakfilosofische en klinische aspecten* [Concepts of anxiety and anxiety disorders: Philosophical and clinical aspects]. Lisse/Amsterdam: Swets & Zeitlinger.

Glas, G. (2001). *Angst – beleving, structuur, macht.* Amsterdam: Boom.

Glas, G. (2003a). Anxiety – animal reactions and the embodiment of meaning. In: K.W.M. Fulford, K. Morris, J. Sadler, and G. Stanghellini (Eds.). *Nature and Narrative: An Introduction to the New Philosophy of Psychiatry.* International Perspectives in Philosophy and Psychiatry, pp. 231–249. Oxford/New York: Oxford University Press.

Glas, G. (2003b). A conceptual history of anxiety and depression. In: S. Kaspar, J.A. den Boer, and A. Sitsen. *Handbook on Anxiety and Depression*, 2nd ed., revised and expanded, pp. 1–47. New York: Marcel Dekker.

Glas, G. (2006). Person, personality, self, and identity. *Journal of Personality Disorders*, 202): 126–138.

Glas, G. (2008a). *Psychiatry in 3-D.* Inaugural address. University of Leiden.

Glas, G. (2008b). Over het psychiatrisch ziektebegrip. In: J.A. den Boer, G.Glas, and A.W. M. Mooij (Eds.). *Kernproblemen van de psychiatrie*, pp. 328–370. Amsterdam: Boom.

Glas, G. (2010). Christian philosophical anthropology: A reformation perspective. *Philosophia Reformata*, 75: 141–189.

Glas, G. (2013). Anxiety and phobias: Phenomenologies, concepts, explanations. In: K.W.M. Fulford, M. Davies, R. Gipps, G. Graham, J. Sadler, … and T. Thornton (Eds.). *Oxford Handbook of Philosophy and Psychiatry*, pp. 551–573. Oxford: Oxford University Press.

Glas, G. (2017a). Dimensions of the self in emotion and psychopathology. *Philosophy, Psychiatry, Psychology*, 24(2): 143–155.

Glas, G. (2017b). On the existential core of professionalism in mental health care, *Mental Health, Religion & Culture.* (Published online 12 November 2017.)

Glas, G. (2018). Psychiatric education. In: J.R. Peteet, M. Lynn Dell, and A. Fung (Eds.). *Ethical Considerations at the Intersection Between Psychiatry and Religion*, pp. 259–274. Oxford: Oxford University Press.

Glas, G. (forthcoming). An enactive approach to anxiety and anxiety disorders. *Philosophy, Psychiatry, Psychology.*

Glas, G. (2019). Psychiatry as normative practice. *Philosophy, Psychiatry, Psychology*, 26 (1), 33–48.

Godfrey-Smith, P. (1998). Functions: Consensus without unity. In: D.L. Hull, M. Ruse (Eds.). *The Philosophy of Biology*, pp. 280–291. Oxford/New York: Oxford University Press.

Goldenberg, M.J. (2006). On evidence and evidence-based medicine: Lessons from the philosophy of science. *Social Science & Medicine*, 62: 2621–2632.

Goldie, P. (2000). *The Emotions: A Philosophical Exploration.* Oxford: Clarendon Press.

Goldie, P. (2002). Emotions, feelings and intentionality. *Phenomenology and the Cognitive Sciences*, 1: 235–254.

Gorovitz, S., MacIntyre, A. (1976). Toward a theory of medical fallibility. *Journal of Medicine and Philosophy*, 1: 51–71.

Goudzwaard, B. (1978). *Capitalism and Progress: A Diagnosis of Western Society.* Toronto: Wedge Publishing Foundation.

Gould, S.J., Lewontin, R. (1979). The spandrels of San Marco and the Panglossian paradigm: A critique of the adaptationist programme. *Proceedings of the Royal Society*, B205: 581–598.

Gould, S.J., Vrba, E.S. (1998). Exaptation – a missing term in the science of form. In: D.L. Hull, M. Ruse, (Eds.). *The Philosophy of Biology*, pp.52–71. Oxford/New York: Oxford University Press.

Gray, J.A. (1982). *The Neuropsychology of Anxiety: An Enquiry in to the Functions of the Septo-hippocampal System*, 1st ed. Oxford: Oxford University Press.

Gray, J.A., McNaughton, N. (2000). *The Neuropsychology of Anxiety: An Enquiry into the Functions of the Septo-hippocampal System*, 2nd ed. Oxford: Oxford University Press.

Gremmen, B. (1993). *The Mystery of the Practical Use of Scientific Knowledge*. Doctoral dissertation: University of Twente.

Gross, J.J. (1999). Emotion regulation: Past, present, future. *Cognition and Emotion*, 13: 551–573.

Gupta, M. (2014). *Is Evidence-based Psychiatry Ethical?*Oxford: Oxford University Press.

Gustavsson, A., Svensson, M., Jacobi, F., Allgulander, C., Alonso, J., … and Olesen, J. (2011). Cost of disorders of the brain in Europe 2010. *European Neuropsychopharmacology*, 21(10): 718–779.

Hafferty, F.W. (2006a). Viewpoint: The elephant in medical professionalism's kitchen. *Academic Medicine*, 81: 906–914.

Hafferty, F.W. (2006b). Professionalism – The next wave. *New England Journal of Medicine*, 355(20): 2151–2152.

Hammer, D., Anderson, M.B., Brunson, W.D., Grus, C., Heun, L., Holtman, M., et al. (2012). Defining and measuring a construct of interprofessional professionalism. *Journal of Allied Health*, 41(2): e49–e53.

Hansen, M.T., van Oetinger, B. (2001). Introducing T-shaped managers: Knowledge management's next generation. *Harvard Business Review*, 3: 106–116.

Harding, C.M., Brooks, G.W., Ashikaga, T., Strauss, T.S., and Breier, A. (1987). The Vermont longitudinal study of persons with severe mental illness: II. Long term outcome of subjects who retrospectively met DSM-III criteria for schizophrenia. *American Journal of Psychiatry*, 144: 727–735.

Hargreaves, D.H. (1994). The new professionalism: The synthesis of professional and institutional development. *Teaching & Teacher Education*, 10(4): 423–438.

Hart, H. (1984). *Understanding Our World: An Integral Ontology*. Lanham, MD: University Press of America.

Haslam, N. (2002). Kinds of kinds: A conceptual taxonomy of psychiatric categories. *Philosophy, Psychiatry, Psychology*, 9: 1031–1058.

HaslamN. (2014). Natural kinds in psychiatry. In H. Kincaid, J. Sullivan (Eds.). *Classifying Psychopathology: Mental Kinds and Natural Kinds*, pp.11–28. Cambridge/London: MIT Press.

Havenaar, J.M. (1996). *After Chernobyl. Psychological Factors Affecting Health after a Nuclear Disaster*. Doctoral dissertation: University of Utrecht.

Hegeman, J., Edgell, M., and Jochemsen, H. (2011). *Practice and Profile: Christian Formation for Vocation*. Eugene, OR: WIPF & Stock.

Hempel, C.G. (1961). Introduction to problems of taxonomy. In: J. Zubin (Ed.). *Field Studies in the Mental Disorders*, pp. 3–22. New York: Grune & Stratton.

Hengeveld, M.H., Vleugel, L., van der Gaag, R.J., Stek, M., and Glas, G. (2009). *Herziening Opleiding en Onderwijs Psychiatrie (HOOP)*. Utrecht: De Tijdstroom.

Henry, M. (1973/1963). *The Essence of Manifestation*, trans. G. Etzkorn. Den Haag: Nijhoff.

Hermans, H.J.M. (2002). The dialogical self as a society of mind: Introduction. *Theory & Psychology*, 12: 147–160.

Hermans, H.J.M., Kempen, H.J.G. (1993). *The Dialogical self: Meaning as Movement*. San Diego, CA: Academic Press.

Herrle, S.R., Corbett, E.C., Fagan, M.J., Moore, C.G., and Elnicki, D.M. (2011). Bayes' theorem and the physical examination: Probability assessment and diagnostic decision-making. *Academic Medicine*, 86(5): 618–627.

Hobson, P. (2004). *The Cradle of Thought: Exploring the Origins of Thinking*. Oxford: Oxford University Press.

Hobson, P. (2010). Emotion, self/other-awareness, and autism: A developmental perspective. In: P. Goldie (Ed.). *The Oxford Handbook of Philosophy and Emotion*, pp. 445–472. Oxford: Oxford University Press.

Hobson, R.F. (1985). *Forms of Feeling: Heart of Psychotherapy*. London: Routledge.

Hodgson, G.M. (2006). What are institutions? *Journal of Economic Issues*, 40(1): 1–25.

Hofstadter, D. (2007). *I Am a Strange Loop*. New York: Basic Books.

Holm, S. (1995). Not just autonomy: The principles of American biomedical ethics. *Journal of Medical Ethics*, 21: 332–338.

Holtman, M.S., Frost, J.S., Hammer, D.P., McGuinn, K., and Nunez, L.M. (2011). Interprofessional professionalism: Linking professionalism and interprofessional care. *Journal of Interprofessional Care*, 25: 383–385.

Hood, B. (2012). *The Self-illusion. How the Social Brain Created Identity*. Oxford: Oxford University Press.

Hood, L., Friend, S.H. (2011). Predictive, personalized, preventive, participatory (P4) cancer medicine. *Nature Reviews Clinical Oncology*, 8(3): 184–187.

Hoogland, J., Jochemsen, H. (2000). Professional autonomy and the normative structure of medical practice. *Theoretical Medicine and Bioethics*, 21(5): 457–475.

Horwitz, A.V., Wakefield, J.C. (2007). *The Loss of Sadness: How Psychiatry Transformed Normal Sorrow into Depressive Disorder*. Oxford: Oxford University Press.

Horwitz, A.V., Wakefield, J.C. (2012). *All We Have to Fear: Psychiatry's Transformation of Natural Anxieties into Mental Disorders*. Oxford: Oxford University Press.

Huber, M. (2014). *Towards a New, Dynamic Concept of Health. Its Operationalisation and Use in Public Health and Healthcare, and in Evaluating Health Effects of Food*. Doctoral dissertation: University of Maastricht.

Huber, M., Knottnerus, J., Green, L., van der Horst, H., Jadad, A.R., Kromhout, D., et al. (2011). How should we define health? *British Medical Journal*, 343: 235–237.

Huber, M., van Vliet, M., Giezenberg, M., Winkens, B., Heerkens, Y., … and Knottnerus, J.A. (2016). Towards a "patient-centred" operationalisation of the new dynamic concept of health: A mixed methods study. *British Medical Journal Open*, 5: e010091.

Huddle, T.S. (2005). Teaching professionalism: Is medical morality a competency? *Academic Medicine*, 80(10): 885–891.

Huddle, T.S. (2013). The limits of social justice as an aspect of medical professionalism. *Journal of Medicine and Philosophy*, 38: 369–387.

Hull, D.L., Ruse, M. (Eds.) (1998). *The Philosophy of Biology*. Oxford/New York: Oxford University Press.

Hunsley, J., Mash, E.J. (2007). Evidence-based assessment. *Annual Review in Clinical Psychology*, 3: 29–51.

Ikkos, G. (2010). Psychiatry, professionalism, and society: A note on past and present. In: D. Bhugra, A. Malik (Eds.). *Professionalism in Mental Healthcare*, pp. 9–22. Cambridge: Cambridge University Press.

Illich, I. (1976). *Limits to Medicine: Medical Nemesis: The Expropriation of Health*. London: Marion Boyars.

Immordino-Yang, M.H. (2011). Me, my "self" and you: Neuropsychological relations between social emotion, self-awareness, and morality. *Emotion Review*, 3(3): 313–315.

Insel, T. (2013). Director's blog: Transforming diagnosis. http://www.nimh.nih.gov/about/director/2013/transforming-diagnosis.shtml [retrieved 06-03-2015].

Insel, T.R., Wang, P.S. (2010). Rethinking mental illness. *Journal of the American Medical Association*, 303(19): 1970–1971.

Irvine, D. (2001). Doctors in the UK: Their new professionalism and its regulatory framework. *Lancet*, 38: 1807–1810.

Irvine, D. (2003). *The Doctors' Tale: Professionalism and Public Trust.* Abingdon: Radcliffe Medical Press.

Jablensky, A., Sartorius, N., Ernberg, G. (1992). Schizophrenia: Manifestation, incidence and course in different cultures. A World Health Organization ten-country study. *Psychological Medicine Monograph*, Supp. 20: 1–97.

James, W. (1884). What is an emotion? *Mind*, 9(34): 188–205.

James, W. (1890). *Principles of Psychology*, Vols. I and II. New York: Henry Holt & Co.

Jameson, J.L., Longo, D.L. (2015). Precision medicine — Personalized, problematic, and promising. *New England Journal of Medicine*, 372(23): 2229–2234.

Jaspers, K. (1913/1953). *Allgemeine Psychopathologie*, 6th ed. Berlin: Springer-Verlag.

Jaspers, K. (1997). *General psychopathology*, trans. J. Hoenig, M.W. Hamilton. Baltimore, MA: Johns Hopkins University Press.

Jochemsen, H. (2006). Normative practices as an intermediate between theoretical ethics and morality. *Philosophia Reformata*, 71: 96–112.

Jochemsen, H. (2008). Medical practice as the primary context for medical ethics. In: D.N. Weisstub, G. Diaz Pintos (Eds.). *Autonomy and Human Rights in Healthcare: An International Perspective*, pp. 189–204. Dordrecht: Springer.

Jochemsen, H., Glas, G. (1997). *Verantwoord medisch handelen. Proeve van een Christelijke medische ethiek.* Amsterdam: Buijten & Schipperheijn.

Jochemsen, H., ten Have, H. (Issue Eds.) (2000). The autonomy of the health profession: An introduction. *Theoretical Medicine and Bioethics*, 21(5): 405–408.

Joyner, M.J., Paneth, N. (2015). Seven questions for personalized medicine. *Journal of the American Medical Association*, 314(10): 999–1000.

Kalsbeek, L. (1970). *De wijsbegeerte der wetsidee. Proeve van een christelijke filosofie.* Amsterdam: Buijten & Schipperheijn.

Kandel, E. (1998). A new intellectual framework for psychiatry. *American Journal of Psychiatry*, 155: 457–469.

Kandel, E. (2006). *In Search of Memory. The Emergence of a New Science of the Mind.* New York: W.W. Norton & Company.

Kanes, C. (2010). Challenging professionalism. In C. Kanes (Ed.). *Elaborating Professionalism: Studies in Practice and Theory 5*, pp. 1–16. Dordrecht: Springer.

Katon, W., Von Korff, M., Lin, E., Simon, G., Walker, E., ... and Ludman, E. (1995). Collaborative management to achieve depression treatment guidelines. *Journal of the American Medical Association*, 273(13): 1026–1031.

Kaul, A.J. (1986). The proletarian journalist: A critique on professionalism. *Journal of Mass Media Ethics*, 1(2): 47–55.

Kendell, R.E. (1975). *The Role of Diagnosis in Psychiatry.* Oxford: Blackwell.

Kendell, R.E. (1988). Priorities for the next decade. In: J.E. Mezzich, M. von Cranach (Eds.). *International Classification in Psychiatry: Unity and Diversity*, pp. 332–340. New York: Cambridge University Press.

Kendler, K.S. (2008a). Explanatory models for psychiatric illness. *American Journal of Psychiatry*, 165: 695–702.

KendlerK.S. (2008b). Book review of *The Loss of Sadness: How Psychiatry Transformed Normal Sorrow into Depressive Disorder* (Horwitz A.V. and Wakefield, J.C.). *Psychological Medicine*, 38: 148–150.

Kendler, K.S. (2009). An historical framework for psychiatric nosology. *Psychological Medicine*, 39: 1935–1941.

Kendler, K.S. (2012). The dappled nature of causes of psychiatric illness: Replacing the organic-functional/hardware-software dichotomy with empirically based pluralism. *Molecular Psychiatry*, 17: 377–388.

Kendler, K.S. (2015). Toward a limited realism for psychiatric nosology based on the coherence theory of truth. *Psychological Medicine*, 45: 1115–1118.

Kendler, K.S. (2016). The nature of psychiatric disorders. *World Psychiatry*, 15: 5–12.

Kendler, K.S., Myers, J., and Halberstadt, L.J. (2010). Should the diagnosis of major depression be made independent of or dependent upon the psychosocial context? *Psychological Medicine*, 40(5): 771–780.

Kendler, K.S., Zachar, P., and Craver, C. (2011). What kind of thing are psychiatric disorders? *Psychological Medicine*, 41: 1143–1150.

Kenny, A. (1984). *Action, Emotion, and Will*. London/Henley: Routledge & Kegan Paul.

Kernberg, O.F. (1984). *Severe Personality Disorders. Psychotherapeutic Strategies*. New Haven, CT/London: Yale University Press.

Kessler, R.C., Merikangas, K.R. (2004). The National Comorbidity Survey Replication (NCS-R): Background and aims. *International Journal of Methods in Psychiatric Research*, 13(2): 1360–1368.

Kessler, R.C., Berglund, P., Demler, O., Jin, R., Merikangas, K.R., and Walters, E.E. (2005). Lifetime prevalence and age-of-onset distributions of DSM-IV disorders in the National Comorbidity Survey Replication. *Archives of General Psychiatry*, 62(6): 593–602.

Khushf, G. (2013). A framework for understanding medical epistemologies. *Journal of Medicine and Philosophy*, 38: 461–486.

Kierkegaard, S. (1846/1992), *Concluding Unscientific Postscript to Philosophical Fragments*, ed. and trans. V. Howard and Edna H. Hong, Princeton, NJ: Princeton University Press. [Page references are to *Søren Kierkegaard Skrifter*, Part VII, edited by Niels Jørgen Cappelørn, Joakim Garff, Jette Knudsen, and Johnny Kondrup, Copenhagen: Gads Forlag, 2002.]

Kierkegaard, S. (1848/1980), *The Sickness Unto Death: A Christian Psychological Exposition for Upbuilding and Awakening*. Princeton, NJ: Princeton University Press. [Page refererences are to *Søren Kierkegaard Skrifter*, Part XI, edited by Niels Jørgen Cappelørn, Joakim Garff, Anne Mette Hansen, and Johnny Kondrup, Copenhagen, Gads Forlag, 2006.]

Killaspy, H., Rosen, A. (2011). Case management and assertive community treatment. In: G. Thornicroft, G. Szmukler, K.T. Mueser, and R.E. Drake (Eds.). *Oxford Textbook of Community Mental Health*, pp. 142–150. Oxford: Oxford University Press.

Kim, N.S., Ahn, W. (2002) Clinical psychologists' theory-based representations of mental disorders predict their diagnostic reasoning and memory . *Journal of Experimental Psychology: General*, 131(4): 451–476.

Kincaid, H., Sullivan, J. (Eds.) (2014). *Classifying Psychopathology: Mental Kinds and Natural Kinds*. Cambridge/London: MIT Press.

Kincaid, H., Sullivan, J. (2014). Classifying psychopathology: Mental kinds and natural kinds. In: H. Kincaid, J. Sullivan (Eds.). *Classifying Psychopathology: Mental Kinds and Natural Kinds*, pp. 1–1). Cambridge/London: MIT Press.

Kircher, T., David, A. (2003). *The Self in Neuroscience and Psychiatry*. Cambridge: Cambridge University Press.

Kistler, M., Gnassounou, B. (Eds.) (2016). *Dispositions and Causal Powers*. London: Routledge (1st ed. 2007, Ashgate).

Kitano, H. (2002). Systems biology: A brief overview. *Science*, 295(5560): 1662–1664.

Kitcher, P. (1998). Function and design. In: D.L. Hull, M. Ruse (Eds.). *The Philosophy of Biology*, pp. 258–279. Oxford/New York: Oxford University Press.

Kleinman, A. (1982). Neurasthenia and depression: A study of somatization and culture in China. *Culture, Medicine and Psychiatry*, 6(2): 117–190.

Kleinman, A. (2004). Culture and depression. *New England Journal of Medicine*, 351: 951–953.

Kleinman, A. (2010). Four social theories for global health. *Lancet*, 375(9725): 1518–1519.

Kleinman, A., Good, B. (Eds.) (1985). *Culture and Depression: Studies in the Anthropology and Cross-cultural Psychiatry of Affect and Disorder*. Berkeley/Los Angeles, CA: University of California Press.

Koole, S.L. (2009). The psychology of emotion regulation: An integrative review. *Cognition & Emotion*, 23(1): 4–41.

Koolhaas, J., Bartolomucci, A., Buwalda, B., de Boer, S.F., Flügge, G., Korte, S.M., et al. (2011). Stress revisited: A critical evaluation of the stress concept. *Neuroscience and Biobehavioral Reviews*, 35(5): 1291–1301.

Krause, E.A. (1996). *Death of the Guilds: Professions, States and the Advance of Capitalism, 1930 to the Present*. New Haven, CT: Yale University Press.

Kupfer, D.J., First, M.B., and Regier, D.A. (Eds.) (2002). *A Research Agenda for DSM-V*. Washington, DC: American Psychiatric Press Inc.

Kurzweil, R. (2001). The law of accelerated returns. http://www.kurzweilai.net/the-law-of-accelerating-returns [retrieved 18-03-2015].

Lambie, J.A. (2009). Emotion experience, rational action, and self-knowledge. *Emotion Review*, 1(3): 272–280.

Larson, M.S. (1977). *The Rise of Professionalism. Monopolies of Competence and Sheltered Markets* (2013 ed. with a new introduction by the author). New Brunswick/London: Transaction Publishers.

Larson, M. (2003). Professionalism: The third logic. *Perspectives in Biology and Medicine*, 46(3): 458–462.

Latour, B. (1987). *Science in Action*. Cambridge: Harvard University Press.

Law, I., Widdows, H. (2008). Conceptualising health: Insights from the capability approach. *Healthcare Analysis*, 16(4): 303–314.

Lazarus, R.S., Folkman, S. (1984). *Stress, Appraisal, and Coping*. New York: Springer.

Leary, M.R., Tangney, J.P. (2003). The self as an organizing construct in the behavioural and social sciences. In: M.R. Leary, J.P. Tangney (Eds.). *Handbook of Self and Identity*, pp. 3–14. New York/London: Guilford Press.

LeDoux, J. (1996). *The Emotional Brain*. New York: Simon & Schuster.

LeDoux, J. (2012). Rethinking the emotional brain. *Neuron*, 73: 653–676.

LeDoux, J. (2015). *Anxious. Using the Brain to Understand and Treat Fear and Anxiety*. New York: Penguin Books.

Lee, M.J.H. (2010). The problem of "thick in status, thin in content" in Beauchamp and Childress' principlism. *Journal of Medical Ethics*, 36: e525–e528.

Legrand, D. (2007). Pre-reflective self-consciousness: On being bodily in the world. *Janus Head*, 9: 493–519.

Legrand, D. (2011). Phenomenological dimensions of bodily self-consciousness. In S. Gallagher (Ed.). *The Oxford Handbook of the Self*, pp. 204–227. Oxford: Oxford University Press.

Levinson, W., Ginsburg, S., Hafferty, F.W., and Lucey, C.R. (2014). *Understanding Medical Professionalism*. New York: McGraw-Hill.

Lewis, G.H., Errazuriz, A., Thomas, H.V., Cannon, M., and Jones, P.B. (2011). The application of epidemiology to mental disorders. In: G. Thornicroft, G. Szmukler, K.T. Mueser, and R.E. Drake (Eds.). *Oxford Textbook of Community Mental Health*, pp. 37–49. Oxford University Press.

Lewis, M.D. (2002). The dialogical brain: Contributions of emotional neurobiology to understanding the dialogical self. *Theory and Psychology*, 12(2): 175–190.

Lewis, M.D. (2005). Bridging emotion theory and neurobiology through dynamical systems modelling. *Behavioral and Brain Sciences*, 28: 169–245.

Lewis, T. (1940). *Soldier's Heart and the Effort Syndrome*, 2nd ed. London: Shaw & Sons.

Loughlin, M. (Ed.) (2014). *Debates in Values-Based Practice: Arguments For and Against*. Cambridge: Cambridge University Press.

Macdonald, G. (1992). Reduction and evolutionary biology. In: D. Charles, D., K. Lennon (Eds.). *Reduction, Explanation, and Realism*, pp. 69–96. Oxford: Clarendon Press.

MacIntyre, A. (1967). *A Short History of Ethics*. London: Routledge & Kegan Paul.

MacIntyre, A. (1984). *After Virtue: A Study in Moral Theory*, 2nd ed. Notre Dame, IN: University of Notre Dame Press.

MacKenzie, J. (1916). The soldier's heart. *British Medical Journal*, i: 117–119.

MacKenzie, J. (1920). The soldier's heart and war neurosis: A study in symptomatology. *British Medical Journal*, i: 491–494, 530–534.

Margolis, J.D. (2015). Professionalism, fiduciary duty, and health-related business leadership. *Journal of the Medical Association*, 313(18): 1819–1820.

Marmor, T.R., Gordon, R.W. (2014). Commercial pressures on professionalism in American medical care: From Medicare to the Affordable Care Act. *Journal of Law, Medicine & Ethics*, 412–419.

Marzano, L., Bardill, A., Fields, B., Herd, K., Veale, D., ... and Moran, P. (2015). The application of health to mental health: Opportunities and challenges. *Lancet Psychiatry*, 2: 942–948.

Matthews, E. (2007). *Body-subjects and Disordered Minds: Treating the Whole Person in Psychiatry*. Oxford: Oxford University Press.

Mayr, E. (1988). *Toward a New Philosophy of Biology: Observations of an Evolutionist*. Cambridge/London: Harvard University Press.

McCrossin, R. (2005). Why clinicians are natural Bayesians: Clinicians have to be Bayesians. *British Medical Journal*, 330(7504): 1390–1391.

McNaughton, N. (2004). The conceptual nervous system of J.A. Gray: Anxiety and neuroticism. *Neuroscience and Biobehavioral Reviews*, 28: 227–228.

Menninger, K., Mayman, M., and Pruyser, P. (1963). *The Vital Balance. The Life Process in Mental Health and Illness*. New York: Viking Press.

Merleau-Ponty, M. (1945/1962). *Phenomenology of Perception*, trans. C. Smith. London: Routledge.

Mezzich, J.E. (2007). Psychiatry for the person: Articulating medicine's science and humanism. Editorial. *World Psychiatry*, 6(2): 65–67.

Mezzich, J.E. (2011). The Geneva Conferences and the emergence of the International Network for Person-centered Medicine. *Journal of Evaluation in Clinical Practice*, 17: 333–336.

Mezzich, J.E., Appleyard, J., Botbol, M., Salloum, I.M., and Kirisci, L. (2016). Conceptualization and metrics in person centered medicine. *International Journal of Person Centered Medicine*, 6(4): 213–218.

Mezzich, J.E., Snaedal, J., van WeelC., Botbol, M., and Salloum, I. (2011). Introduction to person-centred medicine: From concepts to practice. *Journal of Evaluation in Clinical Practice*, 17: 330–332.

Miles, A., McLoughlin, M. (2011). Models in the balance: Evidence-based medicine versus evidence-informed individualized care. *Journal of Evaluation in Clinical Practice*, 17: 531–536.

Miles, A., Mezzich, J.E. (2011). The care of the patient and the soul of the clinic: Person-centered medicine as an emergent model of modern clinical practice. *International Journal of Person Centered Medicine*, 1: 207–222.

Mischel, W., Morf, C.C. (2003). The self as a psycho-social dynamic processing: A meta-perspective on a century of the self in psychology. In: M.R. Leary, J.P. Tangney (Eds.). *Handbook of Self and Identity*, pp. 15–43. New York: Guilford Press.

Mitchell, D.E., Ream, R.K. (2015a). Summarizing the lessons: Shaping a blueprint. In: D.E. Mitchell, R.K. Ream (Eds.). *Professional Responsibility, Advances in Medical Education 4*, pp. 329–337. Dordrecht/New York: Springer.

Mitchell, D.E., Ream, R.K. (Eds.) (2015b), *Professional Responsibility: The Fundamental Issue in Education and Healthcare Reform*. Advances in Medical Education, Vol. 4. New York: Springer.

Mol, A. (2008). *The Logic of Care. Health and the Problem of Patient Choice*. London/New York: Routledge.

Monroe, S.M., Simons, A.D. (1991). Diathesis-stress theories in the context of life stress research: Implications for the depressive disorders. *Psychological Bulletin*, 110(3): 406–425.

Montgomery, K. (2005). *How Doctors Think: Clinical Judgment and the Practice of Medicine*. Oxford: Oxford University Press.

Moore, W.E. (1970). *The Professions: Roles and Rules*. New York: Russell Sage Foundation.

Mouw, R.J., Griffioen, S. (1993). *Pluralisms and Horizons: An Essay in Christian Public Philosophy*. Grand Rapids, MI: W.B. Eerdmans Publishing Co.

Mumford, S. (1998). *Dispositions*. Oxford: Oxford University Press.

Murphy, D. (2006). *Psychiatry in the Scientific Image*. Cambridge: Cambridge University Press.

Murphy, D., Woolfolk, R.L. (2000). Conceptual analysis versus scientific understanding: An assessment of Wakefield's folk psychiatry. *Philosophy, Psychiatry, Psychology*, 7: 271–293.

Murray, C.J. L., Vos, T., Lozano, R., Naghavi, M., Flaxman, A. D., ... and Abdalla, S. (2012). Disability-adjusted life years (DALYs) for 291 diseases and injuries in 21 regions, 1990–2010: A systematic analysis for the Global Burden of Disease Study 2010. *Lancet*, 380(9859): 2197–2223.

Muynck, B. de, Hegeman, J.Vos, P. (Eds.) (2011). *Bridging the Gap: Connecting Christian Faith and Professional Practice*. Dordt: Dordt College Press.

Nasca, T.J. (2015). Professionalism and its implications for governance and accountability of graduate medical education in the United States. *Journal of the American Medical Association*, 313(18): 1801–1802.

Nordén, T., Eriksson, A., Kjellgren, A., Norlander, T. (2012). Involving clients and their relatives and friends in psychiatric care: Case managers' experiences of training in resource group assertive community treatment. *PsyCh Journal*, 1: 15–27.

Nordén, T., Ivarsson, B., Malm, U., and Norlander, T. (2011). Gender and treatment: Comparisons in a cohort of patients with psychiatric diagnoses. *Social Behavior and Personality*, 39: 1073–1086.

Nordenfelt, L. (2007a). The concepts of health and illness revisited. *Medicine, Healthcare and Philosophy*, 10: 5–10.

Nordenfelt, L. (2007b). Establishing a middle-range position in the theory of health: A reply to my critics. *Medicine, Healthcare and Philosophy*, 10: 29–32.

Norman, G.R. (2000). The epistemology of clinical reasoning: Perspectives from philosophy, psychology, and neuroscience. *Academic Medicine*, 75(10 Suppl.): S127–S135.

Norman, G.R. (2005). Research in clinical reasoning: Past history and current trends. *Medical Education*, 39(4): 418–427.

Northoff, G., Qin, P., and Feinberg, T.E. (2011). *Brain* imaging of the self – Conceptual, anatomical and methodological issues. *Consciousness and Cognition*, 20: 52–63.

Nussbaum, M.C. (2001). *Upheavals of Thought: The Intelligence of Emotion*. Cambridge: Cambridge University Press.

O'Connor C., Rees, G., and Joffe, H. (2012). *Neuroscience* and the public sphere. *Neuron*, 74: 220–227.

Oppenheimer, B.S., Levine, S.A., Morison, R.A., Rothschild, M.A., St. Lawrence, W., and Wilson, F.N. (1918). Report on neurocirculatory asthenia and its management. *Military Surgeon*, 42: 409, 711.

Pakman, M. (2000). Disciplinary knowledge, postmodernism and globalization: A call for Donald Schon's "reflective turn" for the mental health professions. *Cybernetics and Human Knowing*, 7: 105–126.

Palsson, B.O. (2011). *Systems Biology: Simulation of Dynamic Network States*. Cambridge: Cambridge University Press.

Parsons, T. (1964/1939). The professions and social structure. In: T. Parsons (Ed.). *Essays in Sociological Theory*, rev. ed., pp. 34–49. New York: Free Press.

Pellegrino, E.D. (2008). The Philosophy of Medicine Reborn. A Pellegrino Reader. In: H. T. Engelhardt, F. Jotterand (Eds.). Notre Dame IN: University of Notre Dame Press.

Perlis, D. (1999). Consciousness as self-function. In: S. Gallagher, J. Shear (Eds.). *Models of the Self*, pp. 131–147. Exeter: Imprint Academic.

Peterson, C., Seligman, M.E. (2004). *Character Strengths and Virtues: A Handbook and Classification*. New York: Oxford University Press.

Petryna, A. (2002). *Life Exposed*. Princeton, NJ: Princeton University Press.

Petryna, A. (2004). Biological citizenship: The science and politics of Chernobyl – Exposed populations. *Osiris*, 19: 250–265.

Phillips, J., Frances, A., Cerullo, M.A., Chardavoyne, J., Decker, H.S., First, M.B., et al. (2012). The six most essential questions in psychiatric diagnosis: A pluralogue part 1: conceptual and definitional issues in psychiatric diagnosis. *Philosophy, Ethics, and Humanities in Medicine*, 7: 3.

Polanyi, M. (1958). *Personal Knowledge: Towards a Post-critical Philosophy*. Chicago: University of Chicago Press.

Polder, J.J., Hoogland, J., and Jochemsen, H. (1996). *Professie of profijt?* Amsterdam: Buijten & Schipperheijn.

Polder, J.J., Hoogland, J., Jochemsen, H., and Strijbos, S. (1997). Profession, practice and profits: Competition in the core of healthcare system. *Systems Research Behavioral Science*, 14(6): 409–421.

Polder, J.J., Jochemsen, H. (2000). Professional autonomy in the healthcare system. *Theoretical Medicine*, 21: 477–491.

Porter, M.E. (2009). A strategy for healthcare reform — Toward a value-based system. *New England Journal of Medicine*, 361(2): 109–112.

Porter, M.E. (2010). What is value in healthcare? *New England Journal of Medicine*, 363(26): 2477–2481.

Porter, M.E., Teisberg, E.O. (2006). *Redefining Healthcare: Creating Value-Based Competition on Results*. Boston, MA: Harvard Business School Press.

Porter, M.E., Teisberg, E.O. (2007). How physicians can change the future of healthcare. *Journal of the Medical Association*, 297: 1103–1111.

Priester, R. (1992). A values framework for healthcare reform. *Health Affairs*, 11: 84–107.

Puolimatka, T. (1989). *Moral Realism and Justification*. Helsinki: Suomalainen Tiedeakatemia.

Ralston, A. (2019). *Philosophy of Psychiatric Practice*. Doctoral thesis: Vrije Universiteit, Amsterdam.

Ratcliffe, M. (2008). *Feelings of Being: Phenomenology, Psychiatry and the Sense of Reality*. Oxford: Oxford University Press.

Ratcliffe, M. (2010). The phenomenology of mood and the meaning of life. In P. Goldie (Ed.). *Oxford Handbook of Philosophy of Emotion*, pp. 349–371. Oxford: Oxford University Press.

Rauprich, O. (2008). Common morality: Comment on Beauchamp and Childress. *Theoretical Medicine and Bioethics*, 29: 43–71.

Ream, R.K., Cohen, A.K., and Lloro-Bidart T. (2015). Whither collaboration? Integrating professional services to close reciprocal gaps in health and education. In: D.E. Mitchell, R. K. Ream (Eds.). *Professional Responsibility. The Fundamental Issue in Education and Healthcare Reform. Advances in Medical Education*, Vol. 4, pp. 287–307. New York: Springer.

Ricoeur, P. (1990). *Oneself as Another*, trans. K. Blamey. Chicago: University of Chicago.

Rissmiller, D.J., Rismiller, J.H. (2006). *Evolution* of the antipsychiatry movement into mental health consumerism. *Psychiatric Services*, 57: 863–866.

Roberts, G., Wolfson, P. (2004). The rediscovery of recovery: Open to all. *Advances in Psychiatric Treatment*, 10: 37–49.

Royal College of Physicians and Surgeons of Canada. (2015). *CanMEDS Framework 2015.* http://www.royalcollege.ca/rcsite/documents/canmeds/canmeds-full-frame-work-e.pdf [retrieved 08-09-2017].

Rueschemeyer, D. (1983). Professional autonomy and the social control of expertise. In: R. Dingwall, P. Lewis, *The Sociology of the Profession*, pp. 38–53. London: Macmillan.

Ryle, G. (1949). *The Concept of Mind.* Chicago: University of Chicago Press.

Sackett, D.L., Richardson, W.S., Rosenberg, W., and Haynes, R.B. (1997). *Evidence-based Medicine: How to Practice and Teach EBM.* New York: Churchill Livingstone.

Sackett, D.L., Rosenberg, W.M.C., Gray, J.A.M., Haynes, R.B., and Richardson, W.S. (1996), Evidence-based medicine. What it is and what it isn't. *British Medical Journal*, 312: 71–72.

Sadler, J.Z. (Ed.) (2002). *Descriptions and Prescriptions. Values, Mental Disorders, and the DSMs.* Baltimore, MA/London: Johns Hopkins University Press.

Sadler, J.Z. (2005). *Values and Psychiatric Diagnosis.* Oxford: Oxford University Press.

Sadler, J.Z. (2007). The psychiatric significance of the personal self. *Psychiatry*, 70(2): 113–129.

Sartre, J.P. (1943). *L'être et le néant. Essai d'ontologie phénoménologique.* Paris: Gallimard.

Satel, S.L., Lilienfeld, S.O. (2013). *Brainwashed: The Seductive Appeal of Mindless Neuroscience.* New York: Basic Books.

Schechtman, M. (1996). *The Constitution of Selves.* Ithaca, NY/London: Cornell University Press.

Schmutzler, D.J., Holsinger, J.W. (2011). New professionalism. In: D. Bhugra, A. Malik (Eds.). *Professionalism in Mental Healthcare*, pp. 115–126. Cambridge: Cambridge University Press.

Schon, D.A. (1983). *The Reflective Practitioner: How Professionals Think in Action.* New York: Basic Books.

Schumann, G., Binder, E.B., Holte, A., de Kloet, E.R., Oedegaard, K.J., … and Wittchen, H.U. (2014). Stratified medicine for mental disorders. *European Neuropsycho-pharmacology*, 24: 5–50.

Sciulli, D. (2005). Continental sociology of professions today: Conceptual contributions. *Current Sociology*, 53(6): 915–942.

Seikkula, J., Olson, M.E. (2003). The open dialogue approach to acute psychosis: Its poetics and micropolitics. *Family Process*, 42, 118–403.

Seligman, M.E.P., Csikszentmihalyi, M. (2000). Positive psychology: An introduction. *American Psychologist*, 55(1): 5–14.

Selvini-Palazzoli, M., Boscolo, L., Cecchin, G., and Prata, G. (1960). Hypothesizing circularity-neutrality: Three guidelines for the conductor of the session. *Family Process*, 19: 3–12.

Selye, Hans (1978). *The Stress of Life*, rev. ed. New York: McGraw-Hill.

Sen, A. (1979). *Equality of What?* The Tanner Lecture on Human Values, delivered 22 May, Stanford University.

Sen, A. (1992). *Inequality Re-examined.* Cambridge: Cambridge University Press.

Sen, A. (1993). Capability and well-being. In: M. Nussbaum, A. Sen (Eds.). *The Quality of Life*, pp. 30–54. Oxford: Clarendon Press.

Shephard, B. (2000). *A War of Nerves: Solders and Psychiatrists 1914–1994.* London: Pimlico/ Random House.

Shoemaker, S. (1968). Self-reference and self-awareness. *Journal of Philosophy*, 65: 555–567.

Simmons, L.A., Dinan, M.A., Robinson, T.J., and Snyderman, R. (2012). Personalized medicine is more than genomic medicine: Confusion over terminology impedes progress towards personalized healthcare. *Personalized Medicine*, 9(1): 85–91.

Slaby, J., Stephan, A. (2008). Affective intentionality and self-consciousness. *Consciousness and Cognition*, 17: 506–513.

Slade, M. (2009). *Personal Recovery and Mental Illness: A Guide for Mental Health Professionals*. Cambridge: Cambridge University Press.

Slade, M. (2010). Mental illness and well-being: The central importance of positive psychology and recovery approaches. *BMC Health Services Research*, 10: 26.

Slade, M., Davidson, L. (2011). Recovery as an integrative paradigm in mental health. In: Thornicroft G., Szmukler G., Mueser K.T., and Drake R.E. (Eds.). *Oxford Textbook of Community Mental Health*, pp. 26–33. Oxford: Oxford University Press.

Slade, M., Thornicroft, G., Glover, G., and Tansella, M. (2011). Measuring the needs of people with mental illness. In: G. Thornicroft, G. Szmukler, K.T. Mueser, and R.E. Drake (Eds.). *Oxford Textbook of Community Mental Health*, pp. 80–86. Oxford University Press.

Sober, E. (1998). Six sayings about adaptationism. In D.L. Hull, M. Ruse (Eds.). *The Philosophy of Biology*, pp. 72–85. Oxford/New York: Oxford University Press.

Solomon, M. (2008). Epistemological reflections on the art of medicine and narrative medicine. *Perspectives in Biology and Medicine*, 51(3): 406–417.

Solomon, R.C. (1983). *The Passions*. Notre Dame, IN: University of Notre Dame Press.

South London and Maudsley NHS Foundation Trust and South West London and St George's Mental Health NHS Trust. (2010). *Recovery is for All: Hope, Agency and Opportunity in Psychiatry. A Position Statement by Consultant Psychiatrists*. London: SLAM/SWLSTG.

Speed, E. (2006). Patients, consumers and survivors: A case study of mental health service user discourses. *Social Science & Medicine*, 62: 28–38.

Stanghellini, G. (2004). *Disembodied Spirits and Deanimated Bodies: The Psychopathology of Common Sense*. Oxford: Oxford University Press.

Stein, L.L., Santos, A.B. (1998). *Assertive Community Treatment of Persons with Severe Mental Illness*. New York: Guilford Press.

Stephan, A. (2012). Emotions, existential feelings, and their regulation. *Emotion Review*, 4(2): 157–162.

Stern, D.T. (2006). *Measuring Medical Professionalism*. New York: Oxford University Press.

Stern, D.T., Papadakis, M. (2006). The developing physician: Becoming a professional. *New England Journal of Medicine*, 355: 1794–1799.

Stolper, E., Van de Wiel, M., Van Royen, P., Van Bokhoven, M., Van der Weijden, T., and Dinant, G. J. (2011). Gut feelings as a third track in general practitioners' diagnostic reasoning. *Journal of General Internal Medicine*, 26(2): 197–203.

Strauss, D.F.M. (2009). *Philosophy: Discipline of Disciplines*. Grand Rapids, MI: Paideia Press.

Strawson, G. (2009). *Selves: An Essay in Revisionary Metaphysics*. Oxford: Clarendon Press.

Strelau, J. (2001). The concept and status of trait in research on temperament. *European Journal of Personality*, 15: 311–325.

Strijbos, D.W., Glas, G. (2018). Self-knowledge in personality disorder – Self-referentiality as a stepping stone for psychotherapeutic understanding. *Journal of Personality Disorders*, 32(3): 295–310.

Sullivan, W.M. (2004). Can professionalism still be a viable ethic? *The Good Society*, 13(1): 15–20.

Swick, H.M. (2000). Toward a normative definition of medical professionalism. *Academic Medicine*, 75: 612–616.

Szasz, T.S. (1961). *The Myth of Mental Illness*. New York: Hoeber-Harper.

Tallis, R. (2004). *Hippocratic Oaths: Medicine and Its Discontents*. London: Atlantic Books.

Taylor, C. (1989). *Sources of the Self: The Making of the Modern Identity*. Cambridge: Cambridge University Press.

Theodoridou, A., Hengartner, M.P., Gairing, S.K., Jäger, M., Ketteler, D., ... and Rössler, W. (2015). Evaluation of a new person-centered integrated care model in psychiatry. *Psychiatric Quarterly*, 86: 153–168.

Thomas, S.P. (2011). Open-dialogue therapy: Can a Finnish approach work elsewhere? *Issues in Mental Health Nursing*, 32(10): 613–613.

Thompson, E. (2007). *Mind in Life: Biology, Phenomenology, and the Sciences of Mind*. Cambridge, MA: Belknap Press of Harvard University Press.

Thornicroft, G., Szmukler, G., Mueser, K.T., and Drake, R.E. (2011). *Oxford Textbook of Community Mental Health*. Oxford: Oxford University Press.

Thornton, T. (2007). *Essential Philosophy of Psychiatry*. Oxford: Oxford University Press.

Toulmin, S. (1976). On the nature of the physician's understanding. *Journal of Medicine and Philosophy*, 1: 32–50.

Tournier, P. (1940). *Médicine de la Personne*. Neuchatel: Delachaux et Niestle.

Van de Camp, K,. Vernooij-Dassen, M.J.F.J., Grol, R.P.T.M., and Bottema, B.J.A.M. (2004). How to conceptualize professionalism: A qualitative study. *Medical Teacher*, 26: 696–702.

Van der Kooy, T.P. (1953). *Op het grensgebied van economie en religie*. Wageningen: N.V. Zomer en Keuning's Uitgeversmaatschappij.

Van der Laan, A.L., Boenink, M. (2015). Beyond bench and bedside: Disentangling the concept of translational research. *Health Care Analysis*, 23, 32–49.

Van der Stoep, J. (2011). Religion, globalization and journalism. In B. Muynck, J. de Hegeman, and P. Vos (Eds.). *Bridging the Gap: Connecting Christian Faith and Professional Practice*, pp. 289–298. Dordt: Dordt College Press.

Van Dunné, J.M., Boeles, P., and Heerma van Voss, A.J. (1977). *Acht civilisten in burger*. Zwolle: Tjeerd Willink.

van Os J., Verhagen S., Marsman A., Peeters, F., Bak, M., Marcelis, M., Drukker, M., et al. (2017). The experience sampling method as an mHealth tool to support self-monitoring, self-insight, and personalized healthcare in clinical practice. *Depression and Anxiety*, 34: 481–493.

van Veldhuizen, J.R. (2007). FACT: A Dutch version of ACT. *Community Mental Health Journal*, 43: 421–433.

van Woudenberg, R. (2003). "Aspects" and "functions" of individual things. *Philosophia Reformata*, 68: 1–13.

Varela, F.J., Thompson, E., and Rosch E. (1991). *The Embodied Mind: Cognitive Science and Human Experience*. Cambridge, MA: MIT Press.

Veatch, R.M. (1983). The physician as stranger: The ethics of the anonymous patient–physician relationship. In: E.E. Shelp, *The Clinical Encounter. The Moral Fabric of the Patient–Physician relationship*. Dordrecht: Reidel Publishing Co., pp. 187–207.

Verkerk, M. (2004). *Trust and Power on the Shop Floor. An Ethnographical, Ethical, and Philosophical Study on Responsible Behavior in Industrial Organisations*. Doctoral dissertation: Delft, Eburon Academic Publishers.

Verkerk, M.A., de Bree, M.J., and Mourits, M.J.E. (2007). Reflective professionalism: Interpreting CanMEDS' "professionalism." *Journal of Medical Ethics*, 33: 663–666.

Verkerk, M., Hoogland, J., van der Stoep, J., and de Vries, J. (2015). *Philosophy of Technology: An Introduction for Technology and Business Students*. London: Routledge.

Vilhelmsson, A. (2017). Value-based healthcare delivery, preventive medicine and the medicalization of public health. *Cureus*, 9(3): e1063.

Wakefield, J.C. (1992a). Disorder as harmful dysfunction: A conceptual critique of DSM-III-R's definition of mental disorder. *Psychological Review*, 99: 232–247.

Wakefield, J.C. (1992b). The concept of mental disorder: On the boundary between biological facts and social values. *American Psychologist*, 47: 373–388.

Wakefield, J.C. (1999a). When is development disordered? Developmental psychopathology and the harmful dysfunction analysis of mental disorder. *Development and Psychopathology*, 9:269–290.

Wakefield, J.C. (1999b). Evolutionary versus prototype analyses of the concept of disorder. *Journal of Abnormal Psychology*, 108: 374–399.

Wakefield, J.C. (2000). Spandrels, vestigial organs, and such: Reply to Murphy and Wollfolk's "The harmful dysfunction analysis of mental disorder." *Philosophy, Psychiatry, Psychology*, 7: 253–269.

Warner, R. (2004). *Recovery from Schizophrenia: Psychiatry and Political Economy*, 3rd ed. New York: Brunner-Routledge.

Wear, D., Aultman, J.M. (Eds.) (2006). *Professionalism in Medicine: Critical Perspectives*. New York: Springer.

Weston, A.D., Hood, L. (2004). Systems biology, proteomics, and the future of healthcare: Toward predictive, preventative, and personalized medicine. *Journal of Proteome Research*, 3(2): 179–196.

Wilkes, M. (2015). Hidden agendas teaching and learning in medicine. In: D.E. Mitchell, R. K. Ream (Eds.). *Professional Responsibility: The Fundamental Issue in Education and Healthcare Reform*, pp. 141–156. Advances in Medical Education 4. New York: Springer.

Wood, P. (1941), Da Costa's syndrome (or effort syndrome). *British Medical Journal*, 767–772, 805–811, 845–851.

Woodbridge K., FulfordK.W.M. (2004). *Whose Values? A Workbook for Values-based Practice in Mental Healthcare*. London: Sainsbury Centre for Mental Health.

Woodward, J. (2003). *Making Things Happen: A Theory of Causal Explanation*. Oxford: Oxford University Press.

World Health Organization (WHO). (2008). *The Global Burden of Disease: 2004 Update*. Geneva: World Health Organization.

Wulff, H.R., Pedersen, S.A., Rosenberg, R. (1986). *Philosophy of Medicine: An Introduction*. Oxford: Blackwell Scientific Publications.

Wynia M.K., Latham S.R., Kao A.C., Berg J.W., and Emanuel L.L. (1999). Medical professionalism in society. *New England Journal of Medicine*, 341(21): 1612–1616.

Zachar, P. (2000). Psychiatric disorders are not natural kinds. *Philosophy, Psychiatry, Psychology*, 7: 167–182.

Zachar, P. (2014). *A Metaphysics of Psychopathology*. Cambridge, MA: MIT Press.

Zachar, P., Kendler, K.S. (2007). Psychiatric disorders: A conceptual taxonomy. *American Journal of Psychiatry*, 164: 557–565.

Zahavi, D. (2005). *Subjectivity and Selfhood: Investigating the First-person Perspective*. Cambridge, MA: MIT Press.

Zahavi, D. (2013). Unity of consciousness and the problem of self. In S. Gallagher (Ed.). *The Oxford Handbook of the Self*, pp. 316–335. Oxford: Oxford University Press.

Zerhouni, A. (2005). Translational and clinical science — Time for a new vision. *New England Journal of Medicine*, 353(15): 1621–1623.

Zuckerman, M. (1983). The distinction between trait and state scales is not arbitrary: Comment on Allen and Potkay's "On the arbitrary distinction between traits and states." *Journal of Personality and Social Psychology*, 44: 1083–1086.

INDEX

Page numbers in **bold** refer to diagrams

3-D view 5–6

Abbott, A.D. 92
abnormality, threshold for 129
aboutness 35
absolutization 4, 160–161
abstraction 3–4, 11
acceptance commitment therapy 25
accountability 86, 146, 147, 164
action tendencies 32–33
adaptation syndrome 49
ADHD 127–128
administration 146–147
administrative duties 83, 147
Adorno, T.W. 161
altruism 114–115, 163–165
American Board of Internal Medicine
    (ABIM) Foundation 120
American Civil War 141
American College of Physicians (ACP)
    Foundation 120
anorexia nervosa 35
Anthony, W.A. 177
Anti-Climacus 13, 14, 66
antidepressants 117
antipsychiatry movement 148–149
anti-stigma programs 2
anxiety 58
appraisal mechanisms 49
appropriateness 102
Aristotle 101, 104, 158

artificial isolation 11
aspects 111–112
assertive community treatment (ACT) 181
atherosclerosis 58
attention 4
attitudes 28
Augustin, St 66
authority 96, 97
auto-affection 69–70
autonomy 121, 122, 129, 161, 162–163;
    patient 109
awareness, definition 32

Bakhtin 181
Bayes' theorem 52
Beauchamp, T.L. 162
beauty 155–156
Beck, Ulrich 146
Belar, Cynthia 187
Belsky, J. 50
beneficence 113, 114, 162–163, 168
benevolence 113, 114
Bennett, M.R. 3
biological citizenship 143
biological dysfunction 21
biomedical approaches 128
biomedical reductionism 1
biopower 142, 144
biosensors 187
Bloom, D.E. 92–93, 130
body awareness 70

body image 35
Borsboom, D. 58–59
brain, production of mental phenomena
    154–155
bridging strategies 53
Brint, S. 188
British Medical Council 186
bureaucracy and bureaucratic control
    90–91, 109, 110, 146–147

Canadian Medical Educational Directives for
    Medical Specialists 82, 86, 89–90, 131
capabilities 137–139
care 114
Cartesian-style philosophy 68–69
Cartwright, Nancy 57
Castellani, B. 92–93, 179
causal network modeling 60
causal processes 4
causal relations 56
CEO, role of 136
character 15; and self-referentiality 75
Chernobyl disaster, psychosocial aftermath
    143, 144
children 4
Childress, J.F. 162
citizens' panels 183
civic partnership 148, 165, 188
civic responsibilities 131
civil society 188
classical disease model 47
classification systems 8, 56; symptoms 5
Climacus 67
clinical judgment 9, 187
clinical knowledge 11, 52–54, 104;
    conceptual status 7–9
clinical perspective 44
clinical practice 42; diagnostic process
    45–47; value-ladenness 5–7
clinical understanding, and normative
    practice 100
co-communicating 190
codes of conduct 91, 120–121
cognitive artefacts 116
coherence 157, 158–159, 160
collaboration 131
collaborative care 165
collaborative care model (CCM), 181
collaborative civic professionalism 131
collaborative communities 131
commitment 96
Committee Innovation Healthcare
    Professions & Education 185
communication 118–119, 191; indirect 67,
    72, 189–190

communicative competence 23
communitarianism 164–165
competence 102, 104
complexity 102–103
complexity theory 1
conceptual issues 2
conceptual stratification 44, 124
conditioning norms 118–120
confidentiality 86
consciousness 29, 68–69
consequentialism 161
constitutive characteristics 101
constitutive rules 106–107
constructivists 48
consumerism 98
content, and form 67
context and contextual factors 83, 86,
    124–149, **125**, 168–169, 188–189;
    clinical perspective 41–42; conceptual
    stratification 44–61, 124; environmental
    127; individual level 125, 126–131;
    influence 21, 21–22, 24; institutional
    level 125–126, 131–139, **134**; and
    knowledge 95–97; macro-level 126,
    139–149, **140**; meso-level 125–126,
    131–139, **134**; micro-level 125, 126–131;
    and normative practice approach 109;
    professional role 129–131; relevance 129;
    role 42, 128; service needs 132–134;
    societal factors 139–149, **140**; societal
    level 126, 139–149, **140**; stratification 42
context-boundedness, scientism and 11–12
context dependence 4
context sensitivity 4, 94
contextual embeddedness 143
continuity of care 181
contract theory 163–165
control 121; paradox of 123
coping mechanisms 30, 49–50, 127
costs 147, 172
covenantal relationships 181
critical philosophy 161
cultural influences, and symptoms 142

Damasio, A.R. 63
data-mining 187
decision making 6, 9, 122, 170
demoralization 22–24, 26
deontology 161, 162–163
depression 5, 22–27, 35, 36, 42, 46,
    129, 142
deprofessionalization 92
Descartes, Rene 68–69, 72
descriptive ethics 100
determinants 4; mental disorder 1

devaluation 95
developmental psychological perspective 68
Diagnostic and Statistical Manual of Mental
    Disorders 5, 54, 56
diagnostic expertise 23, 47–48
diagnostic formulations 45–46, 47–48
diagnostic process 5, 45–47
diagnostic reasoning 45
diagnostic statements 23–24
diathesis 48
dictatorial regimes 143
dimensional disease model 47
direction 108–111
direction interaction 110–111
disease 44–61; background assumptions
    47–48; classical model 47; classification
    system 56; concept roles 54; dimensional
    model 47; dysfunctions 57–58, 61;
    epistemic gap 52–54; implicit models 48;
    natural kinds 54–57, 61; network
    approaches 58–61, 61; psychometric
    approach 59; role of models 47–48; and
    science/practice distinction 54–61;
    stress-diathesis model 46, 48–52, 61;
    systems model 47
dispositions 52, 53
distinctness 152–153
distributive justice 120, 145, 168
diversity 138, 157, 159, 160, 171
division of labor 90–91, 121, 130
Dooyeweerd, Herman 2, 13, 15–16, 94,
    105–106, 109, 113, 115, 116–117, 119,
    150, 151–161; on absolutization 160–161;
    and entities 153–155; on the heart 151,
    159–160, 166; on laws 155–157, 157–158;
    and mental phenomena 153–155; modal
    analysis 153; modal aspects 151, 151–153,
    155–156; relevance 157–159; and
    transcendental order 157
duties 179
duty ethics 161, 162–163
dysfunctions 57–58, 61

economic context 83
economic frameworks 119
economic sphere 135, 138
efficiency 110, 121
effort syndrome 139–140, 141
emotions 5, 30; distorted 76; embedded
    nature of 77; felt tendencies 32; implicit
    aspects 31; intrinsic aspects 31; meanings
    31; person behind 28; recognition 33;
    regulation 49; role 75; secondary reactions
    to 33, 33–34; and self-referentiality 72–73,

75; self-referring capacity 28; signifying
    aspects 31; signifying role 31
emotivism 164
endophenotypes 59
enrichment 113–114
entities 151, 153–155
environmental factors 4
essentialism 55
ethics 100, 103–104, 104–105, 162–163
ethos 108
European Federation of Internal
    Medicine 120
everyday knowledge 10
evidence-based medicine 2, 23, 52, 170,
    171, 184; role of 8–9
excellence, standards of 89, 130
existential motivations 189
expectations 101; shaping 142
experience sampling 59–60
experimental design 11
expert knowledge 88, 91, 93–94, 95–97
explanandum 51, 52, 57
explanans 51, 52, 57
explanatory factors 3
explanatory models 8
explicit reflection 72–73

fallibility 96
Federatie Medisch Specialisten 185
feedback 60
feelings, interpreting 29–31
felt tendencies 32
fiduciary duty 98
financial control 146
First World War 141
flexible assertive community treatment
    (FACT) 170, 181
Folkman, S. 49
form, and content 67
Foucault, Michel 142
foundational norms 115–118
Frankfurt, Harry 64
freedom 161
free market 92
Freidson, E. 88–89, 91
Friedman, Milton 92
Fulford, K.W.M. 170, 171
functionalism 98, 122

Gadamer, H.G. 104
generalizations 104
genes 59, 60
gestures 28
Glas, G. 103

goods 143; patient–physician interactions 130–131; relative value of 137
Gordon, R.W. 92
Gorovitz, S. 96
Goudzwaard, B. 118, 119
governmental agencies 145
grief 29–31, 33
guidelines 116
gut feelings 53

Hacker, P.M.S. 3
Hafferty, F.W. 92–93, 179
Hansen, M.T. 186–187
Hargreaves, D.H. 186
Haslam, N. 55–56
health advocacy 122, 131
healthcare needs 126
health education 134
health, positive approach 184–185
health problems 42
heart 151, 159–160, 166
Henry, Michel 69–70, 72
hermeneutics 104
heuristic framework 99
Hippocratic Oath 90
Hobbes, Thomas 163
holism 102
Holsinger, J.W. 180
Hoogland, J. 103
Horkheimer, M. 161
Horwitz, A.V. 142
Huber, Machteld 184–185
human functioning 159–160

ICT, role of 185–186, 187
idem (sameness) 15
identity 15, 47; formation of 14; medical 143–144; numerical 72, 166–167; personal 68, 72, 166–167; professional 6, 83, 94; qualitative 72, 166–167; and the self 71
Illich, I. 91
illness, patient relationship to 2
illness role 15
immanence philosophies 160–161
immanent reflexivity 64
implicit disease model 48
inclusion 171, 179
independence 129
indirect communication 67, 72, 189–190
individuality 11
individuality structures 151
individualized care 182
information provision 180
informed consent 86, 130
innate capacities 50

insight 104
institutions, role of 6, 131–139, **134**
integrated care 170, 181
intentionality 74
interests 6
International Classification of Diseases 5
interprofessional professionalism collaborative (IPC) 186
ipse (oneself or self-reference) 15
irritability 29
Italy 148–149

James, William 64
Jaspers, Karl 2
Jochemsen, H. 103
jurisdictions 179
justice 113–114, 119–120, 145, 162–163, 168

Kandel, Eric 12–13
Kant, Immanuel 107–108, 155, 162
Kaul, A.J. 92
Kendler, K.S. 54, 56
Kierkegaard, Sören 2, 13–15, 66–67, 72, 189–190; Sickness unto Death 13, 66, 77
Kleinman, A. 142
knowing; clinical and scientific forms of 53; order of 10
knowledge 178; clinical 7–9, 11, 52–54, 104; and context 95–97; epistemic gap 52–54; everyday 10; expert 93–94, 95–97; instrumentalist approach 94; role 111; scientific 6–7, 8, 10, 23, 52–54, 103; tacit 13; use of 104
Koolhaas, J. 49
Krause, E.A. 92
Kuyper, Abraham 152–153

language 118–119, 135
Larson,M.S. 91
laws 155–157, 157–158, 163
law spheres 151
Lazarus, R.S. 49
leading aspects 113
LeDoux, Joseph 12–13, 58
Lee, M.J.H. 163
legal framework 119–120, 124
legislation 1, 90
legitimacy 122–123, 168, 169, 188
Lewis, Thomas 141
lifestyle politics 144
life style programming 144
lived experience 44
Loughlin, Michael 184
love 114

MacIntyre, Alasdair 2, 13, 16, 96, 101–102, 150, 162–163, 164
macro-contextual interactions 144–146
managerialism 98, 109, 110, 146
mandate, public 91
manipulability worry 103–104
Margolis, J.D. 98, 162, 163
markets 147
Marmor, T.R. 92
Marx, Karl 90, 91
mechanistic property cluster (MPC) approach 54, 56
mediating factors 50
medical identity 143–144
medicalization 142, 144, 148
medical practice, underlying model 6
Medical Professionalism in the New Millennium: A Physician Charter 120, 122
medical virtues 82
memory 4
mental capacity, assessments of 131
mental disorder: determinants 1; lived experience 44; role of models 47–48; technicistic view 7
mental healthcare: boundaries 141; crisis in 121–123; paradoxes of 1–2
mental illness, conception of 42
mentalization 72–73
mental life, layered 28
mental phenomena 28; Dooyeweerd and 153–155
mereological fallacies 3–4
metaethics 100
metaphors 58
Mezzich, J.E. 183–184
micropolitics 182
Milan school of family therapy 181–182
Miles, A. 184
mind–body dualism 153–154
mind-brain-in-context 1
mindfulness 25
mineness 64, 65, 66, 73–74, 77
Mitchell, D.E. 147
modal analysis 153
modal aspects 151, 151–153; and laws 155–156
modal functions 152
model of integrated care (MIC) 181
models, role of 47–48
moderating factors 50
modernization 121–122, 165–166, 190
Moore, W.E. 88
moral issues 86
moral principles, guiding role 115
moral subject, the 16
multilayered systems, individuals as 182–183

natural kinds 54–57, 61
needs 137; assessment of 133–134
nervous system 154–155
network analysis, personalized 182–185
network approaches 58–61, 61
network medicine 185–186
neural abnormalities 59
neurocentrism 111, 115
neurocirculatory neurasthenia 141
neuroessentialism 111, 115
neurology 1
new professionalism 186
NIMHE (National Institute for Mental Health in England) *Values Framework* 171
nomenclature 3
nominalism 48, 158
non-conscious inclinations 30
non-objectifying experience 64
non-thematic (non-positional) consciousness 66
normative practice 98; constitutive characteristics 101; definition 101–102; metaethics. 100–101; need for 99; requirements 102–103; scope 100–101
normative practice approach 17, 81, 100–120, 124, 168–169; background 103–106; and bureaucracy 146–147; conditioning norms 118–120; and context 109; and the crisis in mental healthcare 121–123; foundational norms 115–118; institutions in 131–132, 135–137; key conceptual question 105; macro-contextual interactions 144–146; and medical identity 143–144; outline 106–108, **106**; and professional codes 120–121; and professionalism 120–123; professional role 129–131; qualitative norms 111–115; and the recovery approach 179; refinement 176; tensions between structure" and direction 108–111; and VBHC 173–177; and VBP 171; and the virtue-ethical approach 165–167; web of relationships 132
normativity 15–16
norms 6, 101, 102, 103, 104–105; conditioning 118–120; foundational 115–118; meshwork of 145; qualifying 111–115; relationship between 113
numerical identity 72, 166–167
nurse practitioners 83

objective-core-soft-margin concept 6–7
obligations 112–113
OCD 127–128
Open Dialogue 170, 181–182

openness 191–192
organizational competence 23
outcomes 1; and costs 172; measuring 172–173, 176–177; and patient value 176

P-4 medicine 182, 183
panic disorder 35, 37–41
Parsons, Talcott 91, 98
paternalism 148
patient advocacy 180
patient participation 1
patient–physician interactions 180–181; goods 130–131
patients: alienation 121; autonomy 109; capabilities 126; collaboration with 76; inner strengths 37; personal struggle 190; technological sophistication 113; turning point 190; values 9
Pellegrino, E.D. 120, 162
persistent symptomatology 60
personal identity 68, 72, 166–167
personality disorder 129
personalized care 182
personalized network analysis 182–185
personal struggle 190
person-centered care 183–184
person-centered concept 13
person-centered medicine (PCM) 183–185
personhood 166
Petryna, A. 143
pharmacotherapy 7
philosophical framework 2
philosophical resources 13–16
physician assistants 83
Physician Charter, The 120–121, 122
plasticity factors 50, 51
Pluess, M. 50
plurality 130
poetics 182
policymaking 1
pop-science 117
Porter, M.E. 172, 173
positional consciousness 31–32
positive psychology 25, 170, 184–185
power, abuse of 178
practices 15–16
practice, tensions 2
precision medicine 182, 182–183
predispositions 48
preferences 6
pre-reflective consciousness 66, 69, 70–71
pre-reflective self-awareness 73
presentation, three forms of inner 74
pretheoretical intuitions 155–156, 159
Priester, R. 180

primary self-referentiality 35, 37, 42
professional autonomy 90, 121, 122
professional codes 120–121
professional identity 6, 83, 94
professionalism 6, 81, 82, 83, 97–98, 112–113, 131, 143, 148; aspects of 86; assault on 91, 164; conceptualization of 82; criticisms 91–92; definition 88–90; existential dimension 170, 189–192; and expert knowledge 93–94; instrumentalist accounts 165; and normative practice approach 120–123; philosophical reflection 93–97; reappraisal 92–93; sociological perspective 90–93; structural-functionalist phase 90–91; value-oriented framework 180; value-sensitive approaches 179–181
professional–patient relationship 22–24, 86, 96, 105, 112–3, 118, 126–131, 132, 146, 189
professional relationship 81–83, **82**, 97; technicistic view 7
professional role 15, 81, 169, 177, 179–180; attitudes toward 81, 83; complexity 84–85; contextual influences 129–131; devaluation 95; influencing factors 85; new forms 186–187; normative dimension 81, 86, **87**; and professional identity 94; tensions and ambiguities 83–85
profitability 121
proletarianism 92
proportionality 102, 104
proto-professionalization 134
psychiatric classification 56
psychiatric education 185–189
psychiatrists, roles 1–2
psychiatry, object of 125
psychological competencies 86
psychological phenomena, mediation 154–155
psychological vulnerability 21
psychometric approach 59
psychopathological conditions, clinical perspective 21, 22
psychopathology 3; contextual influences 126, 127–131; and self-relatedness 27–41
psychosis 129
psychotherapy 7; biological underpinnings 12–13
Puolimatka, T. 114

qualitative identity 72, 166–167
qualitative norms 111–115
quality-driven healthcare 175
quality of care 146, 147

Ratcliffe, M. 77
rationalism 158–159
rationalization 30
realism 48, 158–159
reality 44, 154, 157
reality distortion 160
Ream, R.K. 147
reasoning 104
recognition, importance of 14
recovery 177–178
recovery movement, the 25, 177–179
recovery-oriented approaches 170, 177–179
recovery rates 177
reduction 3; phenomenological reduction 69
reductionism 1, 7, 47, 161; reductionist
    gaze 10
regulative ideals 107–108, 163
reification 3–4, 10, 11, 46, 155;
    semi-reification 58
relationships: assessment 27; complexity 26;
    definition 135; with illness 24–25;
    interactions 22–27, **22**; and personality
    25; network of 74, 82, 105; with the
    professional 22–24, 86, 96, 105, 112–3,
    118, 126–131, 132, 146, 189; web of 132
relevance 157–159
Research Domain Criteria (RDoC)
    approach 61
resource group assertive community
    treatment (RACT) 170, 181
responsibility 130, 167, 176, 179
Ricoeur, Paul 2, 13, 15, 68, 72, 77,
    165–167
risk society 146
Rogers, Carl 184
role fulfilment 16, 17, 81–84, 170, 191
Rueschemeyer, D. 88
rules 107–108
Ryle, G. 59

Sackett, D.L. 8–9
safety 146, 147
Sartre, Jean-Paul 31–32, 66, 69, 70–71, 72
schizophrenia 177
Schmutzler, D.J. 180
science/practice distinction: dysfunctions and
    57–58; metaphors 58; natural kinds and
    54–57; network approaches and 58–61
science, role of 115–116
scientific input 115–116
scientific knowledge 6–7, 8, 10, 23,
    52–54, 103
scientific laws 156–157
scientism 2, 44, 95, 110–111, 117–118, 161;
    context-boundedness and 11–12; critique

of 9–13; definition 9–10; focus 11;
    self-referentiality and 11–12; values and 10
secondary reactions, to emotions 33
secondary self-referentiality 35–36, 37,
    40, 42
Second World War 151
self- and context-related approach 182–185
self-awareness 21, 29, 29–30, 33, 38, 39,
    40–41, 42, 65–66; application to
    psychotherapy 76; and the body 70;
    emergence of 31–32; lack of 30; minimal
    69, 70–71, 73; non-self-referential forms
    32; and self-referentiality 31–33, 34
self-care 180, 185
self-concept 64
self-confidence 5
self-consciousness 66
self-esteem 64
self-evaluation 28
self-examination 85
selfhood 16
self-interest 147
self-interpretation 21, 29, 29–30, 33, 38, 39,
    42; application to psychotherapy 76;
    internalization of 36–37; role 41
self-management 33, 180–181
self-presentation 74
self-referentiality 2, 5, 11, 12, 15, 21, 28, 42,
    64–65, 71–75, 77–78, 170; application to
    psychotherapy 76; and the body 70; and
    character 75; definition 41, 71–72; and
    emotions 72–73, 75; forms of 15; lack of
    34–35; layeredness 74; loss of 35, 41; and
    personal identity 72; primary 35, 37, 42;
    role 41; scientism and 11–12; secondary
    35–36, 37, 40, 42; and self-awareness
    31–33, 34; and self-relatedness 37–41, 72;
    signification 73–74; tertiary 36–37, 37,
    40, 42; three forms of 33–41
self-referential meaning 31
self-referential signifying 33
self-referring, implicit 65
self-regulation 33, 49–50
self-relatedness 2, 4–5, 13–15, 16, 42, 77,
    167; clinical perspective 21–41, 43; and
    conceptions of self 27–31; definition
    27–28; existential aspects 189; forms of
    67–68; Kierkegaard on 66–67; literature
    62–63; and personal identity 68; and
    psychopathology 27–41; reflection 27;
    and the self 66–71; and self-referentiality
    37–41, 72
self-relating 4–5, 14, 39, 189
self-relating-to-the-illness 27
self-signification 64, 74

self, the 13–14, 15, 42, 62–78, 167; agential use 64; application to psychotherapy 76–77; aspects of 63; and the body 70; Cartesian-style 68–69; definition 62–66; as form of self-experience 63; givenness 71; and identity 71; as integrating device 63; Kierkegaard on 72; literature 62; and personal identity 68, 72; in self-esteem 64; and self-referentiality 71–75; and self-relatedness 66–71; ways of conceiving 27–31
self-understanding, internalization of 36–37
Selye, Hans 49
semantics 57–58
Sen, Amyarta 137–138
serotonin abnormalities 3–4
service needs 132–134, 168
service user movements 148–149
service users, role 148
Shape of Training Review (BMC) 186
shell shock 140
signifying role, emotions 31
skills, transferability 94
Slade, M 177
small world structure 59
smartphones 187
social contexts 118–119
social contract 86, 89, 91, 93, 98, 112, 120, 124, 126, 163, 165, 169
social inclusion 179
social interaction 28, 118–119; withdrawal from 33
social practices 105–106
social recovery 177
social relationships 118–119
social responsibility 187, 188
social spheres 152–153
societal factors 139–149, **140**; bureaucracy 146–147; interplay 139–142; and medical identity 143–144; service users 148
societal reactions 122, 123
specialization 121, 122, 164
specification 113–114
speech acts 28
spheres of interaction 137
sphere sovereignty 152–153
stakeholder perspectives 133
statistical modeling 59–60
stigmatization 2
stratified medicine 182
stress 49, 58
stress-diathesis model 46, 48–50, 61; conceptual aspects 50–52; terminological issues 49
structural givenness 13

structure 108–111
subjectivity 69–70
substantialization 4
subsumption view 104
sustainability 173
symptoms 4; classification systems 5; contextual influences 5, 126, 127–131; cultural influences 142; expression of 4; identification 42; psychometric approach 59; relating to 4–5; threshold for abnormality 129
systems disease model 47

tacit knowledge 13, 178
Taylor, Charles 2, 13, 14, 16, 71, 150, 163–165
technical input 115, 116
technicistic view 7
technocratic control 109, 110
technology overlap 115
technology, role of 116–117, 147, 185–186, 187
Teisberg, E.O. 172, 173
tertiary self-referentiality 36–37, 37, 40, 42
theoretical models, influence 45
theory 104, 158
therapy, turning point 190
Thornton, T. 9
Tournier, Paul 184
tradition 165
training 93–94, 185–189
transcendental conditions 155
transcendental order 157
transcendental philosophy 155–156
translation, problem of 8
translational scientists 8
transparency 1, 121, 147
treatment algorithms 116
treatment planning 26
trust 96, 98, 146–147, 149, 165, 187
trustworthiness 82, 86, 119, 150, 163, 164, 189
truth 67
T-shaped professionals 186–187

unrest 29
utilitarian approach 138
utilitarianism 161, 163–165
utopian longings 117

values 121, 165, 175–176; clinical practice 5–7; patient 9; professionalism 180; scientism and 10
values-based healthcare (VHBC) 138, 170, 172–177
values-based practice (VBP) 170, 170–172

value-sensitive approaches 169, 170–182; assertive community treatment (ACT) 181; collaborative care model (CCM), 181; flexible assertive community treatment (FACT) 170, 181; integrated care 170, 181; Open Dialogue 170, 181–182; positive psychology 170; professionalism 179–181; recovery-oriented approaches 170, 177–179; resource group assertive community treatment (RACT) 170; resource group, assertive community treatment (R-ACT) 181; values-based healthcare (VHBC) 138, 170, 172–177; values-based practice (VBP) 170, 170–172
van der Kooy, T.P. 118
van Oetinger, B. 186–187
Verdinglichung 4
virtue-ethical approach 161–167; accounts of practices 165–167; critique on duty ethics 162–163; critique on utilitarianism 163–165
virtue ethics 105–106
virtues 16, 105, 112–113
vulnerability, definition 51–52
vulnerability factors 45, 46, 50, 51

Wakefield, J.C. 142
Warner, R. 177
wars 139–140, 141
weaknesses 50
Weber, Max 90
well-being 25, 132–133
Wilkes, M. 186
working models, implicit 6
working through 73

Zachar, Paul 55
Zahavi, D. 64, 70, 72